EMOTIONAL ILLNESS AND CREATIVITY

A Psychoanalytic and Phenomenologic Study

Also by Richard D. Chessick, M.D. Ph.D.

Agonie: Diary of a Twentieth Century Man (1976)

Intensive Psychotherapy of the Borderline Patient (1977)

Freud Teaches Psychotherapy (1980)

How Psychotherapy Heals (1969, 1983)

Why Psychotherapists Fail (1971, 1983)

A Brief Introduction to the Genius of Nietzsche (1983)

Psychology of the Self and the Treatment of Narcissism (1985, 1993)

Great Ideas in Psychotherapy (1977, 1987)

The Technique and Practice of Listening in Intensive Psychotherapy (1989, 1992)

The Technique and Practice of Intensive Psychotherapy (1974, 1983, 1991)

What Constitutes the Patient in Psychotherapy (1992)

A Dictionary for Psychotherapists: Dynamic Concepts in Psychotherapy (1993)

Dialogue Concerning Contemporary Psychodynamic Therapy (1996)

EMOTIONAL ILLNESS AND CREATIVITY

A Psychoanalytic and Phenomenologic Study

Richard D. Chessick, M.D., Ph.D.

INTERNATIONAL UNIVERSITIES PRESS, INC.
Madison   Connecticut

Library of Congress Cataloging-in-Publication Data

Chessick, Richard D., 1931–
 Emotional illness and creativity : a psychoanalytic and phenomenologic study / Richard D. Chessick.
  p. cm.
 Includes bibliographical references and indexes.
 ISBN 0–8236–1665–7 (hardcover)
 1. Artists—Mental health. 2. Personality and creative ability.
3. Creation (Literary, artistic, etc.) 4. Pound, Ezra, 1885–1972-
-Mental health. 5. Psychoanalysis and art. I. Title.
RC451.4.A7C48 1999   99–22630
616.89—dc21   CIP

Manufactured in the United States of America

*I dedicate this book to my grandchildren, present and future, to
whom I wish a life immersed in the warmth of loved ones
and in a better experience of Being than we have
all endured in the twentieth century.*

CONTENTS

ACKNOWLEDGMENTS

Among the many wonderful national and international colleagues who have supported my work, patiently listened to my presentations, and offered helpful suggestions and criticisms, I would like to especially acknowledge the kindness and encouragement I received from Dr. Douglas Ingram, currently (1998) President of the American Academy of Psychoanalysis and editor of the *American Journal of Psychoanalysis*, and from Dr. Jules Bemporad, editor of the *Journal of the American Academy of Psychoanalysis*. The late Dr. George Train, Past President of the American Society of Psychoanalytic Physicians, always greeted my efforts with enthusiasm, and I will miss this good friend very much. The same is true of the late Dr. Stanley Lesse, for many years the Editor of the *American Journal of Psychotherapy*, who always welcomed and facilitated the publication of my manuscripts.

I received unusually excellent and gracious cooperation from Ms. Janice Wright, Executive Director of the American Society of Psychoanalytic Physicians, during my presidency of that organization and my five-year service as Editor of their *Bulletin*, and from Ms. Dianne Gabriele in my work as Associate Editor for the International Board of the *American Journal of Psychotherapy*, and from Ms. Edith K. Friedlander, Associate Editor of that journal, who also became a dear friend of many years standing as we worked together on manuscripts for the journal.

This book could not have been written without the dedicated help of Ms. Elizabeth Grudzien, my administrative assistant for many years, who not only typed the manuscript but helped with the many references, library and other errands, and a multiplicity of details that were inevitably required to produce the manuscript. Thank you very much, Betty.

It also could not have been written without the compassion, empathy, and patience of Marcia, my wife of forty-six years, who put up with the preoccupations, midnight rambles, feverish imaginings, and intense concentration this book demanded of me, in addition to the burdens of my psychoanalytic practice. To her I owe all my happiness and no words can sufficiently express my gratitude and love.

Grateful acknowledgment for quotation permission is made to the following:

The Divine Comedy of Dante Alighieri: Inferno translated by Allen Mandelbaum, Translation copyright © 1980 by Allen Mandelbaum. Used by permission of Bantam Books, a division of Bantam Doubleday Dell Publishing Group, Inc.

The Divine Comedy of Dante Alighieri: Paradiso translated by Allen Mandelbaum, Translation copyright © 1984 by Allen Mandelbaum. Used by permission of Bantam Books, a division of Bantam Doubleday Dell Publishing Group, Inc.

The Large, the Small and the Human Mind by R. Penrose, 1997. Used by permission of Cambridge University Press.

Process and Reality by A. Whitehead, 1929. Used by permission of Cambridge University Press.

The Philosophy of Hans-Georg Gadamer edited by Lewis E. Hahn, 1997. Copyright © 1997 by The Library of Living Philosophers. Used by permission of Open Court Publishing Company, a division of Carus Publishing.

The Lantern-Bearers and Other Essays edited by Jeremy Treglown, 1988. Reprinted by permission of the Peters Fraser & Dunlop Group Ltd.

Not Missing Empathy by D. Stern in *Contemporary Psychoanalysis*, Volume 24, pages 598-611, 1988. Reprinted with permission.

A History of Philosophy, Volume 7, Part I: Fichte to Hegel by F. Copleston. Published 1965 by Doubleday. Copyright © 1963 by Frederick Copleston. Reprinted by permission of Paulist Press.

Ezra Pound: The Solitary Volcano by J. Tytell. Copyright © 1987 by John Tytell. Used by permission of Doubleday, a division of Bantam Doubleday Dell Publishing Group, Inc.

The Search for the Self by H. Kohut, 1978. Reprinted by permission of International Universities Press, Inc.

The Analysis of the Self by H. Kohut, 1971. Reprinted by permission of International Universities Press, Inc.

The Restoration of the Self by H. Kohut, 1977. Reprinted by permission of International Universities Press, Inc.

The Origins and Psychodynamics of Creativity: A Psychoanalytic Ap-

proach by J. Oremland, 1997. Reprinted by permission of International Universities Press, Inc.

History and Anti-History in Philosophy edited by T. Lavine and V. Tejera, 1989. Copyright © 1989 by Kluwer Academic Publishers. Reprinted with kind permission from Kluwer Academic Publishers.

Psychotherapists Who Transgress Sexual Boundaries with Patients by G. Gabbard in *Bulletin of the Menninger Clinic*, Volume 58, pages 124-135. Reprinted with permission.

Excerpts from "The Garret" and "Hugh Selwyn Mauberley I, E. P. Ode Pour L'election de son Sepulcre" by Ezra Pound, from PERSONAE. Copyright © 1926 by Ezra Pound. Reprinted by permission of New Directions Publishing Corp.

This Difficult Individual Ezra Pound by E. Mullins, 1961. Reprinted by permission of Noontide Press.

The Interpersonal Theory of Psychiatry, by H. Sullivan, 1953. Reprinted by permission of W.W. Norton & Company, Inc.

War and Peace by Leo Tolstoy, 1868, translated by A. & M. Maude. Published by Oxford University Press, 1933 and reprinted by permission of Oxford University Press.

How Proust Can Change Your Life: Not a Novel by A. de Botton, 1997. Copyright © 1997 by Alain de Botton. Reprinted by permission of Pantheon Books.

Object Concept and Object Choice by J. Arlow in *The Psychoanalytic Quarterly*, Volume 49, pages 109-133, 1980. Reprinted with permission.

Power, Authority, and Influence in the Analytic Dyad by J. McLaughlin in *The Psychoanalytic Quarterly*, Volume 65, pages 201-235, 1996. Reprinted with permission.

Psychoanalytic Approaches to Artistic Creativity by W. Niederland in *The Psychoanalytic Quarterly*, Volume 45, pages 185-212, 1976. Reprinted with permission.

Form Creation in Art: An Ego-Psychological Approach to Creativity by P. Noy in *The Psychoanalytic Quarterly*, Volume 48, pages 229-256, 1979. Reprinted with permission.

From *The Decline of the West* by Oswald Spengler, trans. Charles Francis Atkinson. Copyright 1926 and renewed 1956 by Alfred A. Knopf, Inc. Reprinted by permission of the publisher.

Facing Mount Kenya by J. Kenyatta, 1938. Reprinted by permission of Random House UK Limited.

From *The Life of Ezra Pound* by Noel Stock. Copyright © 1970 by Noel Stock. Reprinted by permission of Pantheon Books, a division of Random House, Inc.

On Transience by Sigmund Freud in *Standard Edition*, Volume 14, pages 305-307. Reprinted by permission of Random House UK Limited and Basic Books.

Beyond Good and Evil by F. Nietzsche (1886), in *Basic Writings of Nietzsche* edited and translated by W. Kaufmann. Copyright © 1966, 1967, 1968 by Random House, Inc. Reprinted by permission of Random House.

Falling in Love by F. Alberoni, 1983. Translation copyright © 1983 by Lawrence Venuti. Reprinted by permission of Random House.

Being, Determination, and Dialectic: On the Sources of Metaphysical Thinking by W. Desmond in *Review of Metaphysics*, Volume 48, pages 731–769, 1995. Reprinted with permission.

The Family and Individual Development by D. Winnicott, published 1965 by Routledge (Tavistock Publications Ltd.) and reprinted with permission.

Unpopular Essays by B. Russell, published 1969 by Simon & Schuster. Reprinted with permission of the Bertrand Russell Peace Foundation.

Ezra Pound by P. Ackroyd. Published 1987 by Thames & Hudson and reprinted with permission.

Thinking Fragments: Psychoanalysis, Feminism, and Postmodernism in the Contemporary West by Jane Flax. Copyright © 1989 The Regents of the University of California.

Poems of Tennyson, A Selected Edition by Alfred Tennyson. Edited/Translated by Christopher Ricks. Copyright © 1989 Longman Group.

The Family Idiot: Gustave Flaubert 1821-1857, Volume I by J. Sartre, 1981. Copyright © 1981 by The University of Chicago. Published by The University of Chicago Press and reprinted with permission.

The Story I Tell Myself by H. Barnes. Copyright © 1997 by The University of Chicago. Published by The University of Chicago Press, 1997 and reprinted with the permission of The University of Chicago Press and the author.

The Complete Greek Tragedies: Volume II. Sophocles edited by D. Grene & R. Latimore. Copyright © 1954 by The University of Chicago. Published by The University of Chicago Press, 1959 and reprinted with permission.

The American Ezra Pound by W. Flory, 1989. Copyright © 1989 by Yale University. Published by Yale University Press and reprinted with permission.

Developmental Theory and Clinical Process by F. Pine, 1985. Copyright © 1985 by Yale University. Published by Yale University Press and reprinted with permission.

Excerpts from *Illuminations* by Walter Benjamin, copyright © 1955 by Suhrkamp Verlag, Frankfurt a.m., English translation by Harry Zohn copyright © 1968 and renewed 1996 by Harcourt Brace & Company, reprinted by permission of Harcourt Brace & Company.

Autobiography by W. Stekel, 1950. Reprinted by permission of Liveright Publishing Corporation.

Love and Friendship by A. Bloom, 1993. Reprinted by permission of his estate.

Excerpts from *A Serious Character: The Life of Ezra Pound* by Humphrey Carpenter. Copyright © 1988 by Humphrey Carpenter. Reprinted by permission of Houghton Mifflin Company. All rights reserved.

From *It All Adds Up* by Saul Bellow, 1994. Copyright © 1994 by Saul Bellow. Used by permission of Viking Penguin, division of Penguin Putnam, Inc.

From *The Cantos of Ezra Pound.* Copyright © 1934, 1948 by Ezra Pound. Reprinted by permission of New Directions Publishing Corp.

The End of Physics by D. Lindley, 1993. Reprinted by permission of Basic Books.

Doing Psychology by M. Basch, 1980. Reprinted by permission of Basic Books.

Boundaries and Boundary Violations in Psychoanalysis by G. Gabbard and E. Lester, 1996. Reprinted by permission of Basic Books.

The Essential Order by R. Galatzer-Levy and B. Cohler, 1993. Reprinted by permission of Basic Books.

Things Fall Apart by Chinua Achebe, 1961. Published by Heinemann Educational Books and reprinted with permission.

The Autobiography of Henry VIII by Margaret George, 1986. Copyright © 1986 by Margaret George. Reprinted by permission of St. Martin's Press, Incorporated.

Excerpts from "Thus Spoke Zarathustra" by Friedrich Nietzsche, from *The Portable Nietzsche* by Walter Kaufmann, editor, translated by Walter Kaufmann. Translation copyright 1954 by The Viking Press, renewed © 1982 by Viking Penguin Inc. Used by permission of Viking Penguin, a division of Penguin Putnam Inc.

The Actual by Saul Bellow. Copyright © 1997 by Saul Bellow. Used by permission of Viking Penguin, a division of Penguin Putnam Inc.

Excerpt from *The Late Summer Passion of a Woman of Mind* by Rebeca Goldstein. Copyright © 1989 by Rebecca Goldstein. Reprinted by permission of Farrar, Straus & Giroux, Inc.

"Love Song" from *New Poems* [1907] by Rainer Maria Rilke, translated by Edward Snow. Translation copyright © 1984 by Edward Snow. Reprinted by permission of North Point Press, a division of Farrar, Straus & Giroux, Inc.

Preliminary versions of chapters 13 and 14 as well as short drafts of passages from other chapters have appeared in *The Journal of The American Academy of Psychoanalysis*, especially Volume 25, pages 665-702, 1997. Reprinted with permission.

Only one who is truly climbing can fall down.

— *Martin Heidegger,* Basic Questions of Philosophy

*For those who in some sense live apart, alienated, disconnected or unin-
vited, philosophy provides a fulcrum, a viewer's box, an Archimedean plat-
form.*

— *Karnos and Shoemaker,* Falling in Love with Wisdom

*The older man admonished his son: "No matter how lofty your pursuits,
you must never fail to hear the cry of a child"*

— *Menachem Schneerson,* Toward a Meaningful Life

*Ah, we are odd, wretched creatures, and if we merely look back over our
lives, there's no lack of occasions to amaze or horrify ourselves.*

— *Albert Camus,* The Fall

*Falling in love with a married woman, the protagonist behaves badly and
weakly. His subsequent life is destroyed by "remorse not for what he had
done, but for what he had not done." His life and the book end with unrelieved Hawthornian gloom:*

> *Amidst the wasted ruins of his life, where the bare bleak soil
> was strewn with wrecked purposes and shattered creeds, with
> no hope to stay him, with no fear to raise the most dreary
> phantom beyond the grave, he sunk down into the barren
> waste, and the dry sands rolled over him where he lay.*

— *Robert Richardson,* Emerson

1 INTRODUCTION

Do you not hear the anguish in his cry?
Do you not see the death he wars against
upon that river ruthless as the sea?

—*Dante,* Inferno, Canto II

Underneath it all is being-towards-death.

Nietzsche claimed that logic and reason can never lead the human mind to the ultimate secret of all things. When the inquiring mind realizes this, he said, it is seized by a feeling of the tragic; it overcomes this feeling by turning to art as the only true justification of our existence. Nietzsche was seeking a new meaning and project for human life and a new basis for ultimate values. He suggested in *The Birth of Tragedy* (1872) that it is to be found in art and in the continual renewal of art (a theme he later rejected). The problem he faced in the wake of the death of God was how to establish values and justify a reverence for human existence in the absence of God and of any hope for absolute knowledge.

In *The Birth of Tragedy* he insisted the world can be justified aesthetically and in no other way. I take this statement to imply that the work of the artist becomes of central and ongoing importance. This includes artists who have created or at least elaborated the innumerable myths we call religions as well as other mythologies and ideologies that found cultures. Creative artists present us with ourselves both individually and collectively, point out new possibilities, and herald future trends as Culture declines into Civilization (see Chapter 11).

In this book I study the complex interplay of psychodynamic factors, inborn talents (or lack of them), and social pressures in the production of the clinical phenomena that characterize

1

mental illness, and I investigate the connections between pathological mental conditions and creative activity. Using the phenomenologic as well as the psychoanalytic approach, I offer careful developmental studies and continually juxtapose the history of the quasi-psychotic genius Ezra Pound with that of "Barry" (a personality whose "history" and "writings" I have invented from a composite of my experiences with several of my psychoanalytic patients), a neurotic failure who had a disordered personality and very limited talents, in order to illustrate the dynamic interplay of their psychopathology with their creative production.

I also use this phenomenologic and psychoanalytic investigation to demonstrate that there are no fixed pathological intrapsychic structural organizations and no such conditions as specific mental "diseases." The psychic state of patients with pathological psychiatric symptoms engages in a dynamic fluctuation and interplay as the ego moves back and forth regressively and progressively in its attempts to deal with its three harsh masters (the id, the superego, and external reality) under the various conditions, vicissitudes, and developmental stages of life.

Here I am utilizing Sadow's (1969) concept of "the ego axis in psychopathology," a schematic framework in which the ego is thought to shift back and forth on a continuum, with each shift resulting in either the various *DSM-IV* (American Psychiatric Association, 1994) symptoms of psychoses, borderline states, neuroses, personality disorders, or in relatively conflict-free capacities as it moves in a regressive or progressive direction. Thus, "the successful interpretation and working through of a psychoneurotic conflict would result in movement to the right, into the conflict-free zone. Ego depletion, whether etiologically based on illness, fatigue, neurotic conflict, object loss, etc., would be depicted by movement to the left" (Sadow, 1969, p. 18). Although Sadow believed the psychotic character has only a restricted range of movement on the ego axis while the borderline character has the capacity to function at various times all along the ego axis, this is a questionable generalization, as we shall see from the cases presented in this book. Sadow's (1969) orientation remained consistent with Freud's structural theory and emphasized that "any individual can be conceived of as exhibiting in his varying psychic manifestations some portion of the entire range. He can be described at any given moment and for any drive as being at a given point of the horizontal axis and as moving in one or the other direction" (p. 22).

Throughout the present book I illustrate and discuss the concurrent development of psychopathology and the unique creative capacities of both a successful and an unsuccessful individual, and the interweaving of their creative efforts and psychopathological manifestations. I hope the old, fallacious notion that psychoanalysis removes or inhibits the creative capacity of an artist will be put to rest for once and for all, because one can see in the case histories related here how patients' psychopathology often actually ruined the products of their creative capacities. The removal of this psychopathology would have liberated these capacities and enabled them at the same time to develop a more successful and fulfilling existence. I discuss a variety of influences that go into the formation and shaping of the psyche, especially both the supraordinate sense of self and the person's ego and superego. With Freud, I regard the id as constitutionally and biologically based and a "given" in each unique individual, along with that individual's inherent skills and talents.

Because of the incredible interdigitation of psychopathology, creativity, and the search for a sense of Being, I conclude this book with a discussion of Truth in art, a discussion which is logically derived from what I label Pound's metaphysical failure, a failure that will be apparent after I describe my view of the background and the status of creativity in metaphysics and philosophy today. After explaining how the psychoanalytic process itself is a form of mutual creativity, I then proceed to investigate the vital selfobject function of art and the polemical issues of whether Truth can be expressed in art, and whether art can bring us into contact with a sense of Being in spite of the fact that concepts like Truth are inherently ambiguous and the grasp of the Being of beings is ineffable. It is clear from phenomenologic and psychoanalytic investigation, however, that experiencing art as a manifestation of Truth depends on one's sociocultural horizon and that the sense of Being depends on one's earliest interactions with one's caretakers. In the postmodern era (Chessick, 1995b, 1996e) we are perhaps always dealing with limited rather than absolute, essential, and eternal truths, and we face the problem of how these absolutes are to be conceived of, and, if they have any meaning, how it is to be expressed.

Focus on the Ego

One need not adhere to Freud's drive theory (although contrary to the current fashion, I am inclined to employ it as a "heuristic viewpoint" [Fölsing, 1997, p. 136] to utilize the concept of the ego axis described earlier. For example, one could use Fairbairn's (1994) object relations theories and characterize the ego as functioning for better or for worse, depending on how much "libido" (in Fairbairn's use of the term) is available for the "central ego" to function. Alternatively, one could use the language of the psychology of the self (Chessick, 1993a), viewing ego functioning as dependent on the relative cohesiveness or fragmentation of the self at a given time. But anyone who works phenomenologically as well as psychoanalytically soon discovers that the relationship between the self, the ego, and consciousness is a very complex and controversial one. The reader will not find me conversant on this topic throughout this book, since it is a subject that deserves a book all of its own. In general, I tend to adhere to the contemporary post-Freudian, post-ego-psychological (Wallerstein, 1995) view, with additional reference to the "sense of self" and other concepts used by Kohut (1977) in his self psychology.

A sharply contrasting phenomenologic view was presented by Sartre, for the purpose of establishing the possibility that a person can form his or her own project deliberately and live an authentic life by choice rather than by simply being a personality determined through compromises among conflicting unconscious forces. This of course was the essential idea of Sartre's original version of "existentialism." Sartre claimed that a free, prepersonal consciousness forms a self or an ego by imposing a unity on its own experiences and reactions to them, both past and present. In her autobiography, Sartre's translator Barnes (1997) wrote, "That we make ourselves by our own pattern struck me as descriptively correct. The notion that the self belongs to an ego which consciousness creates is, of course, complex and controversial" (p. 147). For Sartre, consciousness and not the ego is the active agent, the ego is a passive structure (in Lacan's [1977] even more extreme view, the ego is a self-delusion altogether). Consciousness, for Sartre, determines actions and is "always capable of taking a new point of view on the psychic structures, or self—on the 'I' that it has created. This self, the ego, is what Sartre refers to in the famous pronouncement 'Man makes himself'" (Barnes, 1997, p. 293). Consciousness must create a self, according to Sartre, or the person would be insane.

The essential point of Sartre's argument is that consciousness creates the ego rather than the ego creating what we experience as consciousness, in the traditional Freudian view. Sartre's approach allows the ego to be expanded or restructured by the continuing activity of consciousness. But, as Barnes (1997) admitted, "To tell the truth, Sartre's concept of the ego is a bit slippery" (p. 294). It is nevertheless important to realize that in Sartre's view consciousness is not identical with the ego that it has the capacity to reflect on. Consciousness can review previous conscious acts and various attempts it has made to impose a unity on these acts in order to constitute the person as an ego or self; furthermore, "It can pass judgement on that self, but this judgement itself becomes part of the self that consciousness will next reflect on" (Barnes, 1997, p. 311).

In studying Ezra Pound and Barry from a psychoanalytic point of view, I have leaned heavily on standard, psychodynamic conceptions from Freudian psychoanalysis, object relations theory, and self psychology. When taking the phenomenologic point of view, I have utilized the approach favored by Sartre in his various biographical studies. Sartre conceived of every individual's fundamental project as a gradually evolving unity. There is usually some sort of crystallizing or consolidating moment in early life that points the individual toward a specific orientation. This in turn may be modified (Sartre is not consistent about this) by later important choices, causing an individual's project to unfold not in a predetermined straight line but with many spirals, retrogressions, and progressions. In Sartre's view, it is the task of consciousness to be continually reflecting on this evolution and as a consequence of this reflection make further choices and constructions of the personality.

In order to illustrate this complex interplay of psychodynamics, developmental phases, project consolidation, conscious choices, psychopathology, and what Sartre calls the "practico-inert," that is, the various forces in the milieu with which the individual is forced to contend, I unfold this book in the following manner. The first nine of the *even* numbered chapters will focus primarily on the comparative development, psychopathology, and creative efforts of Ezra Pound and "Barry." As mentioned earlier, "Barry" is an amalgamated imaginary patient whose life and "works" I made up based on disguised clinical material I collected during the psychoanalytic treatment of a number of potentially creative individuals over my forty years of clinical experience. These were patients who had not actualized or lived up to their creative capacities, or whose creative work was spoiled or interfered with by their psychopathology.

The first nine of the *odd* numbered chapters more generally describe the various issues encountered in the even-numbered chapters, such as the fundamentals of the creative process, the relation of falling in love and creativity, and the function of artistic striving, as well as delineate the details of the practico-inert in the era of Ezra Pound and Barry, the ambience of the twentieth century. Along with Sartre, I believe it is *not possible* to understand individuals without at the same time achieving a thorough recognition of what they were attempting to do and why, and what forces they were having to work against in the attempt— their "historicity" (Heidegger, 1962).

What Does Creativity Create?

The closing chapters deal with creativity as a process inextricably involved in psychoanalytic work as well as in the production of art and metaphysics. I have dared to close the book with my own views on Truth that expresses itself through art, Truth that cannot express itself through the traditional methods of science. What art provides for us, in a way that cannot be articulated, helps us "to represent, understand, interpret, come to terms with, and perhaps master our experience and our environment, and to orient ourselves within them, and to communicate with our fellow creatures about them" (Magee, 1997, p. 110). There are several methods through which Truth is approached, and if one wishes to understand creative work and the springs of it, one must be open to all of these possible methods. It was Freud's error to try to reduce creative expressions in the arts, religious mythology, metaphysics, and other manifestations of the attempt to reach transcendence, or even Rolland's "cosmic feeling" (Freud, 1930a) to regressive infantile states. Due to this error he missed the possibility of obtaining information from these creative activities that could not be obtained through the traditional method of science. This caused Freud to contradict himself, because he was actually very sensitive to the psychological insights of such creative geniuses as Nietzsche and Shakespeare, and responsive to the expressions of such artists as Leonardo da Vinci and Michelangelo, although he had little use for modern art and claimed a disinterest in music. He (Freud, 1930a) also freely expressed his own value system without questioning the origin of it as, for example, in the beautiful opening paragraph of *Civilization and Its Discontents*, even though elsewhere he maintained that life had no meaning and that to ask questions about the meaning of life indicates that psychopathology is present.

Holt (1975) delineated the continual tension in Freud between his attempt to be a nineteenth-century strictly empirical scientist and his natural inclination to be a humanist and seek philosophical knowledge. He called our attention to the pervasive, unresolved tension in Freud's writings between two antithetical images of humans. First, there is the prevailing image of humans conveyed by the humanities, in which the person is seen as both an animal and a creature with aspirations to divinity, thus having a dual nature. Each human being is considered to be unique, even though all are members of the same species. Each person is worthy to be respected, helped if in trouble, and encouraged to live up to the extent of his or her capacities. In this tradition, the human is conceived of as a creature of longings and a producer and processor of subjective meanings, including the need to find life meaningful. The complexity of human sexual love as compared to that of animals is stressed, and the human is viewed as an intensely social creature whose life becomes abnormal if it is not immersed in a web of relationships with other people. The human is not static but always changing, and a person's most important motives are unconscious and derived from childhood. The human is seen as both the active master of his or her own fate and the plaything of his or her passions.

In contrast, the school of Brücke and Helmholtz presented the mechanistic image of the human as the proper subject of natural science, no different from any other object in the universe. In this view the differences among people are scientifically negligible, and the person is fundamentally motivated by an automatic tendency of the nervous system to keep itself in an unstimulated state (now known to be neurophysiologically incorrect). Values and meanings are left out of this scientific investigation and consciousness is an epiphenomenon of trivial interest compared to the busy activities of neurotransmitters and the nervous system. In this view, a person's behavior is strictly determined by his or her past history, and free will is a fallacious illusion; the processes known as love are nothing more than disguises and transformations of the sexual instincts. Thus, relationships as such are not real and other people are objects and important only insofar as they provide stimuli that set the psychic apparatus in motion, leading to a reduction of internal pressures. Freud's magnificent literary style obscures this fundamental, unresolved tension in his writing.

I try to avoid Freud's reductionism by approaching the creative work and developmental histories of Ezra Pound and "Barry" both phenomenologically and psychoanalytically, and by using multiple listening (Chessick, 1992a) and exploratory channels. I hope to illustrate the universal and historically all-pervasive human striving to find meaning, to explain what Jaspers (1932c), in the third volume of his *Philosophy*, called "ciphers"— those suggestions of transcendence experienced phenomenologically in our brief lives—and to focus on the universal human yearning to be part of something greater than ourselves that is not simply a regressive desire to return to fusion with one's mother. I view this universal human yearning as a source of motivation for important creative activities of our artists, historians, psychologists, and psychoanalysts, all of whom attempt to produce individual or collective mythologies that humans in a given culture can utilize to organize their lives and activities. The innumerable religions created over the centuries by gifted individuals are the most well known examples of these, as are the various political ideologies. In the last two chapters of the book I attempt to deal with the issue of how to evaluate the relative truth of these mythologies, and in the body of the book I hope to illustrate how the production of these artistic stories and expressions of all art-works in general are interfered with by psychopathology. I view the artist as driven to communicate to us truths about ourselves, — our culture, and our existential plight, the scandal of death, its absurdity and absolute contingency. "Art does not describe; it makes visible" (Safranski, 1998), so that things lose their indifference and commonplaceness (Heidegger, 1971a). In this sense Truth expresses itself in art. I believe we can experience the phenomena that shine forth through the artwork as manifestations of fundamental perhaps inarticulated aspects of the Being of beings (Heidegger, 1962).

The Ego and the Sense of Being

The phenomenologic approach demonstrates that we are not dealing with either "mental diseases" or specific fixed personality structures or disorders, but rather with much more complicated and ever-shifting attempts by the ego to get along in the world — and mediate among conflicting intrapsychic components. Sometimes the ego is laboring very badly indeed, in which case we experience psychotic phenomena, what Kohut (1971) called "fragmentation." Under other conditions the ego is enabled to sublimate, create, or worse, produce neurotic or characterologic symptomatology in a kind of distorted creativity. All humans are in a state of dynamic equilibrium or disequilibrium, which can be influenced by a variety of internal or external factors ranging from constitutional or biological impairment, organic disease, or psychopharmacologic agents, through psychoanalytic psychotherapy and the vicissitudes of life events. The resultant vector of all these internal and external forces impinging on the ego at once produces by means of various compromise formations the phenomena of the particular unique individual that we encounter at any given moment.

Federn (1952), in an interesting but largely neglected view, claimed that the ego is more than simply the sum total of the usual ego functions that psychoanalysts talk about. Federn's editor, Weiss, explained, "It includes the subjective psychic experience of these functions with a characteristic sensation" (p. 6). For the purposes of this discussion let us with Federn label this subjective experience the ego has of its own function the ego experience *(Icherlebnis).*

The phenomenon of the ego's experience of itself cannot be clearly explained. As long as the ego functions normally, one may ignore or be unaware of its functioning. To use Federn's metaphor, normally there is no more awareness of the ego than the air one breathes; only when respiration becomes burdensome or impaired is the lack of air recognized. The subjective ego experience includes the feeling of unity and continuity, contiguity, and causality in the experience of the individual. In waking life the sensation of one's own ego is omnipresent, but it undergoes continuous changes in quality and intensity.

Federn attempted to distinguish within the subjective ego experience *(Icherlebnis)* between ego feeling *(Ichgefühl)* and ego consciousness *(Ichbewusstsein).* Ego consciousness represents an enduring awareness and knowledge that our ego is continuous and persistent despite interruptions by sleep or unconsciousness, because we feel that processes within us, even though they may be interrupted by forgetting or unconsciousness, have persistent origin within us, and that our body and psyche belong permanently to our ego. It is the entity generating the sense of continuity of a person with respect to time, space, and causality. Ego consciousness in the pure state remains only when there is a deficiency in ego feeling. So the mere empty cognitive knowledge of oneself without ego feeling is already a pathological state known as estrangement or depersonalization.

Ego feeling, in contrast, is the totality of feeling that one has of being one's own living person. Federn (1952) explains,

> It is the residual experience which persists after the subtraction of all ideational contents—a state which, in practice, occurs only for a brief time. . . . Ego feeling, therefore, is the simplest and yet the most comprehensive psychic state which is produced in the personality by the fact of its own existence, even in the absence of external or internal stimuli. (pp. 62-63)

Ego feeling is the sensation constantly present of one's own person, the ego's own living perception of itself. (To avoid confusion I should mention that Freud, 1917, used the same term, ego feeling [*Ichegefühl*] in "Mourning and Melancholia," but he used it to mean something akin to self-esteem, which is of course quite different.)

Federn maintained that ego feeling is quite different from mere knowledge of one's self or of consciousness of the ego at work; it is primarily a *feeling* or *sensation,* normally taken for granted. This seems to be a psychodynamic parallel to Heidegger's (1962) explanation that the Being of beings is the most apparent, and yet, we normally do not see it——and if we do, only with difficulty. Remarkably, Federn pointed out, and he certainly had not read the philosopher Heidegger who said the same thing, that the classical Greek language, in contrast for example to English, is necessary in order to get an intuitive verbal concept of ego feeling. This is because in the classical Greek language there is a middle voice, a neutral objectless form. The middle voice implies action involving one's self and not passing over to other objects. In contrast to classical Greek, in English the middle voice is expressed by certain intransitive phrases such as I grow, I drive, I live, I prosper, I develop, I perish, I age, I die.

Our intuitive conviction or grasp or foreknowledge of the Being of humans comes from our inner ego feeling. But our inner sense of existence, of being alive, our capacity to develop a state of relatedness to both the human and nonhuman environment, and of life having some sense of meaningfulness, also requires what Winnicott described as good-enough mothering. Winnicott (1965a) postulated that good enough holding facilitates the formation of a psychosomatic partnership in the infant:

> This contributes to the sense of "real" as opposed to "unreal." Faulty handling militates against the development of muscle tone, and that which is called "coordination," and against the capacity of the infant to enjoy the experience of body functioning and of BEING. (p. 19). . . if the environment behaves well, the infant has a chance to maintain a sense of *continuity of being*: perhaps this may go right back to the first stirrings in the womb. When this exists the individual has a stability that can be gained in no other way. (p. 28)

Searles (1960), in his book *The Nonhuman Environment in Normal Development and Schizophrenia*, claimed, there is within the human individual a sense, whether at a conscious or unconscious level, of *relatedness to his nonhuman environment,* that this relatedness is one of the transcendentally important facts of human living, that—as with other very important circumstances in human existence—it is a source of ambivalent feelings to him, and that, finally, if he tries to ignore its importance to himself, he does so at peril to his psychological well-being. (p. 6)

Searles pointed out how the process and products of technology tend to cause the individual to lose sight of the basic kinship between human and nonhuman, referring to this as "divorcement," which he contrasted to the pantheistic paganism of ancient Greece that imagined the revered deities as often taking the form of various members of the animal kingdom or even the vegetable kingdom.

Searles argued that a chronic inability during infancy and early childhood to relate oneself to a relatively stable, relatively realistically perceived, relatively simple rather than overwhelmingly complex, world of inanimate objects may have much to do with one's ability in adult life to find fundamental, graspable realities and a tangible meaning in life. Conversely a mature relatedness with the nonhuman environment is very fruitful in the assuagement of anxiety, the fostering of self-realization, the deepening of feeling of one's reality, and the fostering of one's appreciation and acceptance of one's fellow men.

Phenomenology

For those readers unfamiliar with phenomenology, a brief review of the concept is provided here. The term "phenomenology" has a difficult history, and over the years has come to have many meanings. It was first introduced into philosophy by Lambert, a German philosopher who was a contemporary of Kant, and who used the term simply to pertain to illusions. Kant (1781) called phenomenology the study of what appears to us in our experience, and he contrasted experience, or "phenomena," with objects and events as they are "in themselves," a dichotomy Kant took for granted but which was broken down by the German idealists.

For Hegel (1807), phenomenology represented the discovery of Absolute Spirit through a study of various stages in the historical development of the mind's experience of the phenomena of self-consciousness.

In the middle of the nineteenth century, phenomenology came to have the wider meaning of an attempt at a purely descriptive study of any given set of experiences. For example, Peirce in 1902 used the term "phaneroscopy" (Brent, 1993, p. 324) to mean a descriptive study of whatever appears before the mind, such as perceptions of so-called reality, dreams, imaginings, and even misperceptions. This was his phenomenologic attempt to approach what he called "prelogical notions" (Brent, 1993, p. 324).

Phenomenology as employed by Husserl (1913) attempted to return to the alleged primordial data of experience, that which shows itself in the manner in which it shows itself. Phenomena so defined are always prior to our theories and concepts; they are immediate data but they are not simply "appearances," for appearances are always appearances *of* something, whereas phenomena *are* that something which shows itself: They are primary, they are what is.

The phenomenology of the definition of "phenomenology" is that one cannot find philosophers in agreement on the definition or use of the term. The use of it always carries the very real danger that it may be employed as a tool for proving what one already believes, in the way "reason" was used in classical philosophy and still is in theology. Also, whether there can be such an experience of "phenomena" entirely free of our preconceptions is certainly a debatable question.

Various applications of phenomenology by philosophers, each in their own way, stimulated the continental European psychiatric investigation of the self and its three important aspects of being in the world, modes of "being-with," as Heidegger (1962) called them: (1) *Umwelt*, our environment; (2) *Mitwelt*, our fellow humans; and (3) *Eigenwelt*, our relationship to ourselves. All of these modes can be described phenomenologically and all are interlocked with our constituted self, so that no hidden essences or entities need to be postulated. This eliminates the whole super-structure of metapsychology, the "disorder" classifications of *DSM-IV* (American Psychiatric Association, 1994) and, above all, the classical notion of an independent neutral subject (e.g., the psychiatrist) observing the outside world (e.g., the patient) as a nineteenth-century scientist collecting data and developing empirical and quantitative laws of cause and effect.

From the point of view of the psychotherapist, the phenomenologic stance is to examine one's reaction to what is simply there in felt experience; the therapist using phenomenology does not disconnect, isolate, or interpret aspects of this experience. *Epoché,* the bracketing of experience, demands refraining from judgment about morals, values, causes, background, and even from separating the subject (patient) and objective observer (therapist). One pays special attention to one's experience or state of consciousness in the presence of the patient. The therapist attempts to continue to observe and listen, staying with the patient's manifest material, and must try to directly experience the patient rather than searching for hidden processes or meanings, or latent content.

Psychiatrists influenced by phenomenology warn that a distance can be created between the therapist and the patient by the standard interviewing technique, a gap that may be unproductively filled by abundant verbal material and analytic ideas, conceptions, and theories. Among the most prominent of psychiatrists concerned with this problem was R. D. Laing (1969), who advised focusing on the emotional interchange, staying strictly with the phenomena presented by the patient, and concentrating on the experienced interaction with the patient. Phenomenological reduction of the cognitive and emotional distance between the patient and the therapist, according to the philosopher and psychiatrist Karl Jaspers (1972), is the crucial procedure in psychotherapy, leading to a true meeting or encounter. This is hard to define and articulate, but such an encounter is something we have all experienced. The application of phenomenology to psychotherapy raises the valid question of whether we as therapists can be sure that we are seeing and hearing our patients as they really are, rather than as projections of our theories about them. The aim of phenomenologic study is to rediscover the whole living person and how being-in-the-world is experienced by that person and those around that person.

Regardless of the various conceptions of phenomenology in philosophy—a dispute still going on today—I believe phenomenology has a useful application in psychiatry and psychoanalysis. We know that the phenomena of the encounter between one person and another, including that between the therapist and the patient, are always interactively or dialectically constituted, and that diagnoses and the postulation of psychic entities commonly made on the basis of the phenomena generated in that encounter are therefore relative to both the observer and the observed, or the therapist and the patient.

As a clinical example, Pao (1979) urged us to consider the diagnosis of schizophrenia not so much on the basis of Bleuler's famous criteria, but as a function of the kind of phenomenologic ambience the therapist experiences, that peculiar sensation of relating to someone who is both there and not there, which generates our considerable personal discomfort. I do not know whether Pao was familiar with Heidegger, but he employs here Heidegger's (1962) distinction between the "hermeneutic as" and the "apophantic as." Self psychologists as well as Sullivanians like Pao recognize the patient through both observation and participation, through experienced interaction subjected then either to Kohut's method of empathy or to Sullivan's interpersonal process, and subsequently to hermeneutic exegesis. A shrug, a gesture, a facial expression, a reaction—the totality of such interpersonal phenomena directly conceptualizes the patient for them.

In contrast to this, for example, Kleinians employ the "apophantic as." They make judgments about what goes on *inside* of the patient, from which they attempt to explain the interaction without direct reference to the therapist; the patient is judged as "projecting," using "projective identification," "splitting," enduring an unresolved "depressive position," and so on. For Heidegger this latter sort of theorizing is removed from the reality of the encounter and sets up a false subject-object (therapist-patient) dichotomy, often with the "therapist-scientist" as the sole arbiter of what is "reality."

There are two somewhat related forms of phenomenologic investigation utilized in psychoanalytic study. The first of these involves a focus on the patient's viewpoint, the so-called "analytic surface," which provides a counter to the analyst's tendency to provide answers and closures. For the therapist to keep returning to and trying to sustain a stance of exploratory openness to the patient's viewpoint also helps to expand and deepen the patient's own search for fresh understanding. It is as if the analyst offers to listen to anything the patient may wish to say and attempts to understand the patient's meaning and viewpoint with the least possible imposition of the analyst's own views or preconceptions. As McLaughlin (1996) puts it:

> I will be alert to and inquire about your nonverbal behaviors and shifts of affect, in order that I may help you sense the many levels of meaning that you have connected with what you are speaking about. I will listen for allusions to how you perceive and react to my behavior, out of my aim to help you articulate the validity and logic of how you have come to see your world and me in it. Through looking at how you see me I will help you try to see yourself, at surface and depth, hoping thereby to strengthen your capacities to find even more of yourself to authenticate and own. (pp. 212-213)

This kind of phenomenologic stance, focusing on the analytic surface, is consistent with Freud's (1905a) view of the "not-knowing analyst" and with his early notion of the primacy of addressing the analytic surface by making contact with the patient's own concerns and states of being.

In a second use of phenomenology, one which is followed by subsequent hermeneutic exegesis, ideally there is a better recognition by patients of how others may experience them and how their difficulties in living come about through their generation of maladaptive interactional phenomena. Focusing on the phenomena of the interaction between the therapist and the patient removes for the latter the onus of being diagnosed as having secret malevolent representations carried about in one's psyche like some sort of poison that threatens to reach out and contaminate those around one. A focus on the phenomenology of the interaction allows the patient to preserve self-esteem during the investigation rather than to feel primitive and contemptible. It preserves the humanity of the patient and the vital sense of wholeness or autonomy of the self even during the investigation.

The greatest weakness of phenomenology is its neglect of the unconscious realm of the psyche as envisioned by Freud. It is possible to maintain there is a similarity in phenomenology between Freud's concept of the "preconscious" and the manner in which some phenomenologists speak of "unconscious," using it as a descriptive adjective. Husserl (1989), in *Ideas* II, a work that underwent revision after revision for about twenty years with a last revision in 1928, discussed the "unconscious" to some small extent. But in my opinion he was curiously ambivalent on the topic and his discussion is ambiguous and open to several interpretations. In *The Crisis of European Sciences* Husserl (1970) specifically stated his disagreement with depth psychology. There remains a profound conceptual gap between Freud's concept of the unconscious and that of the phenomenologic (Husserl) and existential (Sartre) traditions. At the present time there seems to be a consensus among psychoanalysts that a serious disjunction exists between the phenomenologic method and the method of exploring the unconscious that is used in psychoanalytic clinical work.

I (Chessick, 1992a) have located the phenomenologic stance as one of five disjunctive channels of psychoanalytic listening, as I explain more fully in Chapter 3. The other channels I employ are those of the classical Freudian drive/conflict/defense mode, the modified Kleinian object relations theory, Kohut's self psychology, and focus on the here-and-now interpersonal interaction. The phenomenologic stance I have just described I also use as the fifth channel, employing phenomenology in the sense one of my (Chessick, 1999) teachers, the psychiatrist and philosopher Erwin Straus (1958) used it. I (Chessick, 1996b) have found this channel especially useful in situations of impasse or even impending failure in psychoanalytic treatment.

The basic premises and epistemologic assumptions of all five of these approaches or channels are not compatible with each other and remain seriously opposed. Psychoanalysts today are in the same position in their study of the data of the psychoanalytic process as physicists were at the time the corpuscular and wave theories of light were proposed. Each seemed to explain some of the phenomena of optics, but no resolution for the disjunction between the two theories was apparent on the horizon. The same kind of conflict is going on today between advocates of the relativistic and quantum theories of gravity in physics, so in each field, as well as in other disciplines, there is a similar problem. We in psychoanalysis humbly await the appearance of a great mind who will find a way to combine these various channels of psychoanalytic listening into some sort of super-theory. But this is the current state of the art in psychoanalysis.

The foundation or basic psychological constitution of an individual is formed, as Sartre (1981) said in his phenomenologic study of Flaubert, by both the prehistory and the protohistory of that individual. The prehistory includes the structure and history of the entire family, their social situation and its vicissitudes, the sibling order, the characteristics of the parents and grandparents, their expectations from the yet unborn child, their attitudes toward gender, and so forth. The protohistory contains the early events that are truly or falsely constructed by the child, the preverbal relationships that the child has, and of course the love or lack of love for the infant.

Sartre wrote that the baby must be given a mandate to live; he or she must be here for something, and the mother's love does this. The parents engender a sense of meaning and of purpose in life, and society can support or oppose it. If there is no parental love, the result is that one experiences an empty, passive, boring self and life, and tends toward the realm of the imaginary, bathed in low self-esteem. One solution to this, if one has the talent, as in the life of Flaubert depicted by Sartre, is to recreate the world in the arts. In short, the child is fashioned "in his irreducible singularity" (Sartre, 1981, p. 50), by what the mother is. With these considerations in mind, let us turn now to our two central characters.

2 PREHISTORY

*The whole of great art is a struggle for communication. All things that op-
pose this are evil, whether they be silly scoffing or obstructive tariffs. . . .
And this communication is not a leveling, it is not an elimination of differences. It is a recognition of differences, of the right of differences to exist,
of interest in finding things different.*

— *Ezra Pound,* Literary Essays

Pound went through a number of alternative choices of his
middle name, "variously signing himself as Ezra Weston Pound,
Ezra Weston Loomis Pound, and what seemed to be his first
choice, Ezra Loomis Pound. That choice is probably due to admiration for his Loomis ascendants, some of whom had fought in
the Revolution, and some of whom became notorious in upstate
New York as 'the Loomis gang.' They were horse thieves" (Heymann, 1976, p. 6). As a child he was called "Ra" (pronounced
Ray), which he later associated with the Egyptian sun-god, an association with obvious narcissistic implications. Like my composite patient, "Barry," Pound had no siblings and was the sun in
his mother's sky.

Ezra Pound's Prehistory

Ezra Pound was born on October 30, 1885, in the frontier town
of Hailey, Idaho, to Homer Loomis Pound and Isabel Weston
Pound. Homer (an allusively appropriate name for the poet's father) was employed in a government land office as a minor bu-
reaucrat. When Pound was three years old his father was
appointed assayer to the United States Mint in Philadelphia, so
the family moved to the East. Mullins (1961) claimed that

Pound's lifelong interest in money as a phenomenon rather than as something to use for consumption of goods perhaps goes back to his paternal grandfather, Thaddeus Coleman Pound, a pioneer railroad builder and lumberman in Wisconsin who served several terms as a congressman "and became an ardent advocate of monetary reform" (p. 30). In addition to that, Pound's father "sometimes allowed Ezra to stroll through the Mint, and he has described to me one of his earliest memories, when he watched men stripped to the waist as they shoveled heaps of gold coins into large sacks" (p. 31). I will discuss another version of this memory in Chapter 4.

Pound grew up in a comfortable middle-class home of the 1890s. A friend of Pound described his parents as "the quiet, old-fashioned, and extremely pleasant type of American" (Mullins, 1961, p. 31); Homer Pound was a civil servant at a time when that occupation was not as scorned as it is today. The family moved to Philadelphia in 1889 and settled in Wyncote, a small town nearby, when Pound was seven years old. This moving about was critical in Pound's early life, beginning when he was either eleven months or eighteen months, or three to four years old, depending on the biographer. Later he claimed, based on some sort of fantasy, that it tore him away from his "roots." Ackroyd (1987) explained, "both in his life and his work he tried to reconstruct the mythical America from which he imagined he had come" (p. 5). He described Pound's mother as "rather more aloof" than his father, and a person who was deeply ambitious for her son (p. 7). Later Pound complained that the suburb has no roots, no center of life, and Ackroyd reported that on his release from St. Elizabeth's in 1958, "Pound returned here (Wyncote) and walked the streets alone" (p. 7).

Stock (1976) also offered details of the various moves that the Pound family made during the period when they came from Hailey, Idaho, until they finally settled in Wyncote. He claimed that when Pound was eighteen months old, mother and baby moved to New York. From there they lived briefly in Newport and, when Pound was three years of age, they went to live with his grandfather Thaddeus in Wisconsin, finally ending up with Homer in Philadelphia in 1889, when Pound was nearly four years old.

The prehistory on his mother's side was that of the rather aristocratic colonial family with its respect for tradition. On his father's side it was the pioneer family manifesting the most rugged kind of nineteenth-century ruthless idealism. Flory (1989) wrote that Pound's mother "kept her fair share of grand airs. She was very concerned with appearances and cultivated formality of dress and manner" (p. 16). He quoted a comment that "one was inclined to be embarrassed and baffled by her little witticisms, her epigrams, as one so often was by Ezra's" (p. 16).

Pound claimed he was much closer to his father than his mother. The strongest apparent influence on him seems to have been his father's father, Thaddeus Pound, and, as Ezra Pound (Tytell, 1987) correctly said, "the actions of one's ancestors, especially if recited to one in childhood, tend to influence one's character" (p. 13). Tytell (1987) described Pound's mother as a "stiff Victorian Grand Lady who found herself in a dreadful colony" (p. 14). There is an episode, as described variously by various authors, that Pound's mother precipitously took her son on the train back to New York when he was eighteen months old. They were caught in a snowstorm and then spent the next six months with Pound's maternal grandmother in Manhattan and, as stated above, another six months on the farm of Pound's paternal grandfather Thaddeus.

Obviously, the various biographies of Pound do not agree on details of his prehistory or protohistory, and some tend to be either defensive or critical of Pound. The matter is made even more complicated by the fact that Pound often either deliberately lied or at times distorted his recollections of his early life, so these are not reliable at all. My favorite biographical study of Pound is by Humphrey Carpenter (1988). It is the most balanced and carefully researched. Pound's mother became pregnant once more after his birth, but miscarried and did not try again. Carpenter states that Pound with both his parents left Hailey when he was eleven months old. He describes Pound's father Homer as having "something essentially comic" (p. 10) about him, and claims that in Pound's behavior there was "an element of satirical impersonation of his father" (p. 11).

Pound was the indisputable favorite of his mother and held in awe by his father, a position similar to the situation of Sigmund

Freud. Pound never experienced any overt psychological or adolescent break with his parents and continued to write letters to them as long as they lived, even though he left America for Europe at the age of twenty-three. He wrote to them separately, using different literary styles for each. Carpenter (1988) explained, "Yet it was to his parents, after arriving in Europe, that he gave the most detailed and honest account of his situation, while to friends of his own generation he chose to remain enigmatic and boastful. His parents were the nearest he had to allies, the only people with whom pretense was unnecessary, to whom he could display, at least now and then, the vulnerability that no one else must see" (pp. 12-13).

What emerges with some clarity through the myths, confusion, and conflicting reports around the birth and infancy of Ezra Pound is the psychological schism between his parents. The tension in the house must have been painful, with Isabel and her mother (Pound's grandmother) feeling that she had married beneath her, and with Homer, as Pound described him, rather "naive" and going quietly about his civil service business involving coinage. There is a curious resemblance to Tolstoy's Anna Karenina in this marriage and in the precipitous flight of Isabel, who claimed she could not stand the "altitude" of Hailey, Idaho, any longer. As with Tolstoy's flawed heroine, her flight represents the outcome of the marital schism.

The first few years of Pound's life clearly were psychologically stormy under the surface, and much of his work and writing seems to be a search for renewal, or an attempt to sink roots into something solid and to repair a wobbly foundation (see, for example, Pound's [n.d.] translation and commentary on *Chung Yung — The Unwobbling Pivot*). Consider also the effects of moving from his father to live first with the aristocratic grandmother and then the fiery paternal grandfather (and great-grandfather, who lived with Thaddeus on the farm!).

Barry's Prehistory

I turn now to the prehistory of Barry, my amalgamated imaginary case history counterpart of Ezra Pound. I feel free to do this at last, since both Pound and my "patient" Barry are deceased and

Barry's wife has happily remarried. In contrast to Pound's good old-fashioned Yankee background, Barry's prehistory begins in Europe. The most influential person in his prehistory was his maternal grandmother Helen, a Jewish orphan raised in Hungary by Catholic nuns, and a woman of fierce ambition and drive. Helen in her early life became convinced that the only future for a Jewish male was to become a doctor, and indeed her influence was so powerful that her two male sons became doctors, and three of her five grandchildren became doctors. She was married by arrangement to a simple woodcarver in Hungary at the end of the nineteenth-century, and they settled in a small town near Budapest to raise their family. There was considerable friction in the house because the woodcarver had nothing but contempt for his wife's cultural pretensions, at one point threatening to smash the piano that she had purchased with his wages. She required all of her four children to learn to play the piano, and Barry's mother actually became a piano teacher. Although her two male children gave up musical instruments after they became physicians, her two daughters, who became social workers, continued to play the piano to the end of their lives.

When her oldest son was in the second year of medical school there was a Fascist revolution in Hungary and he was not permitted to continue his studies because he was Jewish. Helen therefore brought the entire family to the United States. She did not like the United States and actually returned for a short time to her native Hungary, but the political situation was so bad there they again emigrated, settling in Chicago, where her sons could attend medical school. The schism in the family was resolved by her husband taking a job in nearby Milwaukee, where he lived during the week, and commuting to Chicago only on the weekends.

Barry's paternal grandfather was an extremely stubborn Russian peasant who swam across the Dnieper River and came by himself all the way across Europe to settle in a London slum when he was a teenager in order to avoid military conscription. The plight of the Jews in the Russian army at the turn of the century was terrible: they were severely persecuted. By a combination of shrewdness and stubbornness, Barry's paternal grandfather accrued sufficient money to be able to emigrate to the United States, along with the woman that he met and married, who was also a Russian immigrant living in London. Like Pound's paternal grandfather Thaddeus, there were stories of shady financial dealings by Barry's paternal grandfather in the London slums. But the latter was an austere and distant figure who was not idealized as was Thaddeus Pound.

Barry's father was the second son of a large group of siblings. The first son was killed at the age of two when a section of a roof fell on his head in the slum. He had been left unattended on the porch. Barry's father was crippled by his father. Not long after they moved to the United States, when Barry's father was about eight years old, he fell and fractured his leg. A cast was put on, but Barry's father's father, for reasons of pride—"No son of mine will wear a cast"—refused to allow it to remain, and took it off himself. The result was that the youth's left femur fused with the pelvis, and there was a noticeable shortening of that leg and loss of movement in the left hip joint. Therefore Barry's father could not run, and he walked with a noticeable limp. Barry's father was the only member of his entire large family who received any education, which he gained for himself by long hours of hard work. He was derisively referred to by his siblings as a cripple, and to add to what must have been his humiliation, the youngest child of the large family, a boy, became a star high school basketball player in Chicago in the 1920s. Barry's father assumed the paternal role in the family, often giving money and help to his sisters and brother; the latter was a ne'er-do-well and was essentially ruined by his basketball stardom because he could never adjust to being an ordinary person after high school. He became very obese and died prematurely from coronary artery disease.

Barry's parents met while his mother was working as a secretary for a firm which utilized Barry's father to audit their accounts. Grandmother Helen was strongly against the marriage, as she feared the crippled leg would somehow be inherited. This was her pattern for all her children; she considered none of their chosen spouses good enough for them, and loudly announced this to everybody. Barry's mother, in her one act of rebellion, married his father anyway. They got along quite well, except on the issue of Barry's father's family. There was constant quarreling because Barry's father was always giving money to various members of his family, and they were always appearing at Barry's father's house, utilizing the kitchen, helping themselves to whatever they wanted, and leaving a mess of unwashed pots, pans, and dishes behind. Behind the quarrel was a very thinly disguised contempt that Barry's mother felt for this uneducated large group of workers and peasants. The situation of Barry's mother was similar to that of Pound's mother Isabel, except that Barry's father functioned actively to keep the peace and was much more supportive of Barry's mother's pretensions and immaturity than Homer Pound was of his wife's.

Barry was an only child, and like the only child of his mother's sister, was designated to be a doctor long before he was born. To add to the pressures, shortly after Barry's parents were married the Great Depression struck the United States and his father was financially ruined. From that time on he was extremely conservative and made only a minimal income, although he spent many hours obsessively doing his accounting chores. Barry's father never recovered from the two main blows of his life, the crippling by his own father and the destruction of his financial hopes by the Great Depression. All this happened before Barry was born. At the same time, his father was not overtly depressed, but rather withdrew into obsessive work habits and his paternalistic reaction formation. There was a similarity between Barry's father and Pound's father in that both were gentle, rather naive individuals, with whom it was easy to be friends.

There was also a similarity between Barry's mother and Pound's mother, in that both were fiercely ambitious for their sons and themselves and had many cultural pretensions that fitted in very poorly with the people among whom they had to live on a day-to-day basis. We are told that Pound's mother had great difficulty in communicating with the frontier folk in Hailey, Idaho, and that her elegant diction sounded strange and almost unintelligible to them. Similarly, Barry's mother, in her choice of oriental rugs, delicate furniture, and the ever-present grand piano, seemed quite out of place among the proletariat of her husband's family. One of Barry's earliest memories was of his uncle, a wallpaper hanger married to one of his father's sisters, sitting in his mother's living room on a delicate woodcarved chair, leaning back on the chair—and then Barry heard a loud crack as the back of the chair broke.

Another vivid memory was of the curious transformation that his father underwent while in the company of his family.

Barry often noticed that his father's civil manners and educated way of talking would be dramatically and regressively replaced by crude speech and boorish mannerisms, even though at the same time Barry's father attempted to maintain a defensive professional demeanor and position when among his siblings.

Barry's mother was a kind of child bride; when he was born she was an immature twenty-five years old. His earliest years were spent in a two-story apartment building in which he and his parents lived upstairs and his mother's sister, her husband, and their only child (a girl) lived downstairs, along with Helen, who was Barry's grandmother and the mother of the two sisters. Thus, Helen was in Barry's childhood a living presence of fiery, driving ambition, just as Thaddeus Pound was a ubiquitous spectral and sometimes living presence that profoundly influenced Ezra Pound's life and thought.

Discussion and Comparison

The prehistories of these two individuals each show an internalization of certain grandparental qualities and ambitions that dominated the family, the family mythology, and the family dynamics by their associated powerful drive and boundless energy. These internalizations set out a path in each case from which neither Pound nor Barry could ever deviate in its essentials from youth to old age. Pound came to be increasingly preoccupied with the intricacies and interlocking of monetary theory and governmental matters in attempting to solve his projected internal problems, and Barry became a physician, driven to achieve greater and greater heights by the prevailing maternal familial ambition until he was destroyed. Neither Pound nor Barry had more than a dim awareness of the roots of their preoccupations, or of the fact that they were in a sense possessed by forces and internalizations not only beyond their control, but even beyond their conscious awareness. When Pound's father said in awe of him that there was nothing that Pound did not know, and Barry's father told him, "we expect great things from you, young man," these statements served only as confirmations

that the nurturing fathers were also in obeisance to and con-
formed with the maternal demand for the sons to achieve the
narcissistic aims of the mothers and grandmothers. Both men
grew up with this burden upon them, saved at least temporarily
from gross insanity by the nurturing presence of the fathers who
were more maternal than the mothers, a situation not uncom-
monly seen in clinical work.

In the case of Barry, there was also a series of maids who took
on the main task of caring for the children when they were very
little. One of his earliest memories was of being enraged because
his mother and aunt, living upstairs and downstairs, respectively,
were chattering in Hungarian and paying no attention to him, expecting the maid to take care of him. He gave only a shadowy representation of these maids, except to say that he was very attached
to the first of them, named Kaye, a young Finnish woman. In fact,
his earliest memory in life was reported to be of standing by the
warm stove early on a winter morning when he was about three or
four years old and being dressed and given breakfast by Kaye; his father was away at work and his mother was sleeping late, as usual
("well-bred" women did not get up early—they had maids to do the
housework). This is a warm, nurturing, preoedipal memory, but expresses the absence of the parents as well.

Pound's primary caretaker, on the other hand, seems to
have been his mother, and regrettably there was not as much
amelioration of his situation. It is not unusual to see cases in clinical practice where a loving maid, "nanny," or even grandmother
or aunt had an important ameliorative effect and generated a
vital internalization that permits some hope and reaching out in
later relationships or in therapy.

We will in Chapter 4 pass on to the protohistory of these individuals, the early events truly or falsely constructed by them,
and their preverbal experiences and early relationships. It is important to stress that this protohistory already is laid down on top
of a prehistory, which in the case of these individuals constituted
a heavy burden placed upon them. This burden may be thought
of as an early wound or as an impediment to the ego as it forms
in the earliest years of life, hampering its optimal development
and creating an internal struggle between the wish of the

person's self to develop in its own autonomous fashion and the equally powerful, if not more powerful, wish to carry out the assigned prehistorical project in order to gain the life-enhancing smile and enthusiasm and attention of the mother.

3 EXAMINING THE PSYCHE

We listen with "evenly suspended attention," but this means only that we do not prejudge the content; rather, we allow it to achieve whatever shape it achieves in any particular hour. We may be a blank screen for the patient's transferences, but our minds are not blank. A truly (conceptually) blank mind will hear nothing in an analytic patient's associations; and a mind with a single set of organizing concepts will hear material only in ways susceptible to being organized by those concepts. It seems to me that we now have a broad array of concepts and, while they make things more complex, they also reflect the actualities of development more fully and therefore we and our patients are the gainers for it.
— *Fred Pine,* Developmental Theory and Clinical Process

In the first part of this chapter I explicate the five-channel multiple concept approach to achieving psychoanalytic understanding that constitutes the psychoanalytic aspect of the methodology used in this book. Then in the second part I briefly review some aspects of psychoanalytic observations on the development and formation of the psyche especially pertinent to our understanding of the protohistory and the personalization or consolidation and identity formation of our two protagonists, Ezra Pound and Barry. I close with a few remarks on psychopathology to provide a brief orientation to concepts that will be expanded and illustrated in later chapters as we investigate the careers of Ezra Pound and Barry in detail.

The Multiple Concept Approach

Pine (1985) maintained that diverse developmental moments lead to phenomena focused on by drive psychology, ego psychology, object relations theory, and self psychology. Need tension and release pertain to drive theory, developmental achievements to ego psychology, and experiences with the mother and father to object relations theory and self psychology. Pine rejected Freud's death instinct and viewed the repetition compulsion as arising from the need for mastery or for providing a better representational world, but resulting, unfortunately, in a drama carried out over and over with interior players from old relations. All behavior comes developmentally to function with respect to drive gratification, conscience, adaptation to reality, repetition of old internalized object relations, and maintenance of self-esteem. The degree of pathology is the degree that adult behavior is determined by the past rather than by current realities. The various psychoanalytic theories each address some aspect of this, and the analyst must have in mind an array of concepts as he or she listens. Thus, the analyst is a "prepared explorer."

The Five Channels

I (Chessick, 1992a) suggested a "five-channel" approach to psychoanalytic listening to maximize our understanding of a patient. For those not familiar with this approach I will now briefly review these five standpoints or channels (models, perspectives, frameworks) from which we can tune in to the transmission from the patient. Each of them, as is well known, is based on premises that are currently conflicting and irreconcilable. The *first* channel was presented by Freud (reviewed by Chessick, 1980) and focuses on the Oedipus complex and the emergence in a properly conducted psychoanalysis of the need for drive satisfaction in the transference. This enables us to study the patient's conflict in terms of defenses against the instinctual drives and the resulting compromise formations produced by the ego in dealing with its three harsh masters—the superego, the id, and external reality. Freud's structural theory, placing the Oedipus complex at the focus, was developed for this purpose. At the core of it are the patient's childhood or infantile fantasies, which repeat themselves over and over again in the patient's mental life and behavior (Arlow, 1985). We carefully listen for the derivatives of these fantasies and look for them to be reenacted in the transference. I believe this to be the primary model, the starting point for all psychoanalytic listening.

The *second* channel utilizes the perspective of object relations theory for its model. The work of Klein and her analysand Bion focuses on the earliest projective and introjective fantasies of the patient as they appear in the object relatedness manifest in the transference and in the process of projective identification as it occurs in the analytic process. Bion (1963, 1967) emphasized the "toilet function" of the analyst, in which the analyst must receive, metabolize, and give back in acceptable form the unacceptable fantasies and affects and expressions of these coming from the patient. Klein (1975) developed the concept of projective identification (defined differently by every author), in which the patient is allowed to place into the analyst whatever representations he or she wishes to place there, with more therapeutic focus on preoedipal fantasies and processes. For Klein (Money-Kryle, 1974), projective identification was also an interactional event in which great pressure is put on the therapist to behave in a manner that corroborates the projection. For Kernberg (1975), aware of Klein's confusion of the intrapsychic and the interactional under one process, it is a very primitive mental event that represents an incomplete projection. A study of projective identification operating in the therapeutic process reveals the patient's earliest internalized object relations and yields data about how the patient as an infant organized these relations into self and object representations and then projected and reintrojected various aspects of these images. Understanding of these processes clarifies the patient's relationships in the present because all such relationships are perceived and reacted to through the spectacles of these early organized self and object representations. Kernberg (1975, 1976, 1980) presented the most thorough theoretical elaboration of this material (reviewed by Chessick 1977b, 1993a, 1993b).

A *third* channel, focusing on the patient's being-in-the-world, is the phenomenologic point of view described in Chapter 1. Here an attempt is made to grasp the facts of the patient's life phenomenologically, without other theoretical preconceptions to organize the data. This approach was elaborated in philosophy by Husserl and then differently by Heidegger, and taken up especially by the pioneer psychoanalysts Boss (1963) and Binswanger (1963)—especially in their effort to understand seriously disturbed and psychotic patients. A corollary of this approach began with Feuerbach and Marx, and was elaborated by thinkers like Fromm, Sartre, and—most recently—Lacan (reviewed by Chessick, 1987, 1992b): Society shapes the individual and we can only understand the individual if we understand the society or culture or world in which he or she must continuously live and interact. So, to understand an individual, we must understand that lived state of being-in-the-world which is unique for the situation of each person.

The *fourth* approach is from self psychology (Kohut, 1971, 1977, 1984; reviewed by Chessick, 1993a), which focuses on the state of the patient's sense of self as it is empathically grasped by the analyst. Important predecessors of this approach were Fairbairn and Winnicott. The latter introduced the notion of the true and the false self that was taken up in detail by R. D. Laing (1969) in his brilliant exposition of schizoid and schizophrenic conditions. Kohut brought the focus on the self into a systematic and elaborate theory; significant alterations in this theory have recently been offered by Gedo (1979, 1984), whose work does not receive the attention it deserves. Although Gedo rejected many of Kohut's premises, often on the basis of careful arguments, his establishment of hierarchies of self organization represents a further elaboration and movement away from traditional psychoanalytic metapsychology.

The *fifth* approach to organizing the transmission from the patient might be loosely termed the interactive, focusing on the countertransference of the therapist or, more generally, on the here-and-now factors in the treatment and emphasizing the analyst's participation. Schwaber's (1981a, 1981b, 1983a, 1983b, 1983c, 1985, 1986, 1987) views represent an extreme example of this approach, although they are infused with Kohut's insistence on the primary role of the analyst's empathic grasp of how the patient experiences the analyst, since for Kohut empathy is a process that constitutes the methodology that distinguishes psychoanalysis from the other sciences.

Many of the numerous and conflicting points of view under this rubric have been developed as a response to our increasing understanding, especially in preoedipally damaged patients, of the patient's need for an experience and not just an explanation — in the treatment. Modell (1976) offered the notion of the psychoanalytic process in the early phase of the treatment of narcissistic or schizoid patients as providing a "cocoon," a holding of the patient until the patient is ready for self-exploration. Langs (1982) emphasized the presence of delineated interactive fields in which the data coming from the patient are loaded with allusions to the therapist's participation and even the therapist's mental state. In this extreme (Chessick, 1982b) but carefully worked-out view, the patient's unconscious is given the capacity for perception of the therapist's personal difficulties as well as a motive to cure the therapist so the therapist may in turn cure the patient.

Gill (1982) emphasized the importance of the therapist's participation in the particular transference manifestations that develop in a given treatment and also focused his interpretation on the here-and-now interaction between patient and therapist. Gill's view is close to Sullivan's (1947, 1953) more extreme "interpersonal" theory of psychiatry, which, however, eschews Freud's crucial concept of "psychic reality" and attempts to study a scientifically delineated interaction in the treatment, one in which the therapist both participates in and observes the interaction at the same time. Sullivan's approach suffered from a metapsychological shallowness because of its emphasis on the interactional without sufficient study of the filtering mechanism through which the patient inevitably experiences this interaction. Sullivan's (1947, 1953) concept of parataxic distortion attempts to make up for this deficiency, but has not received widespread acceptance.

Wolf (1985), from a self psychological channel, pointed out in his notion of "regressive listening" the impact of the therapy situation itself on the analyst and his capacity to listen. This important concept belongs at the margin of the self psychological and the interactive channels, and I hope it will receive greater attention and explication in the future.

Nietzsche, postulating the metaphysical notion of the will to power underneath all human behavior and mentation (reviewed by Chessick, 1983), profoundly influenced the psychoanalytic approach of Adler. Breaking with Freud, Adler attempted to evaluate all the data of psychoanalysis from this principle, but his approach suffered from an intrinsic oversimplification of all explanations. I will not employ the concepts of Adler or of the mystical Jung in this book nor will I refer to the latest extension of Nietzsche's approach, constructivism (see Chessick, 1997b).

An Experience, Not Just an Explanation

Loewald (1986) was a pioneer in developing the traditional psychoanalytic approach, but he also insisted that the patient's experience of the analyst was a major factor in the curative process. How does this experience affect the process of psychoanalytic listening? For example, sometimes the patient's experience in the analytic situation is only communicated in what Gabbard (1982) cleverly called the "exit line" of both the patient and the analyst. At the end of the treatment session, as the patient leaves the room, there may occur a "separate" type of dialogue or interaction, in which material that has been left out of awareness during the period of free association is given direct exposition by the patient. This is also an especially valuable time to study countertransference manifestations. Freud, as mentioned earlier, was aware of this phenomenon, at least as a clue to the transference.

Gedo (1977) sharpened our focus on the archaic transferences, in which the patient forces a response out of the analyst and contaminates the evenly hovering attention stance advocated by Freud. The management of such archaic transferences and their effect on psychoanalytic listening is one of the most important and central issues in modern psychoanalytic therapy because so many patients present with preoedipal damage and rapidly develop such transferences. Gunther (1976) emphasized the converse of the archaic transference, namely, the narcissistic aspects of the countertransference. He pointed out that countertransference manifestations appear often after the therapist's narcissistic equilibrium has been upset; they represent an attempt to restore the therapist's equilibrium, and he urged us to look for these situations in psychoanalytic listening.

The most complete traditional exposition of the interaction between patient and analyst was offered in a series of papers by Lipton (1977, 1979, 1983), who restudied Freud's cases in order to demonstrate how significant aspects of the real interaction between the patient and the analyst profoundly affected the data that were presented for psychoanalytic understanding. Freud in his actual practice (often quite sensibly) violated some of his own admonitions, as published in his (Freud, 1912b, 1913, 1914c, 1915b) papers on technique. Stone (1981) systematized this real interaction under the rubric of the "physicianly vocation" of the analyst and demonstrated compellingly the profound impact of it on the material produced and the process of the treatment itself.

It is likely that Freud's papers on technique were basically aimed at preventing massive acting out by incompletely analyzed or even unanalyzed therapists with their patients, as was common in the early days of psychoanalysis and as remains all too common, with less justification, today (Chessick, 1997a). Freud's admonitions tended in the middle of the twentieth century in the United States to become codified into a rigid set of rules that sometimes produced iatrogenic narcissistic manifestations in patients and led to either an impasse in the treatment or to a surrender of autonomy by the patient, accompanied by a massive identification with the "aggressor" analyst; obviously, these are unsatisfactory outcomes for a lengthy and expensive treatment.

The authors described above were all addressing this danger in their own way, but the conflicting premises behind their approaches again highlights the difference between viewing the patient as suffering from a psychic deficit, with emphasis on experiential repair, and viewing the patient as suffering from psychic conflict that requires explication. In this book I have not tried to reconcile the differing premises on which these various modes of attunement are based, as indeed it is my conviction that they cannot at the present time be reconciled. I have attempted to demonstrate the application of these various modes of attunement to achieve a widening understanding of clinical data, and to illustrate implicitly how the use of these five channels can lead to a deeper and more effective understanding.

Limitations of My Approach

My view differs significantly from that of Gedo and Goldberg (1973) in that their principle of "theoretical complementarity" (p. 4) assumed the different frames of reference or models of the mind may operate only as long as no internal contradictions arose among the various parts of the theory. They believed even Freud did not intend to dispense with his older conceptions as he went forward to propose new ones, and the changeover from one set of Freud's concepts to another did not have to indicate that one superseded the other. These authors claimed that Freud "correctly assumed that a given set of data might be understood most clearly by utilizing one particular frame of reference or model of the mind, whereas another set of data demanded a different set of concepts for its clarification" (p. 4). A careful study of *Freud's Models of the Mind* (Sandler et al., 1998) reveals that Freud was inconsistent about this, leaving important unresolved contradictions as he developed his topographic and structural theories.

But in my approach, theoretical orientations or models are being utilized that *directly conflict with each other* and cannot be thought of as complementary because the basic premises that underlie them, both their epistemological foundations (Chessick, 1980) as well as their basic assumptions about human nature and its motivations (Chessick, 1977a), directly collide. This forces a *radical discontinuity* as we shift from channel to channel in our receiving instrument, rather than, as we would all prefer to do, sliding back and forth between theoretically consistent positions, or at least complementary positions that are consistent with each other.

The worst mistake a beginner can make at this point in the development of psychoanalytic theory is to assume that in some fashion these five various standpoints can be blended or melded into some supraordinate theory that can generate all of them. Careful examination of the premises of these standpoints reveals this to be simply impossible in our current state of knowledge, and we are forced, if we use this shifting of systems, to accept the radical discontinuities. The problem in the human sciences is profound, and some thinkers, such as Foucault (1973a), have claimed that *in principle* no agreement can ever be reached on a single theoretical model for scientific understanding of all human mentation and behavior.

It may seem to some readers that certain other theoretical approaches or models should be added to these channels; what I am offering here is what has proved in my forty years of clinical experience to be of the most value, to be the least speculative (experience-distant), and to generate the least number of arbitrary inferences. The most important requirement of a model is that it be suggested by the very data the patient produces rather than superimposed on the data by experience-distant or arbitrary prior conceptions in the mind of the therapist. This is a relative concept because no theory is truly experience-near, since it is impossible to approach data without some prior conceptions. Our only hope is that our conceptions are not too abstract, generalized, and divorced from the specific material, and that they are capable of being validated by a study of how the patient responds to interventions based on them. Even this is fraught with difficulty, as it is all too human to hear what we wish to hear or, in the depictions in the present book, infer what we wish to infer.

The hardest part of using this approach is to be willing to keep discontinuous and conflicting models in one's mind, which offends the natural and very dangerous human tendency for a neat, consistent, and holistic theoretical explanation of all material, even if it is wrong. Kant (1781) called this tendency the regulative principle of reasoning, and Freud would have based it on the powerful synthesizing function of the ego.

My approach requires tolerance and flexibility on the part of the reader as well as a certain maturity, for it is sometimes the unfortunate result of a personal psychoanalysis that the individual becomes a strong and rigid adherent of the particular theoretical orientation or style of one's analyst. Kohut (1984) suggested that the reasons for this are inherent in a psychoanalysis that has incorrectly and prematurely interpreted certain transference manifestations. Since no data available at present convincingly and decisively prove any of these theoretical orientations to be the one and only best orientation, uncritical adherence to any one of them would have to be a leftover of a misunderstood or unanalyzed transference, just as emerging from one's psychoanalysis with a sense of nihilism about all analytic theories would be a similar indication for further analytic work. In the present book I will not discuss these various theoretical orientations (channels, models, standpoints, frameworks, perspectives) in any further detail, as I (Chessick, 1992a) have done it elsewhere, along with clinical illustrations.

Development of the Psyche

Earliest Years

Next, I briefly review some other concepts taken from the various channels and important to further understanding of Ezra Pound and Barry. Aries (1962) argued that childhood was "discovered" after the end of the Middle Ages, and from then on the family ambience centered around the child and his or her education. Although individualism was held in check by the family and increased the power of the tight-knit family circle, it flourished at the expense of the communal society of earlier times. Winnicott (1965b; Davis and Wallbridge, 1981) stressed the mother-infant interaction as crucial to the psyche and to all development. The mother enables the baby to catch hold of time, to join the present with the past and the future; she institutes a sense of Being out of her interactions with the baby, as described in Chapter 1.

When "eight-month anxiety" appears, it means a true object relation to the mother has now formed and there are reliably stored memory traces. Around the age of eight months there is a crystallization of affective response, beginning ego integration, and the first establishment of a love object. This is because a synthesis of good and bad object representations has started to take place, and the good object representation of the mother predominates if all has occurred advantageously (Spitz, 1965).

Even an utterance, poetic or otherwise, is a product of an interaction; the situation enters into the utterance as a horizon, a common understanding, a common evaluation. Utterances are intertextual, and every utterance is related to previous utterances. Bakhtin (Todorov, 1984) called this "dialogism." The consciousness awakens surrounded by the consciousness of others, and as an example he emphasized the plurality of consciousnesses in Dostoevsky's writings, in which the characters seem to be in a dialogue with the author.

For Erikson (1950), ego identity develops out of the gradual integration of all identifications. A nucleus of separate identity appears early in life. The neurotic ego falls prey to overidentification, which isolates the individual both from his or her budding identity and from his or her milieu. Disturbances in development of the sense of identity in childhood destroy the adult sense of humanity and are crucial to understanding the development of harmful political systems, wars, and other crimes in a society. For Erikson, a study of childhood in a society is the key to understanding the society. Ego identity requires the ability to experience one's self as something that has continuity and sameness and to act accordingly, as we have seen in Chapter 1, even in reference to the work of Federn. When it goes wrong we end up with a predominance of autoerotism and fragmentation.

Horney (1939) correctly pointed out that what is crucial in childhood is the sum total of early experiences, not the specific stages. From these experiences the person receives his or her orientation to the world. The soil out of which a neurosis grows contains feelings of alienation, hostility, fear, and diminished self-confidence. But we should never forget that the child refuses to acknowledge the mother's impairment as a caretaker. The child erects a reaction formation against disappointment, identifies with the mother's pathology as superiority, and splits off rage and disillusionment (see Gedo and Gehrie, 1993).

Due to aggression in the paranoid position, the schizophrenic patient attacks his or her own mental apparatus and shatters it, according to Bion (1967). Then occurs a projection of the fragments. This ruins the patient's capacity for perception, and the psychotic individual feels surrounded by bizarre and dangerous objects. In the psychotic we uncover a primitive catastrophe, not a buried city of repressed infantile wishes as in the neurotic. Failure of the mother-infant interaction results in the destruction of the link between the mother and the child and a developmental arrest in which aggression is employed in an attack even on the child's own mental apparatus. When the archaic "beta" projections are not metabolized by the "alpha function" (Bion, 1967) of the mother, the infant reintrojects nameless dread. This happens when the mother has no capacity for "reverie," and so a misunderstanding object is therefore introjected by the infant.

Similarly, the great difficulties of the autistic children Bettelheim (1950) worked with were not due primarily to regressive or defensive mechanisms, but to a failure to organize their personalities from the very beginning. Living experiences for them failed to coalesce and stayed fragmentary. Their hatred of people prevented the forming of relationships; children totally overpowered by adults engage in hostile procrastination. In the narcissistic personality disorder the role of maintaining the parental self-image has been assigned to the child. The child gets love only when it fulfills parental expectations, so the child's personality develops as a sensitive scanning mechanism (Aronson and Scharfman, 1992). Bettelheim's stated aim was to bring out the best in every child, to enable the child to enjoy life and make it worth living. He hoped to help children to live successfully not only with respect to society's expectations but also to what the individual child enjoyed and to what made life meaningful for that child. Bettelheim's work has come into considerable disrepute today, as illustrated by Sutton's (1996) even-handed biography, and therefore I will not further refer to Bettelheim's theories and approaches in this book.

Most people have a set or repertory of alternative psychological patterns. The compulsive repetition of preexisting behavioral patterns is psychopathology, but besides such repetitions, patients show what Gedo (1988) called "apraxias," failures to acquire basic skills.

Because of compulsive repetitions and apraxias, everyone determines their own unfavorable destiny, as the pre-Socratic philosopher Heraclitus already suspected when he wrote   ἤθos ἄνθρὼπῳ δαίμων (I translate this as "character produces a person's fate"). When a preverbal pattern is present, it is much harder to modify; such patterns did not originally buttress self-esteem but were important as early tension-relieving devices. We must investigate childhood circumstances that prevented the acquisition of the basic skills in the first place, such as identification with a sick parent, anxiety about progress, a safeguarding of autonomy requiring the rejection of external influences, grandiosity (in which the person feels so perfect no skills need be learned), or too much frustration and disappointment in a caretaker.

Personalization

Sartre (1978), utilizing phenomenology, believed you become what you are in the context of what others have made of you.

His concept of "personalization" implies both previous conditioning and historical conditioning. Even an attempt to fight and deny one's background asserts the background. In personalization an individual forms during childhood a basic choice or project, which is the definitive force, although it may be disavowed during the "identity formation" of late adolescence, in producing the direction of the person's life curve. Even the quality of a person's sex life can be a manifestation of his or her basic project, a view similar to Kohut's (1984) depiction of the "sexual drive" as a disintegration product and of adolescent sexuality as being primarily based on issues of self-esteem.

Understanding the quality of a person's sex life as a manifestation of an underlying choice of project is suggested in Sartre's (1973) *Being and Nothingness.* He argued that needs mutually influence each other and there is not a simple hierarchy of one based on another. One cannot reduce the higher needs to the lower, as Freud thought. There is also a superficial resemblance of Sartre's focus on one's basic project to Kohut's (1977) discussion of the program of the nuclear self. Sartre claimed that to live is to project one's self toward one kind of future rather than another.

In Sartre's view, personalization is the building up of an orientation culminating in a choice (Barnes, 1981). The consciousness tries to fit new experiences in with a unity that has already been developed. If it cannot, one of the following may occur: There is (1) a crisis that causes the individual to attempt to make a new choice of being and to make himself or herself over, or (2) a pretense that such a transformation has occurred when it really has not, or (3) a disavowal, which Sartre calls "false distraction," or (4) an imaginary forgetting, or "bad faith."

Sartre (1981) described how Flaubert developed from a child playing imaginary private roles in the family to an adult who chose to objectify the imaginary in art. For Sartre, we do not control our destinies once our projects are chosen. We are not at home in the world. The world is allergic to man. We are alienated and mystified and inserted into the world, but ordinarily we ignore this except when some supposedly familiar object becomes suspect. Then the whole world takes on a suspicious quality. All we took for granted is thrown into question, and "I no longer know who I am."

Remember that for Sartre, children and parents engage in the dialogue of the deaf, and the ego is created by the consciousness (see Chapters 1 and 15 of the present book). The problem of life is what he called contingency, that is, chance or the unexpected. We do not know what our consciousness will be in the future, and we do not know what others and what the physical world will do. Emotional crises, he says, are purposeful and attempt a magical transformation to alter one's relationship to a situation when there is no way out (Sartre, 1948). An active agent carves out his or her being in the world by leaving a mark through action on the surrounding environment, while a passive agent announces through bodily symptoms and behavior what he or she is about to become. A trigger must set off a decisive change, an explosion such as the nervous crisis and "seizure" of Flaubert. This seizure allowed him to be regressive and cared for like a child, provided a release from his father's wishes that he pursue a law career, and was an escape from the bourgeoise lifestyle to that of an artist (Sartre, 1981).

Sartre (1963) also emphasized the great importance of society and cultural tradition, which influences an individual by enhancing or opposing his or her basic project. The "practico-inert," the material and bureaucratic conditions of society, takes the place of his earlier concept of "Being-in-itself" from *Being and Nothingness* (Sartre, 1973); it resists our projects and limits our knowledge, but it is the only instrument we have for living. Notice that a wrong culture can alienate us from our basic project and oppose our struggle to choose and realize ourselves. This was the central argument in Sartre's opposition to Hartmann's (1958) ego psychology, with its stress on the goal of adaptation.

Later in his work Sartre moved from his concept of the "lone man" theory of freedom to social problems, for to be free, he asserted, others around you must be free. He presented an atheistic materialism in which ethics arise from defining whatever is good as useful to human freedom. He insisted, and I agree, that one cannot avoid the political life if one wants freedom for one's self and others. The key task of anyone who wants humans to approach their potential, a common goal of philosophers and psychiatrists, is to allow each person to carve out freely his or her being-in-the-world in that brief interlude between birth and death. This orientation must be based on a principle of reverence for human life defined as beginning at birth. A society should be judged by the degree to which it facilitates or impedes this goal, and by how it treats the poor, the sick, and the mad, its marginal members.

Origin of the Self

Kojéve (1980), in his famous interpretation of Hegel, insisted that for Hegel the primary concern of the philosopher is knowledge of one's self or "self consciousness." The "I" is the key to the human's self-consciousness and is generated by desire, especially by desire for recognition by the other. Recognition as an individual is the crucial issue in Kojéve's interpretation of Hegel. In my (Chessick, 1992b, 1993a) lectures to students on Kohut's work I often ask (1) What thinker first placed the development of the self at the center of his theories, (2) insisted the self can only develop when it receives intense recognition from another self, and (3) tried to show that self-development is ruled by forces out of our conscious awareness, like the unfolding of a seed into a plant, an unfolding that makes rational sense only by looking backward after development has gone as far as it can? The answer, of course, is Hegel (1807). His philosophy is in eclipse now but I believe it will rise again in a modern version in the 21st century as it did around the beginning of the 20th century.

Perhaps the most well known use of the term "self" is that of George Herbert Mead (1962), a pragmatist who tried to eliminate the parallelism between the mind and the body by viewing the mind and the self as arising out of social interaction and having no innate separate existence. For Mead, the self was a social self that formed in two stages. At first, the individual's self is constituted simply by an organization of the attitudes of others toward both the individual and one another in the specific social acts in which the individual participates with them. Then, at the second stage, there is added "an organization of the social attitudes of the generalized other or the social group as a whole to which he belongs" (p. 158). Thus, for Mead the mind or self is formed by "reflexiveness" from social experience, a view that influenced H. S. Sullivan (1953) in forming his "interpersonal school" of psychiatry (Chessick, 1974, 1977a; Greenberg and Mitchell, 1983). I discuss the "self" as it is conceived of in self psychology in Chapter 17.

Adolescence

For Wittgenstein (1972; Schulte, 1992) our world picture is a system of not moved or easily replaced convictions. It is a framework for all discussions and proofs. It is tied to our practice—"This is the way we do it." Our world picture rests neither on empirical knowledge nor verification of hypotheses. Testing must stop at some underlying point. What we are taught as children and take on faith is an organized structure containing conclusions and premises that give each other mutual support. This world picture is not easily shaken by conflicting empirical propositions because it is more like a mythology one decides to adopt, ignoring conflicting evidence. The changeover to another system is a conversion moved more by persuasion than by reason. Psychoanalysts need to keep this in mind.

Even *The Odyssey* is seen (Tracy, 1990) as a search for identity by both Odysseus and Telemachus. Books nine through twelve are the most famous, as Odysseus achieves his identity in a trip to the underworld and in telling his story. In the oedipal period the boy must renounce his early passivity with respect to his mother. Then in preadolescence there is new instinctual pressure of a quantitative type, and a crucial theme of the preadolescent boy is the fear of the castrating mother, which is often defended against by the gang stage (Blos, 1962). Early adolescence has to do with the decathexis of incestuous love objects and the clamor for new ones. Friendships in boys are based on a shared ego ideal. In adolescence proper, or middle adolescence, narcissism predominates, followed by beginning consolidation, but also delaying action, stages of disengagement, and even hypochondria. This is characterized by the striking uniformism of United States adolescents, who all must look and act alike and do and wear the same things. Homosexuality may briefly appear at this stage.

Late adolescence has to do with consolidation, as will be illustrated in Chapter 6. It is a critical and decisive turning point.

Irreversible identifications take place, a "narrowing down" of one's world picture, as well as a delimitation and channeling of ego functions. Postadolescence is ideally characterized by harmony, integration and morality, but adolescent rebellion cannot be terminated until the infantile sexual ties to the parents are resolved, which in some cases never happens. Prolonged adolescence is related to the phenomena observed in narcissistic personality disorders.

Love

When requited passion occurs, there is an unconscious illusion of partial gratification of childhood desires, a momentary escape from the constraints of reality in the passionate embrace. What sets these passionate affairs in motion? In the young it is the flux and instability of their personalities. In middle age, it rises out of the relentless and leaden repetition of experience, a search for an antidote for frustration, disappointment, and repetition, and above all from the wish to attain the unachieved and forbidden childhood wishes (Gaylin and Person, 1988).

Love is the highest human pleasure, and in some ways it is beyond the pleasure principle. There is a tremendous developmental need for the self to be loved for its own sake, to be adored like an infant. Kernberg (1980) claimed that in romantic love there is a union with incestuous objects that helps to overcome the sense of inferiority to parental objects. The ego ideal is not depleted in love as Freud (1914b) thought, but instead there is an increased libidinal investment of the self when one falls in love. Furthermore, culture and history determine our thoughts on love and shape romantic love. I discuss the relationship of love and creativity in Chapters 7 and 9.

Depression

The neurotic or characterologic depressed (dysthymic) person is manifesting an ego state that represents a basic reaction to situations of narcissistic frustration which the ego feels helpless to prevent. The depressed person, severely disappointed in himself or herself, has lost incentive and gives up not the goals but the pursuing of them. This pursuit has until the present proved to be useless, and the depressed person feels fatigue and entrapment.

The most complicated neurotic depression occurs in people who are dependent on external narcissistic supplies (Greenacre, 1953). When these are lacking, depression develops. The incorporation of the object is a recovery mechanism, as Freud (1917) thought, but there are other ways of recovering: (1) goals again appear in reach; (2) modification or reduction of the goals; (3) relinquishment of the goals; and (4) hypomania or depersonalization. However, one must never forget the role of the severe primitive superego in stubbornly maintaining the goals and being perpetually at war with the ego.

Depression is a feeling of the helplessness of the ego due to the tension between highly charged narcissistic aspirations and the ego's shocking awareness of the incapacity to live up to them. Thus, depression arises due to a tension within the ego itself, a basic reaction of the ego to situations of narcissistic frustration. The ego suddenly finds it cannot live up to any or all of the wishes to be worthy and loved, to be strong and secure, and to be good and loving. The result is a feeling of helplessness and inhibition of function, just as anxiety is a reaction to situations of danger (Chessick, 1996c).

The depressed individual has a sense that something is fundamentally wrong with the universe, an awareness of some elemental lack at the core of things. Richardson (1995) supplies us with a phenomenologic quotation from Emerson's friend, the elder Henry James, who once gave the following account of his awareness of emptiness at the center:

> Every man who has reached even his intellectual teens begins to suspect that life is no farce; that it is not genteel comedy even; that it flowers and fructifies on the contrary out of the profoundest tragic depths—the depths of an essential dearth in which its subject's roots are plunged . . . the natural inheritance of everyone who is capable of spiritual life is an unsubdued forest where the wolf howls and the obscene bird of night chatters. (p. 486)

4 PROTOHISTORY

When a mother nurses or cleans an infant, she expresses, like everyone, her integrity of self, which naturally sums up her entire life from birth; at the same time she achieves a relationship that is variable according to circumstances and individuals. . . . But at the same time, by this love and through it, through the very person of the mother—skillful or clumsy, brutal or tender, such as her history has made her —the child is made manifest to himself. That is, he does not discover himself only through his own self-exploration . . . but he learns his flesh through the pressures, the foreign contacts, the grazings, the bruisings that jostle him, or through a skillful gentleness. He will know his bodily parts, violent, gentle, beaten, constrained, or free through the violence or gentleness of the hands that awaken them . . . he internalizes the maternal rhythms and labors as qualities lived with his own body. What is this passivity . . . if, for example, he is abruptly turned on his back, on his stomach, taken too soon from the breast, how will he discover himself? Brutal or brutalized? Will the dissonance, the shocks become the bruised rhythm of his life or quite simply a constant irritability of the flesh, the promise of great future furies, a violent fatality? Nothing is fixed in advance; it is the total situation that is decisive since it is the whole mother who is projected in the flesh of her flesh. Her violence is perhaps only clumsiness, perhaps while her hands bruise him she sings continually to the child who cannot yet speak, and perhaps when he can see, he learns his own corporal unity from his mother's smiles; or perhaps, on the contrary, she does what is necessary, neither more nor less, without unclenching her teeth, too absorbed in an unpleasant job. The consequences will be very different in the two cases. But in either, the infant, wrought each day by the care bestowed upon him . . . internalizes the maternal activity . . . which conditions all the drives and inner appetite-rhythms, promptings, and constants and inexpressible desires—briefly, his own mother, absorbed into his body's innermost depths, becomes the pathic structure of his affective nature.

Jean-Paul Sartre, The Family Idiot

Pound's Earliest Years

In 1890, when Pound was five years old, his mother finally prevailed on his father to move out of the city of Philadelphia, which
she considered flooded with immigrants socially beneath her, to
the borough of Jenkintown, eleven miles north of downtown
Philadelphia. This small town was a rail junction and a shopping
place for the local farm community. As a child he preferred to be
in a group or gang, and avoided close friendships with individuals. The community was anti-Semitic, and there was a general
resentment toward all immigrants.

His mother read to him daily from the classics, even when
he was a young child. Because of his mother's successful accomplishment in educating him at home, he irritated his schoolmates
with his advanced language. Looking back on this earliest period
of his life, one notices many hints that he was deeply uncomfortable as a small boy in school, which he began to hide by a certain
false bravado and exhibitionism.

Two years later the Pounds moved to another area of
housing adjacent to Jenkintown, called Wyncote, where Ezra
Pound lived until he went away to college. Yet he never felt much
sense of home there. His feeling of alienation went back as far as
he could remember. Throughout his life he vituperatively criticized the society in Wyncote as superficial and sciolistic. The picture we have of his mother is that of a person similar to Barry's
mother in that she emphasized a superficial kind of cultural
achievement out of the narcissistic need to feel superior to her
friends and acquaintances.

With the transfer of houses there was a transfer of schools;
he was already being called "professor" by his school fellows. "In
his first school photograph we see a child small for his age, rather
withdrawn and uncommunicative in appearance" (Carpenter,
1988, p. 26). From the ages of about eleven to sixteen he described himself as an earnest Christian who read the Bible daily
and took religion with great seriousness; he apparently fell away
from religious practice because he did not get on with a new minister. By the age of thirteen he could be excited by hearing the
recitation of a passage from Homer and, although his inclina-
tions were toward outdoor activities, he already began to have in-

terests in academic subjects such as Latin. He also enjoyed the game of chess, and showed interest in girls. At the age of twelve his aunt took him for a three-month "grand tour" trip to Europe. We lose track of Pound for a year at the age of fifteen, until he matriculated at the University of Pennsylvania. We do know that by the age of fifteen Pound had determined and articulated his basic project, which was to know more poetry by the age of thirty than any man alive. He set off on a self-education regime, but he often cut corners, so his knowledge was sometimes very profound and sometimes very superficial.

Tytell (1987; also see Chapter 2 in the present book) reported that Pound spent time with his father at his father's place of work, the Mint in Philadelphia:

> When Ezra was eight, there was a recount of the silver coinage and he watched the workers shovel coins into giant counting machines: "all the bags had rotted in these enormous vaults, and they were heaving it into the counting machines with shovels bigger than coal shovels. This spectacle of coin being shoveled around like it was litter—these fellows naked to the waist shoveling it around in the gas flares—things like that strike your imagination." (p. 16)

He was pampered and spoiled by his mother and made to wear his hair in curls even at the age of four in an effort to make him into an object of beauty. At twelve he entered Cheltenham, a military school close to his home. It was already noticed by his classmates that he had an odd way of dressing and a flamboyant arrogance; people made fun of him, as "he was all books."

There is a classic combination here of Pound's poetic ambitions to write the greatest poems ever written and his mother's narcissistic use of his compositions by declaiming them at the Wyncote Ladies' Club: "She may have been the only member of that association who was not wealthy, but her son was a poet!" (Tytell, 1987, p. 19). Although Pound received a lot of support from his easy-going father, who at the same time was depreciated by his narcissistic and ambitious mother, a lot of his rebelliousness was an attempt to get free of his sense of entanglement with her:

It is likely that he took the cue for the formality of his manner from his mother's very studied and rather affected behavior. However, it was clearly his intention to set her values at defiance so that, where it was her intention to impress by overawing people with her rigorousness in observing the proprieties, it was his intention to impress by shocking people with the cavalier way in which he flouted the same proprieties. (Flory, 1989, p. 23)

In summary, Pound was a young boy and adolescent who on the surface appeared to be reasonably well adjusted, but a closer look informs us that he felt alienated from others at a very early age, had great difficulty with intimacy and preferred superficial relationships, and was struggling to actualize some of his mother's narcissistic ambitions as his basic project, one that also allowed him to utilize his remarkable inborn skills and talents. At the same time his deeper instinctual needs as well as his need for the mirroring and nurturance of his own true self remain repressed. The rage and disappointment in the lack of response to him as an autonomous self rather than as an object of showmanship for his mother was split off and directed at Jews, and fueled his identification with Fascists and eventual depreciation of Americans, which occurred when he fragmented and his reality testing broke down (see Chapter 14). Anyone can experience this fragmentation phenomenologically by reading the transcripts of his radio broadcasts from Italy during World War II (Doob, 1952), to be discussed in Chapters 14 and 18.

Pound displayed a mixture of idealization of his father with a sense that his depreciated father was not really part of the divinely royal dyad mother-son (Mother-Ra). He remained on more relaxed terms with his father, and he utilized his experience of his father's profession as a source of information to bring about the magical transformation of the world through the crackpot monetary policies that he embraced in later life. It is perhaps the existence of this unresolved paranoid-schizoid position under the guise of superficial geniality that caused Tytell (1987) to label him "the solitary volcano"; by mid-adolescence it was already clear that he was seething inside. At that point he was able to direct his enormous energies into forming a flamboyant narcissistic personality as a sort of negative identity against his mother's prudishness and primness, and to deliberately embark with all his skills and very considerable talents upon self-education and the pursuit of his basic project of being the world's greatest poet.

Barry's Protohistory

Barry's infancy and childhood can only be described as constituting a profoundly skewed development. Constitutionally he was not physically well coordinated, so he was not able to keep up with the average boy in athletics. In addition to that, his mother had, among other bizarre and sometimes culturally induced fantasies, the idea that a fat child was proof of a good mother. From the beginning of Barry's life there was a strong pressure placed on him to eat, even to the point where if he refused to eat something his mother exploded in a temper tantrum and would strike him. One of Barry's earliest memories was of being forced to eat a dish of peas and annoying his mother because he was hesitant about it; soon after, he vomited. (In Chapter 16, a derivative of this appears in Barry's play.) Throughout his childhood Barry was one of the fattest children in the class and was continuously ridiculed by the other boys and girls because of his appearance.

Another of his mother's narcissistic fantasies, constituting his prehistory as I have discussed it in Chapter 2, was that Barry had to become a doctor. Part of this was the firm conviction (as described earlier) coming from his grandmother that the children in this family all had to be doctors, and part of it came from his mother's frustrated narcissistic aspirations. Because of the family's emigration to the United States, grandmother's two daughters, Barry's mother and aunt, could only attain degrees in social work, for they could not attend medical school. Therefore, Barry, as an extension of the grandiose fantasies of his mother, was destined to medical school, just as Flaubert, according to Sartre (1981), as an extension of his mother's narcissistic aspirations and his father's ambitions, was originally destined to become a physician.

Barry learned early in life to fear his mother's temper. It was not long before, as with Ezra Pound, his ambitions coalesced with his mother's grandiosity, and even in childhood he showed signs of what Kohut (1971) described as presumptive of a narcissistic personality disorder. The competitiveness with which Barry approached all issues in grammar school was ferocious because he was driven by the familial pressure to achieve. At times he was so sure that he would be first in scholastics that he announced in advance he would win a prize, only to find that someone else had come in ahead of him. When this happened there was a profound and painful sense of humiliation and despair as his narcissistic aspirations were frustrated . . . or should I say, his mother's narcissistic aspirations! When Barry did win a prize or win high accomplishments in school there was an unforgettable look of triumph on his mother's face, a look which he saw only in one other place, namely, on his grandmother's face when there was some familial success.

His older cousin, living downstairs at the time (mentioned in Chapter 2), had a brilliant mind. Barry did not. This industrious young girl was invariably first in everything academic, and even as a grammar school child spent many hours studying, becoming the darling of her teachers. None of them recognized how unhappy she secretly was; all were fooled by her "Shirley Temple" smile. She was the star of the family, and Barry, being younger and less intelligent, was a poor second. There was no fair competition because his cousin was older and so much superior, but Barry followed in her academic footsteps, going to the same grammar school, high school, college, and medical school. After that she married and their paths entirely diverged. A successful and affluent doctor, she committed suicide while still a young woman after becoming addicted to barbiturates.

The dominant influence on Barry's early life was clearly his mother, with his maternal grandmother close in the background. Barry's father was a passive and gentle individual who formed the one source of soothing that Barry had, but he saw his father rarely, since the man was working day and night to survive the economic depression of the 1930s and spent what little free time and money he had taking care of his relatives. There was an amiable atmosphere in Barry's house except on the subject of his father's relatives, which invariably produced explosive arguments. During these arguments Barry's mother would use him to soothe her, and Barry would talk about running away with her some day. He remembered this as early as the age of six, late in the oedipal phase of development. She never contradicted him when he expressed this ambition. On the one hand she felt she had married beneath herself, but on the other hand her husband protected and took care of her as he would a child and as he did for the rather primitive members of his family.

The times with his father were generally pleasant, but his father concurred in the family ambitiousness and, except for a few rare occasions, encouraged the same kind of "greatness" of performance. In this sense Barry never formed a basic project; his basic project was formed for him! He was to be a doctor, preferably a surgeon, a man of great standing and authority to whom people would look up and whom they would not dare to oppose. His mother could then bask in the sunshine of his power and fame and announce to all the world that she was, indeed, his mother. Barry often remembered a huge sign in the local library when he was a child that contained what was claimed to be a quotation from Abraham Lincoln: "All I am and ever hope to be I owe to my angel mother." As a child he was not aware that Lincoln had bouts of serious depression and was a profoundly melancholic character.

As one might expect from what I have already described, grammar school was a nightmare for Barry. He was relentlessly teased by the children and pushed around by the class bullies. He was only able to get gratification from the praise of teachers. Remarkably, when he was in the seventh grade, a young science teacher seemed almost to have fallen in love with him. She allowed him to make long lectures to the class, most of which he made up as he went along, and she seems to have believed he was reporting on library research that he had done. The children in the class knew better, but she paid no attention to them. This went on and on through the seventh grade, and he was even accompanied by this teacher on walks after school.

In the eighth grade Barry invited a couple of girls in his class to the first eighth-grade dance, naturally picking the most attractive girls in the class. Of course he was turned down. He went to one eighth-grade party and instructed his father to come to get him at ten o'clock, which he thought was everyone's bedtime. He picked up his date and went to the party; it was going strong when his father appeared. Barry went home with his father, but his date stayed and was taken home later by somebody else. It was clear already at this point that Barry was socially maladjusted, naive, and mixing in a social group that had more money and more experience than he had.

When he went to the University of Chicago he was much happier because many of the very young students who were accepted under the Hutchins plan (see Chapter 5) were socially maladjusted and most of the other students who were not, had just returned from World War II and were much older than he was. In the fierce competition for grades in all courses he was barely able to hold his own, but through many hours of grinding study he achieved high enough grades to be admitted to medical school.

In a sense Barry's college years were tragic because he could not pursue the subjects he was most interested in since he was burdened down with a whole series of premedical courses. In those days many of the premedical requirements were really tests of the students' willingness to memorize enormous amounts of useless trivia; after all, they would have to do a lot of memorization in medical school! So for hours and hours Barry sat and memorized the Latin names of all the plants and all the animals as well as the anatomy of pigs, cats, and sharks. One summer in the boiling heat he took quantitative chemistry, which often required the use of an oven. In that subject he got an "A" in the theory and an "F" in the lab, not because of the heat but because as mentioned, he was not very well physically coordinated and had much trouble with the exacting requirements of laboratory work in quantitative chemical analysis.

At one point on a very hot summer day, after having worked three weeks on an assigned "unknown" compound, he fired it in the oven, carried it toward the scale to weigh it . . . and dropped it. At this point he exploded with a string of expletives, which was not customary for him, but the frustration was overwhelming. To his intense humiliation, from behind a partition there emerged the instructor of the course, who proceeded to give him a terrible dressing down and threatened to fail him. A failure in quantitative chemistry meant a rejection from medical school, and the reader can imagine what Barry went through to apologize, humiliate himself, and make retribution for his behavior.

By this time Barry's life was being lived for him; his real interests were in the humanities and the Platonic ideals or "forms" such as those residing in mathematics, which more suited his poor memory but fair reasoning power. Underlying this was an as yet unarticulated groping for a sense of Being, for an experience of transcendence of the prosaic, material, scientific or "ontic" world (Heidegger, 1962). A schism had developed in Barry's personality that never healed, and his self-esteem was based solely on his capacity to achieve his mother's ambitions. In the area of friendships and sexuality he was unable to be comfortable, and he compensated by many hours of hard memory work. This gave him a sense of superiority to the other students who were having a good time, but it also locked him on an alienated course. The idealized parent imago and the grandiose self formations of early infancy (Kohut, 1971) had been to some extent integrated into the ambitions and ideals poles of his self, but, unfortunately, there was no area of skills, talents, and abilities that allowed a striving from his ambitions pole to his ideals pole that was really true to his own capacities and genuine interests. This led to a sense of despair about life and a kind of chronic depression and sense of emptiness, a condition outlined in Chapter 3.

He was allowed and encouraged by his mother to fantasize himself the victor in an oedipal struggle and to feel superior to his father in both his accomplishments and his mother's love, ignoring the fact that it was his father who slept with his mother. Still, at the core of his being there was a sense of longing for a soothing selfobject. Although his father came the closest to fulfilling this function, Barry did not develop homosexual proclivities, but remained in search of the beloved one who never comes, as described by another narcissist, Rilke (1984b, p. 131).

The sense of inner deadness that Barry suffered from was prior even to these developments, and actually can be traced to the failure of his child-mother in her capacity to provide him with an average expectable maternal environment in which to develop. This unresolved search for a sense of Being remained with him throughout his life and is evidence that Winnicott (1965a; see Chapter 1 in the present book) was correct. I (Chessick, 1996d) have come across this sense of deadness and emptiness in many patients who suffer from a defect in ego feeling, as described by Federn (1952; see Chapter 1 in the present book). Ego feeling, the ego's own perception of itself, of one being one's own person, a residual sense of being alive and existing which is taken for granted when normal, can lead to certain characteristic complaints when it is defective. These are the vague "borderline" complaints of the meaninglessness of life, an inner deadness, a quest for holding, and what Searles (1960; see Chapter 1 in the present book) described as noncherishing relationships to the human and nonhuman environment. Heidegger (1962) would say that ego feeling is related to the quest for Being. It is represented by pre-Socratic thinking wherein the "Being of beings is most apparent" and is especially expressed in poetry. I will elaborate on this theme in later chapters.

Contrasted to problems in ego feeling are pathological defects in ego consciousness, our subjective awareness of our functioning self in time, of being an enduring individual even when we are asleep, that is, our knowledge of our own ego at work, the source of Descartes's "I think, therefore I am." Defects in ego consciousness lead to delirium states, dreamlike states, and feelings of unreality, closer to the problems suffered by Ezra Pound. One must distinguish all this from defects in the ordinary ego mechanisms of defense and efforts at adaptation, which lead to the more stereotyped *DSM-IV* "symptoms" of psychopathology.

Barry received no religious education since his parents were not observant; in some ways he thought of himself as Bazorov in Turgenev's (1948) *Fathers and Sons*. He did experience fleeting feelings of transcendence in his studies of Plato and mathematics, which at times he squeezed around the edges of the premedical courses. For example, as a college junior he wrote a paper on the ecstatic joy of proving a complex geometric theorem in conics, in the tradition of Plato's philosophy (sign on the entrance to Plato's Academy: "Only those who know mathematics may enter here"). So Barry, unlike Sartre, could not be called an atheistic materialist but rather an agnostic who was seeking transcendence but who was locked into a materialist project in life that made it extraordinarily difficult for him to find the truths he was looking for.

Discipline was primarily from his mother and usually consisted of blows to the face when she lost her temper. One of the earliest neurotic symptoms he noted occurred in the third grade. He would have an anxiety attack just before the teacher handed out report cards, hoping there would be no bad marks that he would have to take home to show his mother. Perhaps in connection with the kind of discipline he received, one of the earliest problems he faced was that he could not bring himself to fight back when physically attacked by other boys. He would try to cover himself as well as he could, but he could not get himself to physically punch back; this problem was with him throughout his entire life, and on those few occasions as an adult when he was assaulted he again could not respond with physical force. He was never able to understand the origin of this curious collapse in the face of physical assault. In my clinical experience this is not an uncommon problem in persons who have been primarily cared for by a hot-tempered and physically abusive parent.

Barry passed the usual childhood developmental markers with no other obvious abnormalities. There was an important prekindergarten memory. One night about two o'clock in the morning there was a flap of his window shade due to the wind and he awoke with a start, convinced that he had seen a vivid portrait of the head of the devil on his window shade. It was a light green color and only in outline, resembling a peculiar picture that his parents had hanging on the wall, an embroidered outline of the head of the devil, but red on a black background. The vision of this projected "all bad object representation" (Kernberg, 1976) was so terrifying that he cried out and woke up his mother, who came in and tried to silence him. He could not be consoled, however, and continued to cry, at which point his mother characteristically lost her temper and spanked him soundly. He carried this memory throughout his entire life.

All of this took place against the backdrop of the Great Depression and then World War II. During the Great Depression money was extremely scarce and Barry's father lost all confidence in the markets, preferring to place what he had in government bonds. Because of this action he missed the post-World War II explosion in the stock market entirely, and inculcated in his son a similar fear of the business world and investments. In addition to the financial fears and the background of quarrels over Barry's father giving money to his family against the wishes of his mother, worry over the possibility of victory by the Axis powers in World War II also contributed to the troubled ambience. In 1940, 1941, and 1942 it was not inappropriate to anticipate that the German invasion of Russia would be successful and the Japanese invasion of Southeast Asia would triumph, leading to a merger of the Axis powers on the continent of India and the domination of the Axis powers over the entire Eurasian continent! Liberals like Barry's father and Jewish families would surely have been sent to a concentration camp if subsequent events had led to a German victory over the United States.

Barry's selfobject function of creativity began when he was a young child. Being alone quite a bit, he invented a number of games that he played by taking both sides; this was often accompanied by some fecal withholding and was associated to his father's obsession with daily bowel movements to ensure one's health. Although both of his grandfathers and his father had an important role as soothing selfobjects, unfortunately he did not see very much of them, and they could not overcome the powerful effect of "the mighty trio" (his mother, his mother's sister, and his mother's mother) that formed the overwhelming influence on his life. For example, when he was about five years old his mother called him to lunch, and she was so impatient for him to come that she leaned over and rolled down a few stairs. At this point, although unhurt, she began screaming and kicking and crying like a two-year-old having a tantrum. His mother's sister spanked Barry and then fed him the lunch. This was the second time that Barry saw his mother have an actual infantile tantrum. The first time was when his mother brought a pot of soup to her mother and her mother refused it; at that point Barry's mother, an adult woman, threw herself on the floor and had a tantrum in front of her mother and her little boy. Barry's grandmother, his mother's mother, looked on this impassively and did nothing.

Barry's closest peer relative, the brilliant girl cousin who lived downstairs, was even more completely identified with "the mighty trio" until Barry was about nine years old. At this point his aunt divorced her husband and remarried, moving to another side of the city. After that he still saw them often, and the new uncle became an important influence in his college years, as we shall see in Chapter 6. Grandmother Helen continued to live downstairs. She died when Barry was in adolescence.

5 EDUCATION

The civilization that we are seeking to establish is the civilization of the dialogue. This is the only civilization in which a free man would care to live . . . it assumes that the object of the intellect is the truth, and though the whole truth may never be wholly discoverable, the way to progress toward it is through a free exchange of ideas. It insists upon reason, upon independence, and upon communication.
— *Robert Hutchins,* The Arts of Freedom

To understand Barry's dilemma and Ezra Pound's lifelong rage at American universities one must understand something about so-called "education" in the United States, and the contributions of their contemporary, Robert Hutchins (1936, 1948, 1968). Barry, like his famous peer Allan Bloom (1987), author of *The Closing of the American Mind*, was a product of the special "Hutchins Plan" at the University of Chicago. Under this plan students in the third year of high school were permitted to enter college and get a special degree from the University of Chicago if they could qualify by passing an entrance examination. This enabled superior students to skip over two years of high school and was part of Hutchins's futile attempt to improve the disgraceful United States educational system.

The problems that Hutchins faced then, like those today, were the voracious love of money, the ever-increasing difficulties of the democratic process in the United States, and the prevalent false ideas of "progress" that generate the worship of utility and science. His solution, very much influenced by the philosopher Mortimer Adler, was based on the postulate that the purpose of a university is the study of truth for its own sake. He believed in the existence of a hierarchy of truths that remains unchanged and

59

the same for all. From this point of view, a study of the classics constituting "the western canon" (H. Bloom, 1994) has contemporary relevance and metaphysics becomes a justifiable enterprise and remains the "queen of the sciences," the discipline seeking to unify and correlate all facets of wisdom.

This lofty Aristotelian viewpoint, which still seemed so hopeful and reasonable in the 1930s, at the demoralized time of the Great Depression and before the outbreak of World War II, has of course been replaced in today's fashion by the "postmodern" stance, a diametrically opposed point of view. The educational implications of this postmodern stance motivated Allan Bloom (1987) to write his controversial best-selling polemic, to which no satisfactory refutation has yet been produced.

The Postmodern Stance

The four horsemen of postmodernism, Derrida, Rorty, Foucault, and Lyotard, attacked modernist thinking for committing the three major sins of foundationalism, logocentrism, and specialization. Foundationalism implies that there are certain a priori foundations that are self-evident and that everyone can accept universally and for all time as absolute truth. Logocentrism assumes that the spoken word has a certain priority over the written word and that somehow the name of something indicates information about the reality of it. Modern linguistics, founded by Saussure (1986), has demolished this attitude by showing that the meanings of words are not related to any sort of "reality" existing "out there," but are simply relative to each other. Language therefore needs to be understood as a self-contained system rather than some sort of mirror of reality. Specialization, which has become increasingly necessary in the age of the knowledge explosion, has led to what Kohut (1978) cleverly called "tool-and-method pride" (p. 690), resulting in each specialty having little to do with the others and assuming a kind of arrogant superiority in its claim to be investigating and gathering "knowledge." According to postmodernists, until these flaws in contemporary intellectual life are eradicated, culture will continue to flounder and injustice will characterize the twenty-first century as it has the twentieth century.

Postmodern thinkers wish to reconstruct philosophy. Their attention is focused on the human world, with special attention to the narrative, or "text" as they call it. Human experience is to be understood through investigation of the text or narrative presented by an individual or by a culture. Some postmodernists carry this to an extreme by arguing that there cannot be any form of truth, because truth is the outcome of power arrangements, justice is a matter of conventions, and the historical Western concepts of the good and the beautiful are merely cultural artifacts. Postmodernism flies the flag of "anything goes" (Becker, 1994, p. 177), bidding farewell to a culture that we have cherished since the time of the ancient Greeks.

Postmodernists claim that those once-appealing metanarratives that fueled the hope for the final emancipation of humankind, such as psychoanalysis, are grandiose flops that draw on a concept of reason and rationality that is culturally bound and that suppresses opposition. Any projects of the human sciences, like psychoanalysis, liberalism, Marxism, and so forth, are seen as nothing but illusions based on allegedly a priori concepts of reason, which themselves have no legitimate foundation. Becker (1994) explained,

> For post-modernists this vision is nothing frightening; rather it is the image of the *condition humaine* which is closer to the truth than anything that went before it, *and* it is most liberating. It helps to set free whatever was once irrational. . . . Socio-cultural fragmentation is epistemically insurmountable; diversity, not unity, would be the first transcendental of postmodernism. (p. 177)

Postmodern thinkers, extending and building on the work of Heidegger (White, 1991), have led us to the concept that reality is a social construction and that "meaning" in the psychoanalytic process is jointly created by both the patient and the analyst, as it is in any dialogue. This view rests on the claim that what we humans denote as "objective" knowledge is actually based on social agreements rendered through language and that the so-called realities we live with are actually constituted by the words we use to describe them—the alleged social construction of reality (Berger and Luckmann, 1967).

Flax (1990) offered a clear distinction between the modernist and the postmodern points of view. According to postmodernists, the modernist view arose from the Enlightenment. They describe the Enlightenment as based on the notion of a coherent and stable self in each person; the hope that philosophy could provide an objective, reliable, and universal foundation for knowledge and for the judging of all truth claims; the idea that truth represents something "real" and unchanging; the belief that reason, autonomy, and freedom go together in the progress of humankind; a theory of language in which objects are made directly present to consciousness by naming them or through the proper use of language; the assumption that history has meaning and is a record of the inevitable progressive perfection of humans and the increasing realization of human capabilities; a hopeful attitude toward human nature that tends to blame evil on circumstances and assume that given the proper nurturance humans will turn out to be intrinsically good; and the faith in science as the greatest example of the use of reason in the achievement of progress.

Postmodernists, in contrast to this view, attack any notion that humans have an essence, referring repeatedly to the "decentering" of the subject. They consider all attempts to impose order on "reality" and history as fictional and reconstituted by the needs for power and the satisfaction of desires, implying that history and metaphysics have no end and tell no coherent story. For postmodernists, as Flax (1990) explained,

> Western metaphysics creates a false appearance of unity by reducing the flux and heterogeneity of experience into binary and supposedly natural or essentialist oppositions that include identity/difference, nature/culture, truth/rhetoric, speech/writing, and male/female. The construction of these qualities through and as opposites reveals the philosopher's desire for control and combination. The members of these binary pairs are not equal. Instead, the first member of each is meant to dominate the second, which becomes defined as the "other" of the first. Its identity is determined only by its being as the negative of the first. The other has no independent or autonomous character of its own; for example, "woman" is defined as a deficient man in discourses from Aristotle through Freud. (p. 36)

It is important to see these oppositions as asymmetric because this relationship reveals a very important and crucial hidden premise: "To be other, to be different than the defining One is bad." Women have accepted this premise because "it is better to be defined and determined as the lesser other of the One, than to be outside Being altogether" (Flax, 1990, p. 37).

What follows from the postmodernist argument is that the "real" is always heterogeneous and differentiated. Therefore, whenever a narrative appears unified, clear, and complete, something must have been suppressed in order to sustain the appearance of unity. This insight is extremely important for psychoanalytic clinicians and all students of the human sciences to understand, because the suppressed within the story does not lose its power; it continues to affect the character of the whole. Here lies the value of deconstruction, a radical form of hermeneutics that explores again and again the limits of the narrative in order to reveal the many unresolvable antinomies in a given text. The implication for psychoanalysis is that any interpretation of clinical material or human narratives must suppress some aspects of the material, and that other interpretations are always possible. (In previous publications, I [Chessick, 1995b, 1996e] attempted to find a midpoint between the postmodernist implications of nihilism in the assessment of our interpretive work on the one extreme, and the patriarchical and authoritative attitudes of the early psychoanalysts in their reading of their so-called clinical data, on the other.)

Criticism of Postmodernism

Searle (1995) argued that "the rejection of realism, the denial of ontological objectivity, is an essential component of the attacks on epistemic objectivity, rationality, truth and intelligence in contemporary intellectual life" (p. 197). It must be kept in mind in any discussion of postmodernism that in spite of its rhetoric, postmodernism is still another narrative of the intellectual adventures of humankind. The doctrine that there is no foundation to anything also rests on a foundation and therefore is self-contradictory (Maker, 1994). The value of postmodernism is in reminding us that our theoretical formulations are useful heuristic tools but not proclamations of universal truths, and in helping us to appreciate better and tolerate the "other" of our culture as well as opposing "schools," what we at any specific time in our given culture or institutions consider to be irrational, bizarre, unorthodox, heretical, fantastic, and unacceptable.

The starting point is a plurality of conversations, but the question is whether the dialogue must remain a plurality of crisscrossing and irreconcilable conversations, as Bakhtin might have it, or whether it is possible to rearticulate and transvalue (to borrow Nietzsche's term) the plurality of conversations into a plurality of interlocutors within one common mode of conversation in which their differences could be reconciled. The question is whether, as in Derrida's (1981) concept of "differance," such transvaluation inevitably pushes some patterns in the background or even suppresses them as the price of consensus. If so, we can have no faith in the assertion of transcendental unities, such as the self or "truth." Or perhaps, as Bataille (1988) described it, we are lost among babblers in a night; discourse is impotent and transcendence is found only in moments of intoxication, eroticism, and love.

Logocentrism is Derrida's umbrella term for what he maintained is the principal characteristic of Western thought: its ineradicable tendency to establish an origin, foundation, principle, or center as a guarantee of the truth of our claims to knowledge. He claimed that Western philosophy accords priority to speech, to the spoken word as the natural, transparent, authentic mode of communicating, and subordinates writing by insisting it is derivative and depersonalized, a potentially distorted representation of speech. Lavine (1989) replied that Derrida did not successfully venture an unequivocal reversal of priorities by proving that writing is prior to speech, nor did he consider the prioritizing of speech over writing as a mistake that could have been avoided: Derrida "works only 'in the margins,' to deconstruct the text, to dismantle its reasoned, structural or genetic, arguments, by revealing failed distinctions, insoluble paradoxes, strategic repressions, irrational rhetoricality, blindness to the complex relations of language to philosophy" (p. 102). Lavine (1989) also objected that "Derrida's deconstructions are less than satisfactory. . . . The metaphysics of presence and the prioritizing of speech over writing—which are for Derrida the primary characteristics of logocentrism, appear to be over-generalized as characteristics of western thought" (p. 119). He concluded, and I agree, that we must restore to reason at least to some degree its powers of criticism and evaluation in order to overcome the failures of current culture and the appalling "pathologies of the political world" (Lavine, 1989, p. 121).

Some feminists also challenge postmodernism. For example, Lovibond (1989) pointed out, "If there can be no systematic political approach to questions of wealth, power and labour, how can there be any effective challenge to a social order which distributes its benefits and burdens in a systematically unequal way between the sexes?" (p. 22). The postmodern point of view undermines the foundations of constructive political action, and feminists urge us not to be carried away by postmodern thought into political apathy or to use postmodern thought as an excuse to avoid grappling with the problems of inequality and injustice in our contemporary world. It is inconceivable to me that a psychoanalytic clinician or any adult, for that matter, can be comfortable with these injustices and inequalities and still call himself or herself a mature individual; lack of a social conscience is a significant manifestation of a narcissistic character disorder (see Chessick, 1993a).

Responses to Postmodernism

Shapiro (1989) insisted Derrida has a second point of view that does allow for a certain amount of determinacy in our hermeneutic activities "while envisioning a limit of absolute playfulness as a horizon for these efforts" (p. 185). If this is correct, it enables a certain overlap between the views of Derrida and Gadamer, whose work on hermeneutics I discuss in Chapter 20, for Gadamer (1991) pointed out that interpretation can never be complete or final because it always involves both the demands of the text or subject of study and those of the historical or cultural situation of the interpreter. Gadamer repeatedly emphasized the commonalities of understanding that appear to guarantee unity of meaning, yet Derrida would deconstruct even this, underscoring an irreducible equivocation and undecidability of meaning. But Derrida (1994) insisted, "deconstruction is not an enclosure in nothingness, but an openness toward the other" (p. 360).

Habermas (1971, 1973) offered what I consider to be one of the best antidotes to postmodernism. His basic ideas are at least as sound as any foundationalist propositions can be in this unfortunate era of postmodernist predominance. His thought rests on the notion of an "ideal speech situation." Our normative beliefs can only be formed rationally under the condition of free and unlimited debate. Our current beliefs are not formed that way, but self-reflection, argued Habermas, will liberate us and bring us to consciousness; it will make us aware of the determinants that ideologically produce contemporary praxis and the currently prevalent conception of the world.

For Habermas there are three stages to emancipation. The first is to become aware of the unconscious determinants of our present consciousness, as in the process of psychoanalysis. This first stage, a liberation from ideology, raises us to the second stage, a new cognitive state with more objective knowledge of the world. It finally sets us free in order to ground appropriate political action, the third stage. According to Habermas, the forms of knowledge are technical or scientific knowledge with the goal of control of nature, hermeneutic knowledge with the goal of communication and social orientation, and self-reflective knowledge, produced by such geniuses as Marx and Freud. This latter knowledge produces a new type of understanding and is modeled on psychoanalysis with the goal of enlightenment. The crucial unproven fundamental premise in Habermas's thinking is that the ideal speech situation would lead to a consensus or agreement. There is a certain Enlightenment faith here in the value and ability of reason to overcome evil, which Habermas called the "redeeming power of reflection."

The contemporary tragic loss of the direction of science causes us to pause and reflect, and consequently leads us to consider the forgotten foundations of science residing in the life world, as Husserl (1970) pointed out. The contemporary scientific world is an idealized mathematical world divorced from ethics. The gods do not whisper into the ears of the practitioners of "normal" science. Habermas claimed that we must now go back to the life world and the interests of human beings and bring science under our domination. He attempted to restore the suppressed connection between knowledge and interest, for science and knowledge have ethical implications; they are not "neutral." At present, Habermas (1975) said, we have a crisis of legitimation. In this situation a political system loses the authority it needs to govern; as politics become pragmatic and corrupt, loyalty to political order is lost. This is a crucial contradiction in modern capitalism and leads to new social movements attempting to reinject lost moral values. Although McCarthy (1991) basically criticized Foucault and Derrida and sided with Habermas, he asked whether Habermas's structures, imbued as they are with such universality as the "ideal speech situation," are not simply a thinly disguised Eurocentrism. He claimed that Kant's "ideas of reason" reappear in Habermas as pragmatic presuppositions of communication.

In my view, social action is everything, for to not act, to not resist war and injustice, is also a form of action, of compliance with evil. Lasch (1985) shares my view that Habermas's work focused our attention on the problematic nature and political implications of both modernist and postmodern thought. He reminded us of Foucault's "spacial model" from the 1960s, a binary opposition in which "the space of the Same" is characterized by light and is the space of "rational" discourse, whereas the elements that characterize "the space of the Other" or the realm of darkness are those elements that have been excluded by rational discourse, such as representations of madness, sexuality, desire, and death. This "space of the Other" obviously bears strong resemblances to Freud's unconscious or Harry Stack Sullivan's (1953) "not-me."

Habermas wished to maintain the project of modernity of those Enlightenment philosophers,

> who wanted to utilize the accumulation of specialized culture for the enrichment of everyday social life. While fully aware of the dark side of the dialectic of the Enlightenment perceived by Horkheimer and Adorno, Habermas has

> sought to show that there is still a way of redeeming, recon-
> structing and rationally defending the emancipatory
> aspirations of the Enlightenment—the emancipatory aspi-
> rations that call for autonomy, concrete freedom, justice
> and happiness, embracing all of humanity. (Richters, 1988,
> p. 617)

Lyotard (1984) repeatedly defined postmodernism as incredulity toward metanarratives, that is to say, the rejection of
metaphysical philosophy, philosophies of history, or any form of
general theoretical explanations or systems, such as Hegelianism,
liberalism, psychoanalysis, or Marxism. But Kellner (1988)
pointed out that Lyotard gave no good reason for the rejection of
all grand narratives and suggested that one might counter him
with an injunction to let a thousand narratives bloom, "though
one would need to sort out some differences between these narratives, and perhaps—à la Habermas—distinguish between better
and worse narratives in order to provide a critical position towards conservative, fascist, idealist and other theoretically and
politically objectionable narratives" (p. 254). He points out that
even postmodernism presupposes a master narrative, "a total-
izing perspective, which envisages the transition from a previous
state of society to a new one" (p. 253), posing an unavoidable internal contradiction of the whole postmodern movement.

Liberal Education

In his view of liberal education, Hutchins (1948) leaned on Cardinal Newman's dictum that liberal education is the cultivation of
the intellect as such, the achievement of intellectual excellence.
He did not worry about the pragmatic or financial utility of liberal education and he correctly considered it to be a blessing or
gift in itself, first to the owner of it and then through him or her
to the world. As Cardinal Newman (1852) explained,

> Thus is created a pure and clear atmosphere of thought,
> which the student also breathes.... He profits by an intellec-
> tual tradition which is independent of particular teachers,
> which guides him in his choice of subjects, and duly inter-
> prets for him those which he chooses.... A habit of mind is

formed which lasts through life, of which the attributes are freedom, equitableness, calmness, moderation, and wisdom.... This then I would assign as the special fruit of the education furnished at a university, as contrasted with other places of teaching or modes of teaching. This is the main purpose of a university in its treatment of its students. (p. 82)

The idea of liberal education has a certain elitist implication, for it claims that such an education enables people to become truly human and able to form a genuinely free and democratic community. It is based on Aristotle's definition of the human as a rational animal, a notion that has been largely discredited by the history of the world in the twentieth century. The unspeakable calamities of the two world wars and the Holocaust undermined human confidence in the power of reason and dashed the hopes of the Enlightenment, leading to the relativistic and nihilistic postmodern fashion today. Hutchins (1948) complained about,

the universal willingness to leave decisions to others, which we see in its most acute form in those countries which have allowed themselves to be taken over by dictatorships of one kind or another . . . the hope of any healthy democracy lies in the independence of the individual. The habit of independent decision is one that the University of Chicago seeks to foster. (p. 3)

Following Hutchins, I believe the notion that a great civilized conversation is taking place, beginning in the remotest reaches of both eastern and western antiquity and continuing to our own day. The determination to become a part of that conversation or at least to understand it, should form the motivating force to attain a genuine liberal education. This quasi-Hegelian point of view assumes that the process of dialectic can lead to a better and better approximation of truth, in contrast to the postmodern claim that there are no truths but simply beliefs immersed in a cultural context, having no cross-cultural validity.

Another way to look at this is to utilize Heidegger's conception of inceptive thought, for example as discussed in his little volume titled "Basic Concepts" (1993). This form of thought focuses on the originary decisions that sustained in advance what we consider to be essential in Western history, and it began, he says, with the Greeks. In modern times this has led to the contention that technology and unconditional will or tyranny are essential. Inceptive thinking, a form of reflection on the way our era experiences Being, claims Heidegger, is something that our youth is not prepared to do: "The store of knowledge that today's youth bring with them corresponds neither to the greatness nor to the seriousness of the task" (p. 11). What exists today, he says, is a "degeneration of knowing. For example, "Whether one occasionally 'reads a book' is a measure for the petite bourgeoisie. It does not ask whether today's man, who gets his 'education' from 'charts' and 'magazines,' from radio reports and movie theatres, whether such a confused, dizzy, and purely American man still knows, or can know, what 'reading' means" (p. 11). He adds that it is not sufficient just to declare how much better it was in the old days, because "even the former school and educational system of the last decades was already no longer able to awaken and keep awake the binding power of spirit and the blindingness of the essential, and thus no longer able to force us into reflection" (p. 11).

Both Ezra Pound as a modernist (not a postmodernist) and Barry as a product of the Hutchins plan retained some sense of optimism regarding the possibility of the existence of universal values. The pursuit of these values and what are commonly known as metaphysical truths becomes one of the highest and most worthwhile aims of a human, as Plato and Aristotle insisted. Hutchins (1968) argued that the aim of education is to develop the mind, connect humans with humans, and produce a lofty habit of mind. In contrast to this, our current culture works to make producers and consumers rather than to help its members partake in the great civilized conversation. Hutchins demanded that a university should be restricted to those who want a life of the mind, not to baby-sitting, vocational certification, or scientific research. The discrepancy between this view of the university and our current United States universities, which put their primary investment in football teams, is obvious. How do coed bathrooms and fraternity drinking parties contribute to a lofty habit of mind?

Santayana (1896), whose acquaintance with his fellow expatriate Pound is described in Chapter 14, and whose metaphysics are discussed in Chapter 18, maintained that in the contemplation of beauty we are raised above ourselves (transcendence). Beauty for Santayana is a pleasure regarded as a quality of a thing, an emotion, and a sense of the presence of something good, satisfying a natural capacity. Aesthetic education is to train ourselves to experience the maximum of beauty to which we can repeatedly return with increasing appreciation. Beauty permanently raises the tone of the mind and is an indescribable ineffable experience. Without it, humans are not humans but simply, as so often in our civilization, mechanical and voracious consumers of material goods.

Liberal education is a habit of mind, a philosophical habit. Cardinal Newman (1852) did not feel that it necessarily leads to virtue, but he thought it made an individual into a cultivated lady or gentleman, which he assumed was the way humans ought to be. We hope that the kind of liberal education stressed by Hutchins and most emphasized today at St. John's College in Annapolis, Maryland, and Santa Fe, New Mexico, will lead to producing a humane and empathic individual, because one of the most treasured truths that has emerged from the civilized conversation is the importance of respect for human life beginning at birth, a respect that has been increasingly neglected in a culture inundated by handguns and assault weapons, exposing its children to a daily TV diet of lust and violence.

Unfortunately, study of the humanities does not humanize a person. The most we can hope for, as Steiner (1997) said, is that, "Once a young man or woman has been exposed to the virus of the absolute, once she or he has seen, heard, 'smelt' the fever in those who hunt after disinterested truth, something of the afterglow will persist . . . such men and women will be equipped with some safeguard against emptiness" (p. 49). The reduction of this emptiness is extremely important, as a great deal of sadistic and pornographic behavior in our culture as well as the embracing of fads and cults, road rage, and the movie and television imbecilities are the result of attempts to ameliorate the empty depleted self in our culture of narcissism (Lasch, 1978), as so brilliantly described by Kohut (1991, 1977) in his psychoanalytic self psychology.

Friedrich Schiller (1965), the great German poet and man of letters, claimed that the "aesthetic condition" restores a human to himself or herself and makes free choices possible. Aesthetic education, he said, counteracts the disintegration of the human personality in a highly mechanized civilization. In his view there are two crucial human impulses, the sensuous and the rational. These powers have been torn apart by modern civilization, and no reform is possible until they are brought together again by aesthetic education to act on each other. The artist sets out the ideal, the glowing peaks of humanity. For Schiller aesthetics leads humans to rational morality, and beauty leads spiritual humans back to matter and the world of sense. Beauty also leads sensuous humans to form and thought, producing a harmonious combination of sensuousness and reason that he believed generates moral behavior. According to Schiller there is no other way to make the sensuous individual rational than to first make him or her aesthetic. A human personality separate from the material world emerges only in the aesthetic state.

Schiller admired Plato's idea of education through art; Plato educates us about eternal and mathematical truths through his magnificent artistic dialogues. For Plato a person can live well only if he or she knows the ends of life. Is this true? Barry, a product of the Hutchins plan, thought so. Others consider questioning the ends of life as meaningless nonsense or neurotic. For Thrasymachus, an opponent in Plato's *Republic* (Cornford, 1975), happiness is getting more than your fair share of wealth, pleasure, and power, and this is the prevalent view today. But for Plato the aim of education is insight into κόσμος, the harmonious order of the world. If it succeeds, the pursuits of Thrasymachus fade into insignificance. Plato's classical Greek emphasis is on self-mastery and discipline, with reason deciding the direction in which a human's desires should be set. But Freud showed this decision is always a complex and multidetermined one.

Plato recognized that dreams represent archaic appetites allowed to clamor because reason has been withdrawn. He said the worst type of human behaves as people do in their dreams. Plato claimed poetry is an enemy of philosophy because the pursuit of it is an alternative to intellectual study and it moves one away from ultimate values and eternal Forms. The whole thrust of the civilized conversation since the time of Plato has been in the direction of disagreement with this view as it is expressed in the final book of *The Republic.* Here Plato was wrong, because in his emphasis on mathematical reason he overlooked how truth could shine forth in artworks, such as his own magnificent dialogues.

Nietzsche versus Plato

By way of contrast, the views of Nietzsche are often quoted or, more often, misquoted by postmodernists. For Nietzsche, the Platonic Forms and eternal high values are all dead: God, progress, perfectability of humans, historical destiny, universal morality. But Nietzsche had values also: self-honesty, lack of fear, laughter, despising the petty and mediocre, and, above all, the importance of life and living so that one might will to be able to live every moment of one's life over and over again. Nietzsche's great failing was his lack of empathy and compassion (Cooper, 1983). He opposed social programs aimed at helping the mass of humanity because he felt it diverted our attention from producing the overman. He despised democracy and the common man. Allan Bloom (1987) tended to blame Nietzsche for the nihilism and relativism that pervade today's college classrooms, but this is only one of a number of possible interpretations of Nietzsche's thought, as I explain in Chapters 15 and 17.

Human, All Too Human was Nietzsche's (1878) first fusion of philosophy and psychology. He attempted to explain reality without metaphysical ideas and to understand culture not through God-given higher qualities but through the evolutionary transformation of lower qualities which humans have in common with animals, such as the desire for power, and fear. So, for example, empathy allows alertness to the motives of others and protects against danger, a notion also put forth by Kohut. (Elsewhere, I [Chessick, 1981] discussed the relevance of understanding Nietzsche to the study of Freud and Kohut and I [Chessick, 1983] reviewed Nietzsche's life and work in detail.)

Nietzsche used letter writing as a substitute for personal contact, and he became increasingly isolated and alienated. Hayman (1980) described Nietzsche as having had the terrible habit of "generalizing on the basis of inadequate research" (p. 190). He characterized Nietzsche's writing as "the literary chatter of a man with no one to listen to him" (p. 56), which may account for his increasingly strident tone. The final diagnosis of Nietzsche's madness remains forever elusive; most likely he died from general paresis.

Solomon (1996) maintained that Nietzsche's perspectivism enabled him to use *ad hominem* arguments, since a particular perspective always occurs in the context of "surrounding impressions, influences, and ideas, conceived of through one's language and social upbringing and, ultimately, determined by virtually everything about one's self" (p. 195). Solomon claimed that a radical interpretation of perspectivism is wrong and that "the quality or value of the interpretation depends, in part, on what we think of the interpreter" (p. 197). This is what Solomon called an *ad hominem* approach to philosophy, asking, "Whose interpretation is this?" In Solomon's reading of Nietzsche, "some interpretations and perspectives are superior to others because some people are better educated, more sensitive, more insightful than others" (p. 198). In Chapter 17 I discuss Nietzsche's "perspectivism," which Bloom found so distasteful.

Education Today

Sartre said that we are what we turn ourselves into after a long path of error. Shattuck (1983) claimed that a study of the great classics helps us with this by reducing our groping in the dark. The most powerful complaint about what has happened to education in our current culture was initiated by Allan Bloom (1987). It is not for nothing that his book became a universal best-seller, because it struck a chord in the human heart at a time when there is so much despair about values and truths. For Bloom, bourgeois vulgarity is the true nature of people and the theoretical person is the most threatened human in a democracy such as ours. He correctly pointed out that college offers the only chance civilization has to educate a person in order to make that person human. The inherent crisis of our civilization is that first principles have become incoherent and inconsistent, leading to the current view that natural sciences are all that count and everything else is a matter of taste.

Crucial education comes *after* puberty. Humans in societies invariably need myths and metaphors and ciphers (Jaspers, 1932c) and not only science by which to live. This is a very important point, and it again emphasizes the value of the arts in creating and offering the indispensable truths pointed to in these myths, metaphors, and ciphers. The crucial difference between the philosopher as an explorer of these truths and other people is that the philosopher mixes the inevitability of our death and our constant dependence on chance (Sartre's "contingency") into every thought and deed. Therefore, according to Bloom, the philosopher relates to all others ironically, with empathy, sympathy, and a playful distance.

Freud did not distinguish between culture, an exalted time in which morality was high and education in art and sensibility prevailed, and civilization, a time of practical accomplishments (see Chapter 11). Loewald (1988) explained that sublimation assumes a conversion from a lower to a higher state. Sublimation is not neutralization, for passion is not absent in sublimation. Although in sublimation there is a loss of the freshness and immediacy of bodily pleasure, sublimation has a higher value and purpose because, asserted Loewald, who was a pupil of Heidegger and was a philosopher before he became a psychoanalyst, humans naturally and developmentally tend toward higher organization and further maturation, an appropriation of the id into one's life context. Loewald (1978) reminded us of Heidegger's concept of *Geworfenheit*, our being thrown into the world, leading to *Entwerfen*, the situation in which we develop and take over our basic project. So the human must take his or her nonpersonal beginnings and create a self from them. The concept of sublimation does not imply a kind of sham and metapsychological debunking of our highest values and activities; rather, it denotes a vitally necessary activity that propels us to higher and higher levels of the unique development of our autonomous selves.

A colleague of Bloom's at the University of Chicago, the famous contemporary novelist Saul Bellow (1994), called our attention to "the distracted public," describing distraction as a barrier through which "a writer must force his way" (p. 155):

> Vast enterprises described as the communications industry
> inform, misinform, or disinform the public about politics,

wars, and revolutions, about religious or racial conflicts, and also about education, law, medicine, books, theater, music, cookery. . . . The truth is that we are in an unbearable state of confusion, of distraction. (pp. 155-156)

In this plethora of information, which Bellow feels "simply poisons us" (p. 157), there is not a true picture of the world: "the written word is untrustworthy and the spoken word (radio and TV) irresponsible" (p. 157). Bellow said, "Television has proved that millions of people passionately love lust and violence" (p. 159), and he concluded, "for our peculiar pseudoknowledge of what is happening, for the density of our ignorance, and for the inner confusion and centerlessness of our understanding, for our agitation, the communicators are responsible. Intellectuals and universities, from the ideological side, also have much to answer for" (p. 160). Bellow's solution? "Embrace aesthetic bliss when you can get it" (p. 162). His beautiful essay has a certain echo of Schopenhauer's philosophy in it.

Kojève (1980), an influential interpreter of Hegel, is reported by Bellow to have claimed that man's return to animality appears no longer as a possibility that is yet to come but as a certainty that is already present. The question Bellow (1994) raised is whether our distraction, "the moronic inferno," can be induced to yield to attention. Bellow pointed out that distraction is a by-product of nihilism, and he concluded, "Writers, poets, painters, musicians, philosophers, political thinkers . . . must woo their readers, viewers, listeners, from distraction" (p. 167). Emergence from distraction is aesthetic bliss, argued Bellow: "When you open a novel—and I mean of course the real thing—you enter into a state of intimacy with its writer" (p. 168). That is to say, the reader experiences the distinct and unique human quality of the writer, which Bellow called "more musical than verbal . . . the characteristic signature of a person, of a soul" (p. 168). He believed that people hunger for a knowledge of essences, which cannot be destroyed even by our present experience of moral and intellectual anarchy.

One of the great concerns of Tocqueville was that in a democratic system the public demands larger and larger doses of excitement and increasingly strong stimulants from its sources of communication. We are amusing ourselves to death

(Postman, 1985), posing a serious threat to the future of democracy. Pelikan (1992) emphasized the value of the impact of the university as a civilized community that by example and teaching inculcates personal caring and empathy among the students and faculty. In the next chapter we shall see how the absence or presence of this civilized community affected Ezra Pound and Barry. To the task of the university to produce this impact, we must add the requirement from Cardinal Newman that the university should be dedicated to knowledge as an end in itself. The university must offer an ambience for living in contrast to the distraction, ever-increasing ·stimulation, and ephemeral pleasures in a surrounding civilization all too rapidly declining into barbarism and "the triumph of meanness" (Mills, 1997).

The goal of a university education must be to facilitate civility in discourse, learning to reason and analyze, refinement of taste, skill in the forming of judgments, and a sharpening of mental vision. As Steiner (1997) explains,

> This is the point. To direct a student's attention towards that which, at first, exceeds his grasp, but whose compelling stature and fascination will draw him after it. Simplification, leveling, watering down, as they now prevail in all but the most privileged education, are criminal. They condescend fatally to the capabilities unbeknown within ourselves. Attacks on so-called elitism mask a vulgar condescension: towards all those judged *a priori* to be incapable of better things. (p. 50)

Accordingly, an Oxford don reading Thucydides in Greek claimed, "I *am* western civilization," and the same could be said by Davis Robertson dancing the role of the faun in a revival of Debussy's music with Nijinsky's ballet choreography, *L'aprés Midi d'un Faun*. The problem that we face today, reflected in the poetry of Ezra Pound, is that the longing for the European Enlightenment ideals has disappeared: Europe no longer serves as a theater of self-improvement for the young. For Ozick (Atlas, 1992), "high art is dead: a class of educated citizens that prided itself on knowledge of European culture has dwindled to virtually nothing" (p. 134).

The artist hopes to compensate for the brevity and meaninglessness of our individual existence, for our being-towards-death. American education all too often disables, confuses, and alienates students: no passion for the arts or capacity to understand and appreciate them is instilled in college. As Bloom might have suggested, listen to the kind of junk music that rattles the walls of the average college dormitory. Art does not engage the central energies of humans today; science prevails. Bellow (1994) has said that art in our day has moved to the margins, and instead there is ceaseless crisis and chaos. Can this moronic inferno be bypassed by art? Surely this cannot happen without a major restructuring of the higher educational programs in our country, focusing on the best that has been thought and said in the world (to borrow Arnold's wornout phrase), instilling in the students an aesthetic sensibility enabling them to appreciate and learn from the arts, and demonstrating by the very behavior and ideals of the professors a sense of community, empathy, and concern for others based on a fundamental reverence for human life from birth.

If all this sounds utopian, what is the alternative? Our artists herald the forthcoming vicissitudes of our civilization. The poetry of Ezra Pound and the impotent strugglings of the neurotic Barry need to be not only explained by psychodynamics, but also to be phenomenologically understood on the background of their basic projects, their education, and the disintegration of humanism around them in their contemporary culture. This culture forms what Sartre (1963) called the practico-inert that opposes, as it does for all of us, their ideals and their basic struggle to actualize their projects, dreams, and aspirations.

The importance of all this is not yet recognized in our materialistic culture, but it will be, since the era of rampant global capitalism and multinational corporations contains within it not "the end of history" (Fukuyama, 1992) but the danger of increasing polarization of the rich and the poor and subsequent explosion or implosive collapse. Sooner or later a rethinking will be necessary and fruitful, and the truths in art and metaphysics will once more receive attention. Both Ezra Pound and Barry, each in his own way, were trying to express and overcome the practico-inert in which they were immersed, and grope toward a solution beyond it. Both failed, and their psychopathology contributed to that failure.

6 CONSOLIDATION

Said Abdul Baha: "I said 'let us speak of religion.'
"Camel driver said: I must milk my camel.
"So when he had milked his camel I said 'let us speak of religion'.
And the camel driver said: It is time to drink milk.
'Will you have some?' For politeness sake I tried to join him.
Have you ever tasted milk from a camel?
I was unable to drink camel's milk. I have never been able.
So he drank all of the milk, and I said: let us speak of religion.
'I have drunk my milk. I must dance,' said the driver.

— Ezra Pound, The Cantos

Pound persevered to take two degrees, a Ph.B.[1] at Hamilton College in 1905 and an M.A. at the University of Pennsylvania in 1906. But in June, 1907, for reasons never clearly explained, the University of Pennsylvania discontinued his graduate fellowship, forcing his withdrawal from the doctoral program. Heymann (1976) quoted from Pound's "How I Began" as to how Pound educated himself: "In this search I learned more or less of nine foreign languages, I read Oriental stuff in translations, I fought every University regulation and every professor who tried to make me learn anything except this or who bothered me with 'requirements for degrees' " (p. 10).

Pound as a student in graduate school at the University of Pennsylvania was described by the poet William Carlos Williams, who was studying medicine at the same graduate school: "I was fas-

---

[1]The Bachelor of Philosophy, an older version of the "B.A." degree, was awarded up to 1920 according to phone conversation in 1998 with F. Lorenz, Curator, Special Collections, Hamilton College, Clinton, N.Y.

cinated by the man. . . . He was the liveliest, most intelligent and unexplainable thing I'd ever seen and the most fun—except for his painful self-consciousness and his coughing laugh" (Mullins, 1961, pp. 31-32). Pound seems to have deliberately obscured his finer qualities and put his worst foot forward in all situations. Of course, as is typical of adolescents and students, he had many admirers of his daring, flamboyance, and rebelliousness.

In June 1906 Pound was awarded a traveling fellowship by the University of Pennsylvania for the purpose of going to Europe and gathering material on the work of the poet Lope de Vega. He visited Spain, France, and Italy and returned to the United States the following summer.

As he was not able to get further financial backing he went to Wabash College in Crawfordsville, Indiana to earn money as a teacher in the Department of Romance Languages.

Four months after his arrival there he was fired. A young woman whom he had allegedly fed and lodged because she was penniless was found in his room. He had quarters in the home of a couple of maiden ladies who were scandalized and telephoned the president of the college and several trustees. The incident with the young woman at Wabash College was not sexual but rather a kind of characteristic self-defeating flaunting on the part of Pound, of American traditional conservative midwestern mores (see Carpenter, 1988, pp. 80-81). His detestation of the United States began to flower.

Disgusted, he traveled by cattle boat from New York and in the spring of 1908 reached Gibraltar. "He had $80 in his pocket, a manuscript of poems, the cloying desire to see those poems in print and the determination to reach London by way of Venice" (Heymann, 1976, p. 12). Having arrived in Venice from Gibraltar, he paid for the printing of 100 copies of his first book of poems, *A Lume Spento,* and enjoyed the magnificent little city on the water. Then he set out from Venice on foot for London with dwindling funds and a lack of acquaintances, but with the confidence of youth and his copies of his book of poems. These were reviewed by the *Evening Standard* (London) as "wild and haunting stuff. . . coming after the trite and decorous stuff of most of our decorous poets, this poet seems like a minstrel of Provence at a suburban musical evening" (Mullins, 1961, p. 37).

Pound's Education

Let us examine his education in greater detail. Pound enrolled in 1901 at the University of Pennsylvania shortly before his sixteenth birthday, and at the end of his first university year he went with his parents on his second visit to Europe. During that year he was already busy composing verse. Also in that year he formed his lasting literary friendship with William Carlos Williams, who was several years older than Pound. They remained friends until Williams' death more than half a century later. Williams was already amazed at Pound's knowledge of literature and his determination to devote his life to it; it was already quite clear that Pound had formed a solid basic project. But Pound was not a good student, insisting on studying only what interested him. In 1903, because of his poor academic performance and because his parents did not like the company he kept, he transferred to Hamilton College in upper New York State. Here he spent two years studying various languages and in 1905 he received a "Ph.B." from that school.

Pound preferred intensive study with one or two teachers, something that the University of Pennsylvania's enforced variety did not permit. When he moved to Hamilton College he took forty units of language study: French, Italian, Spanish, Provençal, Anglo-Saxon, English literature, and Hebrew. And of course he immersed himself in Dante. For three centuries Milton's *Paradise Lost* was the dominant single book of English literature. Both Pound and T. S. Eliot recoiled from its diction and syntax and proposed a change of allegiance to Dante, whom Kenner (1993) called arguably the most influential dead White European male of twentieth-century letters.

Pound returned to the University of Pennsylvania in 1905 to study for his master's degree, where he developed an interesting relationship with the poetess Hilda Dolittle (discussed in Chapter 8). He received his master of arts degree in June 1906, along with the fellowship that allowed him, as mentioned earlier, to spend the summer of 1906 in Europe on his own. The alleged reason for the fellowship was research for the thesis on Lope de Vega that he hoped to present in a year or two toward his doctorate. But his fellowship was not renewed and he decided to leave the University of Pennsylvania without completing his doctorate.

It was at Hamilton College that

> Queer spellings and a great variety of dialect voices gradually began to creep into his letters: sometimes, it seems, for emphasis, but often as not for the sheer fun of it. In later years he also developed oddities of typing, with strange spacing, phrasing and line-breaks, often reinforced by an array of underlinings and marginal interpolations in ink. (Stock, 1970, pp. 15-16)

Later sections of the *Cantos* seem to depend on gaps between the lines and indentions, that is, empty space, almost as much as words. By this time he had already imbibed a tremendous amount of classical knowledge and was actively writing poetry. "Lean and erect, he wore his auburn hair in a leonine mass," and his untrammeled hair was a distinguishing feature that "he flaunted as a sign of his non-conformist poet nature" (Tytell, 1987, p. 19).

The title of his 72-page poetry book *A Lume Spento* is translated by Mandelbaum as "With Tapers Spent," taken from line 132 of Canto III of Dante's (1984) *Purgatorio. A Lume Spento* was dedicated to William Brooke Smith, an art student and painter who was friendly with Pound at Hamilton College and who introduced Pound to the self-sufficiency of art and aesthetic appreciation. But Pound did not get along well with his fellow students and was regarded as a restless oddball "nervously rushing with a long stride while declaiming the poetic virtues of Dante" (Tytell, 1987, p. 22).

Wabash College, the site of his first job, was in a small town with 8,500 residents, and had an enrollment of 150 students. Something in the smallness of Crawfordsville, not just its small size but its narrow mental scope, provoked Pound into flamboyance and caused him to say outrageous things in class. Pound as a teacher at Wabash College wore a black velvet jacket, flowing bow tie, patent leather pumps, and a floppy wide-brimmed hat, and he carried a Malacca cane. Although he was a man who energized others, he fit very poorly into a small college and was considered exhibitionistic and self-indulgent. While he was there he remained deeply immersed in the study of Dante and in Provençal studies. As stated earlier, he was dismissed in disgrace and his reputation at home was ruined. He never forgave small-town America for this and he never forgave his professors at the University of Pennsylvania for not considering him worthy of finishing and receiving an advanced degree. Already in 1904 the idea of the long poem, the epic including history, occurred to him and became his ultimate creative aim, developing into the *Cantos*. Ezra Pound's writing from the beginning was characterized by clarity of expression and technical discipline. He was an extremely meticulous worker and in his early days destroyed many of his products.

Pound's Personality

Pound as a college student was aloof from his classmates, indifferent to them, and a person who did not appear to have or care to have any particular friends. Becoming a poet enabled him to get a sense of protection not only against the sneers of his fellow students but against what he considered to be the defect of American education: "it discouraged real thinking and gave rise instead to what he called an 'omnimurkn diarhoea' of sloppy mental habits" (Carpenter, 1988, p. 36). As William Carlos Williams put it, "not one person in a thousand likes him and why? Because he is so darned full of conceits and affectation. He is really a brilliant talker and thinker but delights in making himself just exactly what he is not: a laughing boor" (Carpenter, 1988, p. 42). As a student he tasted little bits of many books but rarely read one through with concentration, and it is clear that all through his life he was not the scholar he pretended to be, even though many people were fooled. He "worked on this principle of judicious selection, deploying his limited knowledge with considerable agility" (Carpenter, 1988, p. 43).

By the time he was in the second year at Hamilton College he began to adopt different masks or characters through which he spoke in his poetry, a style reminiscent of Nietzsche, although there is no evidence that he was a student of Nietzsche. He seems instead to have been interested in the Neo-Platonist philosopher Plotinus; he wrote a poem in 1905 at Hamilton College expressing a wish to experience some kind of mystical-intellectual transcendence: "To be drawn through 'the node of things/Back sweeping to the vortex of the cone'" (Carpenter, 1988, p. 53). The troubadours appealed to Pound because he liked to think of himself as a "combative, aggressive, wandering minstrel, an outcast who nevertheless commanded the attention of a cultured audience" (Carpenter, 1988, p. 56). The pathological aspects of Pound's personality showed themselves to a greater extreme by the time he was at Hamilton College; there was an almost paranoid feeling that the University of Pennsylvania faculty had a personal loathing of him. Yet at intervals over the next twenty years he was still trying to acquire his doctorate from that university by asking permission to submit various bits of writing in lieu of a formal thesis. These requests were either ignored or rejected.

By the time he left Venice for London he had acquired a characteristic style of behavior and developed many of the intellectual themes that interested him for the rest of his life. For a long time his brilliance and his energy enabled him to be interesting to many individuals who would have otherwise been repelled by his exhibitionism, narcissism, and adolescent rebelliousness.

During this period of consolidation of Pound's project one also can get a glimpse of the consolidation of his psychopathology. He was able to form some intellectual friendships and, as described in Chapter 8, some relationships with women, but on the whole he was an alienated, isolated individual who had great trouble getting along with authority figures and an almost paranoid contemptuous loathing of those with a different outlook than his own. The narcissism and exhibitionism were there for everyone to see, as well as the grandiosity involved in projecting an epic poem on the order of Milton, or perhaps Dante. Pound was brilliant enough to make such a project not totally unreasonable, but his superficiality of study and his obsessive need to show off seriously interfered with the prolonged production of the first-rate poetry of which he was certainly capable. He was a fascinating and exciting individual, capable by his brilliance and provocativeness of challenging those around him, but at the

same time he was already hiding by his flamboyant behavior a secret self-doubt that he never allowed himself to get in touch with
until near the end of his life. Both Ezra Pound and Barry, by the
time they had finished their formal education, had embarked on
basic projects that carried them along to the end.

Barry

When Barry's brilliant cousin who lived downstairs was a very
little girl she used a favorite teddy bear as a transitional object.
Her greatest concern at bedtime was to take the teddy bear to
bed with her so she could more easily fall sleep. Her mother,
Barry's mother's sister, very early in this brilliant child's life became addicted to barbiturates. She was very strict and insisted
that the teddy bear be left on top of the dresser at bedtime. One
of Barry's earliest memories was of seeing his cousin crying as she
painfully recounted the episode when she took the teddy bear
from the dresser and brought it in bed with her in spite of her
mother's instructions. When this was discovered she was pun-
ished by spanking. In many ways Barry's personality was a reflection of his attempt to be worthy of the kind of excited attention
and admiration his cousin received; she was continually held up
to him as a model by his mother and her mother. She was not interested in him since he represented simply a nuisance of a little
brother, and she never hesitated to put him down and to display
his ignorance; since she was five years older, brilliant, and knew
much more than he did, this was easy for her to do.

There was a certain lifelong need on Barry's part to flaunt
more learning than he had, a need similar to that of Ezra Pound.
One of his most embarrassing college memories was of taking a
date for the first time to a concert by the Chicago Symphony Orchestra. When she opened the program she said to him, "Oh, they
are playing the *Eroica* tonight." "No," he replied, "They are playing
Beethoven's Third Symphony." Humiliations of this nature plagued
Barry for the rest of his days, and to the end he considered himself
a sciolist and a shameful failure, perhaps as a reaction formation to
his repressed infantile grandiose and exhibitionistic strivings and
perhaps in envious comparison to his cousin, or both.

Like Ezra Pound, Barry entered college at the age of sixteen. This was allowed by the Hutchins plan at the University of Chicago if one could pass the entrance examination. His college experience was quite different from that of Ezra Pound, however, as the move from a Chicago public high school to the University of Chicago in those days represented a move to a different world. In the previous chapter I described the idea of the university and the aims and ambience of a university community as it was conceived of by Hutchins and others at the time. The simple fact that students were courteous to each other was an incredible dramatic change from the public high school bullies that Barry had to endure, and the first two years of his college life were by far the happiest two years of his life.

One of the reasons for this was the required reading canon for all students in the college. They had to read widely in the Western classics and not spend time on secondary sources. The small classes consisted of students sitting around a table with an instructor, discussing the readings. Allan Bloom thrived on this sort of ambience and went on to become a professor in his own right, while Barry could only enjoy two years of it because he had to go on to premedical courses. It was during these first two years that he became aware of a whole world of beauty and timeless patterns, and what the psychiatrist and philosopher Jaspers (1932c) called "ciphers" that point to a transcendence beyond the apparent, materialistic world. In his study of some of the great authors of the Western world Barry was able to experience directly the groping of superior minds toward understanding ourselves and the world around us and to be excited by that very process of groping. It is this same process that the arts have to offer, except that the arts speak to us in a different form, sometimes a form which is more direct, more emotional, and less rational and conceptual. At the University of Chicago under the Hutchins plan Barry was educated to experience both.

The most important interpersonal problem Barry encountered while in college stemmed from his lack of money. Most of the students had considerably more money, drove their own cars, and so were able to entertain girls lavishly. Barry had nothing and was on scholarship. He had to attain very high grades as a condition of the scholarship in order to achieve his aim of being accepted into medical school; since he was not all that bright, this meant he had to immerse himself day and night in study. Like Ezra Pound he had few close friends, but he did not, as Pound did, annoy or provoke his classmates or teachers. He was generally considered the kind of mediocre individual who was not very good at anything and who had no outstanding characteristics or abilities. He was viewed with a certain contempt by his classmates and looked down on by the more wealthy students, but they usually did not actively dislike him. The brilliant students like Allan Bloom just ignored him.

He adjusted to and made the best of his loneliness and he took an inward turn at the time, immersing himself in aesthetic and intellectual experiences. He went to sleep at night to the recorded sound of Tchaikovsky's *Pathetique* symphony. There was a similarity to the plight of Ezra Pound as a college student defending himself against his intrapsychic difficulties by the intensive pursuit of poetry, voraciously reading and writing. Barry wrote a bit of poetry (which never got published), but his aesthetic experiences were passively enjoyed and he was more active in mathematical and chess performance (although he was a weak chess player). One of the saddest memories from his college days was of having to turn down an offer from a mathematics professor to work with him on a dissertation that would have enabled him to graduate with honors in mathematics. The pressure of having to get top grades in the hated premedical courses allowed no time. So Barry had the opposite attitude toward getting an education in college from that of Ezra Pound, who studied only what he wanted to learn.

Barry was able to form an extremely idealizing relationship with his new uncle (see Chapter 4), who was a world-renowned scientist in chemistry, but who also had some outside intellectual interests as a consequence of a European education. This uncle, a refugee from the Holocaust, was the central figure of Barry's adolescence in college and medical school and at the time was a profound influence in keeping Barry at least temporarily enthusiastic about science, a project that as we have seen was really alien to him, although he was only dimly aware of it at the time.

The second two years of college and premedical studies were pure grinding and memorizing, and Barry was indeed admitted to medical school, where he was rewarded by two more years of prolonged grinding and memorizing. Some psychoanalysts have insisted that medical students and doctors all have obsessive-compulsive disorders; I would not agree with such a generalization, but the curriculum in those days at least certainly demanded an obsessive attention to memorizing details rather than emphasizing independent thought.

An important turning point in Barry's life occurred in the third year of medical school, when the students were allowed to go out on the wards dressed as doctors and do physical examinations as well as interact with patients. He passed all of this successfully but with great disappointment. On the whole, Barry was demoralized by his classmates and the medical professors around him. These individuals were extremely narrow, considering themselves scientists and with little other interest in academic and aesthetic pursuits ("Philosophy is bunk," said one of his professors authoritatively). They were willing to work incredibly long hours, which Barry realized often represented an escape from interpersonal and intimate relationships into the laboratory and into the protected situation where one could be a "doctor" with a "patient," a relationship that had strict boundaries around it. The hours were very long and very demanding, and there were only brief periods of rest allowed for the students. In those days medical students were treated very badly and there was no recourse. The competition for grades was ferocious and the professors for the most part were arrogant and unempathic. This was the time of the trial of the Rosenbergs in the United States, and Barry endured some anti-Semitism from some of the professors. He did not dare to challenge their obnoxious comments. His lack of mechanical skills caused him the greatest trouble in anatomical dissection and in surgery; surgical professors were exceptionally intolerant of him, and more than once he was thrown out of the operating room by a hot-tempered surgeon for contamination of himself or the operating field or for cutting a surgical knot incorrectly.

The nightmare of the second two years of medical school was relieved only by occasional rest periods during which most of the students ate their lunch, but Barry read instead over and over again a little volume that he carried with him everywhere, titled

Selected Poems, by Ezra Pound (1949). There was something about these poems that filled Barry with a strange sense of aesthetic stimulation, as if they were signals coming from another world outside the realm of science and technology. Pound (1939) wrote that the starting point of creating or appreciating poetry is to remember that language is a means of communication. "To charge language with meaning to the utmost possible degree," he said, there are three "chief means": (1) "throwing the object (fixed or moving) on to the visual imagination," (2) "inducing emotional correlations by the sound and rhythm of the speech," and (3) "inducing both of the effects by stimulating the associations (intellectual or emotional) that have remained in the receiver's consciousness in relation to the actual words or word group employed" (p. 63). Pound named these, respectively, phanopoeia, melopoeia, and logopoeia. This was the height of Pound's genius, and it displayed itself with a minimum of psychotic interference in his little volume of *Selected Poems.* I hope the reader will look at this volume. See, for example, the poem "Difference of Opinion with Lygdamus," which contains in Section VII one of the most beautiful love poems in the English language. I resist the temptation to quote at length from these various poems; for help with understanding some of Pound's allusions I recommend the text by Froula (1983). The point here is that something about Pound's poetry had a magnetic attraction for Barry, immersed as he was in the long hours of technical medical work that never seemed to end. It was as if during those brief periods allowed for gobbling down one's lunch, a light from another realm of existence briefly flickered in.

One of the things he learned in medical school was that he did not wish to spend his life in the practice of the mechanical arts involved in such specialties as internal medicine and surgery. Nor was he so intellectually and cognitively oriented as to prefer, for example, the role of a noninvasive cardiologist (which also, in those days, was a very limited and frustrating specialty). So, against the wishes of his family, he chose the field of psychiatry, which he erroneously believed would allow him to utilize his long-standing and college-stimulated philosophical interests and attraction to human affairs, along with his basic project of medical practice. The dean of the medical school was also a chemist who regarded Barry's uncle very highly and thought Barry was extremely lucky to have such extra guidance. Near graduation, as was the custom, he called in Barry and other students individually to discuss their choice of specialty. When Barry told him it would be psychiatry, this physician, who was well liked by the students, uncharacteristically turned bright red in the face and exploded with rage at Barry, and saw to it that he did not receive any honors or prizes he had earned at graduation. This was a severe humiliation that Barry never forgot, and it left him feeling even more alienated from the group of regular physicians. There was, and still is, a rejection of psychiatrists by many physicians as "not real doctors," "crazy," and "ineffectual."

Before he was able to go into his specialty training, however, Barry had to put in the required year of internship in order to be licensed as a physician. For this purpose he chose to work in a large, charity community hospital where he got a chance to practice every branch of medicine night and day. Because of the shortage of personnel he was allowed to do every imaginable kind of procedure and developed considerable medical skill before his year was over. For Barry it was an unrelieved nightmare of hard work with insufficient rest or sleep, and of having to endure an utter disregard for the physical and mental needs of the interns. Much of this has changed since those days, but in that era an intern could not take any time off unless so physically ill as to be utterly incapacitated. At times his roommate seriously considered suicide because he was so harassed by the resident surgeons and overtired and overworked, so Barry's first psychiatric experience was in dealing with a depressed colleague and helping him get through the internship (which his roommate successfully did, subsequently becoming a wealthy radiologist).

This was also Barry's first experience with real poverty and ignorance and his first opportunity to observe the dreadful conditions that characterize the lives of a large percentage of humanity even in the richest country in the world. If nothing else, he was confronted with the total failure of the public educational system in those impoverished areas, a failure the politicians blamed on the teachers but which was really a function of the conditions under which people lived. The individuals who came to this community hospital could barely read or write, if at all, and spoke in a grammatically confused jumble of slang words and dialect that Barry had to learn quickly in order to communicate with them. A bit like Pound, he subsequently introduced some of these words into his speech or writing "for fun," but to a much smaller and less noticeable extent.

The worst experience was during the month he served on the pediatric burn unit, where he had to attend to children who were massively burned and hospitalized because of it, the poor things lying ensconced in a bed in this strange place on a ward where there were no parents or parental nurturing figures. It was from the experience of changing the dressings of burned children, which of course had to be done, and being exposed to the intense suffering and disfigurement these children endured, that Barry lost all religious belief. He could never after that time accept the idea that any god could be so cruel. Thus, in Barry we experience an individual who had an almost instinctual yearning for a transcendent realm and a sense of the eternal, but who was convinced that it was not to be found in religion. In the Jewish prayer books and in those of most other denominations there are pages and pages of praise and thanks to God; Barry could never get himself to partake in a prayer like this after his service on the pediatric burn ward.

Barry was now launched almost in spite of himself on a project that was somewhat alien to his true needs. The demands of this project hampered his already diminished social life and kept him from acquiring the social skills that he would have needed to become a financially successful doctor. These social skills should have already been learned in childhood from observing his parents, but their emphasis was on intellectual achievement and social skills were considered irrelevant. The Hutchins plan college experience reinforced this attitude. There was a sciolistic studiousness about him that later caused his colleagues to say something like, "Barry knows a lot, but he thinks he knows everything." They were surprised when he did not make the high grade honor society (A.O.A.) at the end of medical school. The individual who came out first in his class subsequently committed suicide, as did one of the three women in the class, among others. He was known as a poor intern because he suffered much fatigue and could not enthusiastically immerse himself in the reading of electrocardiograms and the suturing of wounds.

Barry was a theoretical man who, in the sense described by Schiller (1965) as mentioned in the previous chapter, needed a combination of an aesthetic education with his cognitive scientific orientation to complete his humanity. He was aware of this even in medical school and yearned for it preconsciously, and he was also vaguely aware that something was wrong, that the life he was living was somehow not his own. Although he tried to immerse himself in his beloved uncle's scientific interests, this gave him only temporary enthusiasms and distractions. Not only was there nobody available with whom he could discuss these matters either in his family or among the medical school faculty, but also he did not have the time or energy available to try to sit down and articulate his concerns. So he went on and on with his project almost automatically.

7 LOVE AND OBJECT CHOICE

In toil, in sweat and grime we're doomed
*   to languish,*
and love—ah! Love itself soon turns
*   to anguish!*
Brief are the pleasures we seek in vain
*   to capture.*
How dark our path, and fraught with pain
*   our rapture.*

The gates of joy we may not enter, all's
*   forbidden!*
And the light of day from our eyes is
*   hidden!*
You've spoken truly: vain is all our striving
and wise is he who bows his head in
*   silence!*

                                                    —Puccini, Il Tabarro

For Heidegger (1962), human being or *Dasein,* thrown into the
world, is being-towards-death. Furthermore, *Dasein* is that being
who thinks the Being-question: Why is there something rather
than nothing at all? For some psychoanalysts *Dasein* is also that
being who seeks transcendence; who at a concert listens enraptured to Beethoven's Fifth Piano Concerto, the "Emperor" Concerto, and watches the lovely lady two rows ahead of him . . . she
in turn is looking at the man adjacent to her with a grey feline expression in her half-closed eyes. *Dasein* thinks ἔραμαι . . . to desire eagerly . . . to love passionately... to lust after—all three
meanings packed into one classical Greek verb.

Freud on Love

Freud's views on love can be organized into three theories
(Bergmann, 1988). The first, expressed in *Three Essays on Sexuality*
(Freud, 1905b), stressed the finding of the love object as a re-

finding of the infantile love object. The second, in the paper "On Narcissism" (1914b), described love as a massive transformation of narcissistic libido into object libido with a subsequent depletion of the ego ideal. The third, in the paper "Instincts and Their Vicissitudes" (1915a), deemphasized the instinctual component and depicted love as a relation of the "total ego" to its object, without any clear definition of "total ego." Freud mistrusted sexual passion as a basis for marriage. He (Freud, 1931) claimed that first marriages, based on falling passionately in love, are often disappointing, while second marriages, assumed to be more dispassionately chosen and more practically determined, turn out better. Whether this is true or not remains highly debatable.

Freud discussed love 130 times in his collected writings (Hitschmann, 1952), but he was not consistent about the subject; he seemed ambivalent and uncertain about the matter of passionate love. Freud (1912a, p. 180) explained that the affectionate and sensual currents had to become properly fused to produce the normal attitude in love. For Freud both of these currents are derived from the sexual instinctual drives; the affectionate current has aim-inhibited goals and the sensual current has an openly erotic intent. But Altman (1977) emphasized the ego and superego aspects of the experience of love and added that love requires good ego and superego functioning—it is far more than the discharge of libido.

For Freud, tender feelings are always transformed sexual feelings. But Bergmann (1982) added, "In real life many traumatized patients fall in love not with the real person who reminds them of their parent, but with the person they hope will heal the wound the parental figures have inflicted. To fall in love with the rescuer or the person one has rescued is a frequent theme of romantic love. It is also an important source of transference love" (p. 107).

Freud (1921) focused on the idealization of the love object, which he believed to diminish with each sexual satisfaction. For Freud, being in love is based on the simultaneous presence of directly sexual impulses and of sexual impulses that are inhibited in their aims, while the object draws a part of the subject's narcissistic ego libido to itself. He quoted Schopenhauer's saying that sexual passion is the most perfect manifestation of the will to live.

Freud (1921) also asserted there is a repressed hostile residue in each love affair which can cause considerable difficulty. He believed that behind the sometimes expressed wish of the couple to die "is the unconscious wish for, expectation of, and belief in life everlasting in reunion with the love objects of childhood" (p. 44). This points again to the ceaseless effort to make good the loss of the preoedipal object, which results in a never-ending quest for love (Bak, 1973). Altman (1977) thought such love is doomed since it is founded on depression and the unconscious wish for a reunion with the mother of infancy. This is close to the view of Melanie Klein, described in Chapter 8.

An important correction to Freud's discussion of the problem of love was made by a number of authors, including Chasseguet-Smirgel (1970). Contrary to Freud's pronouncement, one's ego ideal is not depleted when one falls in love, but there is an increased libidinal investment of the self that accompanies the experience of being in love. The great writer Robert Louis Stevenson (1988) described it quite well:

> It seems as if he had never heard or felt or seen until that moment; and by the report of his memory, he must have lived his past life between sleep and waking . . . a very supreme sense of pleasure in all parts of life—in lying down to sleep, in waking, in motion, in breathing, in continuing to be—the lover begins to regard his happiness as beneficial for the rest of the world and highly meritorious in himself. (pp. 8-9).

Being in Love

Thomas Hardy (1897) claimed in his novel *The Well-Beloved* that falling in love, what he described as a state of being "powerless in the grasp of the idealizing passion" (p. 121), does not tend to occur less after youth as popularly believed, but sometimes even happens more frequently in the third, fourth, and fifth decades of life. Only the aging process, he said, in which some individuals sooner, and some later, reach "the calm waters of philosophy," puts an end to these episodes. So Hardy's protagonist in his sixties can finally relax with a sigh, "Thank Heaven I am old at last. The curse is removed" (p. 202). This, of course, is Hardy's misconception, since individuals in their sixties and older, if they are in good health, can still be driven by very powerful energies. All of Hardy's novels explore this common but perplexing human paradox: With the painful desire and perpetual dissatisfaction that love brings as well as the genuine suffering it often entails, why do humans keep repeating this pattern, bringing unhappiness upon themselves and others?

The Well-Beloved portrays the curious correlation between the capacity for falling in love and the capacity for artistic creativity that I will discuss in Chapter 9. For Hardy's protagonist there is a wraith, a "migratory Well-Beloved," which represents a "sisterly-image" that invests one loved woman after another; when it leaves a person his love for her disappears and she is abruptly abandoned. In Hardy's extreme example we are presented with a rather clear demonstration of Freud's (1914b) notion of narcissistic object choice fused with brother-sister twinship incestuous desires, very similar to the love of Siegmund and Sieglinde in Wagner's *Die Walküre.*

The argument of De Rougemont (1983), the Swiss theologian and essayist, is that the famous lovers Tristan and Isolde are not in love with one another but with love itself, with their "being in love." For De Rougemont their unhappiness originates in a false reciprocity that disguises a twin narcissism. De Rougemont elaborated the Tristan and Isolde legend into a struggle between feudal honor and unlimited passion, describing an inescapable conflict in the West between passion and marriage, but Updike (1963) strongly disagreed, arguing that De Rougemont makes too much of myths and ignores the importance of love in confirming and amplifying each partner's existence.

Bak (1973) suggested that "being in love" is often preceded by separation or by an important object loss—real, imaginary, or threatened, "or by one of the numerous losses of object representations that lead to melancholia." He continued, "To these precipitating causes I might add damage to the self image and lack of fulfillment of strivings of the ideal-ego which indirectly lead to the threat of object loss" (p. 1). For Bak, "being in love" is a way of avoiding melancholia on the one hand or a regression to narcissism on the other, by means of finding a substitute object in order to undo the loss. He pointed out the well-known theme in history and literature where attempts to substitute another love object prove unsuccessful and the lover develops acute melancholia and even commits suicide.

The state of "being in love" emphasizes the irrational, stormy, emotional turmoil or grand passion, such as that of Goethe's (1774) Werther, whose sufferings are described in a literary masterpiece. This is distinguished by Freud from the "epic" phase of love, which is calmer, more rational, and durable, what we usually call mature genital object relations. Being in love, or falling in love, with its characteristic sexual overvaluation of the object is conceived by Bak (1973) as based on an attempt to undo the separation of the mother and child. Balint (1953) postulated "primary love," in which the infant wishes for a tranquil, quiet sense of well-being. The goal is to be automatically loved and satisfied without being under any obligation to give anything in return. Many people spend their adult lives searching for this, and of course are repeatedly disappointed. If it is not forthcoming, a reactive narcissism often appears, in which the individual attempts to love and gratify himself or herself. Another detour would be active object love in which one gets vicarious gratification out of giving to others. This is closer to healthy object love, in which one happily gives and is spontaneously given.

Chasseguet-Smirgel (1985) labeled the "malady of the ideal" as the *"primum movens"* of psychic life. She postulated that when the infant comes to realize that the narcissistic state of perfection is impossible it sets up an image of such perfection in the ego ideal, as described by Freud (1914b). The ego ideal becomes a substitute for the lost object of primary fusion, and all human beings spend the rest of their lives trying to bridge the gap between the ego and the ego ideal, in order to reinstate this primary fusion with the mother. This "malady of the ideal" becomes a central impetus for all the activities of the person, accompanied by a nostalgia for a lost state of perfection. When the person falls in love, at least at first, contrary to Freud's contention that the ego is impoverished, the radiance of the ego ideal falls on the ego, so that the first moments of love "are full of exalted joy, of an expansiveness of the ego" (p. 55). The possibility of a fusion of the two agencies produces the range of phenomena of "the ephemeral plunge into the world of primary narcissism" (p. 56), often experienced as a blinding light, a thunderbolt, and so on, magnificently portrayed by Wagner just after Tristan and Isolde drink the love potion (their excuse for declaring their love).

In discussing Hardy's *The Well-Beloved*, Werman and Jacobs (1983) pointed out that although "infatuation" is common, the psychoanalytic literature pertaining to it is relatively limited. They conceived of infatuation as "a final common pathway, arising from multiple sources and consequently having different aims" (p. 456). Similarly, we should avoid any simplistic interpretation of a legend with so many versions (Gediman, 1981) as the Tristan and Isolde story. Also, the pathological, shifting, repetitive, and compulsive "infatuations" of Hardy's protagonist are of a phenomenologically different quality than the existential, deep, profound, and unique episode of "falling in love" that overwhelmed Tristan and Isolde.

Limerence

The importance of the illusory nature of infantile gratification in passionate love is lent some credence by the work of McClelland (1986), who suggested there are *two* psychologies of love, which he tried to relate to the left brain and the right brain. Whether or not the fanciful neurophysiology is correct, McClelland pointed out that mechanistic explanations of love always seem to fall short of the romantic and phenomenological side of love, and tend to view the latter as a sort of aberration from rational calculations, an unfortunate consequence of physiological arousal. He advocated a second, or "right brain," psychology of love, consisting of the imaginative experiences described by the poets, which are altruistic, irrational, and not explainable by self-serving motives. He would be much less inclined than Viederman (1988) to say that passionate love is destined to fade, but instead he quoted Shakespeare: "Love is not love/ Which alters when it alteration finds,/ Or bends with the remover to remove;/ O no!

it is an ever-fixed mark,/ That looks on tempests and is never shaken" (Sonnet 116). Viederman might retort this is an idealization of the state of being in love. No prediction can be made in any given case about whether or not passionate love will be lasting or an ephemeral state; any sort of resolution or nonresolution is possible.

A more technical way of approaching the state of passionate love was presented by Verhulst (1984), who borrowed from Tennov (1979) the term *limerence* to indicate the state of passionate and romantic love. The "limerent" person is the person who experiences this state and the limerent object is the person with whom the limerent is in love. Tennov (1979) described a long list of symptoms of limerence, converting the phenomena of romantic love into the jargon of academic psychology. One of the most interesting of these "symptoms," beside the emotional dependence of the limerent on the limerent object, is that limerence is characterized by a continuous intrusive preoccupation with the limerent object. Verhulst proposed to look at limerence as an altered state of consciousness and viewed "limerence as an affect dominated state of mind, which contrasts with the ordinary, language-dominated state" (p. 124). Although limerence is defined as an altered state of mind, Verhulst added that early life experiences will influence the form and style of the limerent's experience. Romantic love is not seen simply as an immature form of love based on some sort of developmental arrest; the experience of passionate love can show either or both mature or immature secondary characteristics.

All authors agree that before limerence begins a person may be in a state of readiness and heightened susceptibility for it, caused by biological factors such as the upsurge in hormone levels during adolescence and psychological factors such as preceding loneliness, discontent, and alienation. The higher the level of readiness, the more the choice of a partner or limerent object is contingent upon circumstances rather than personal factors. This introduces an element of chance into partner choice in a way different from Freud's deterministic approach. There are, of course, also specific characteristics of potential partners that constitute their conscious or unconscious "limerence appeal" to the individual.

The duration of the state of limerence according to Verhulst is variable, and depends on such factors as uncertainty about the partner's commitment, external difficulties in the way of the love relationship, and actual physical separation. These interfering circumstances tend to perpetuate limerence, keeping the relationship perfect on a mostly imaginary and fantasized level. Tennov estimated the average limerent duration to be approximately two years. As this state of mind continues alongside of the world of rational language and reality, the unsubmerged part of the ego seems to gradually regain control and the limerent state of mind dissolves.

Complexity of the Phenomena

Arlow (1980) claimed, "there is no clear delineation of any specific syndrome which we call loving or being in love" (p. 122). He objected to those authors (such as Bak, 1973, or Bergmann, 1980) who try to trace the psychology of loving to the wish to reachieve symbiotic fusion with the mother in order to undo primordial separation. Arlow explained that "cultural ambience influences not only how love is expressed, but also how it is experienced" (p. 129), and that love relations integrate complex needs of individuals at a given time, so that "what happens is determined by the nature of the unconscious conflict which the individual is trying to resolve at that particular time of life" (p. 128). In the "oceanic feeling," or the sense of total fusion with the beloved often described by poets in the ecstasy of love, there is still a "concomitant awareness of the existence of the other person as an independent object" (p. 119).

A thorough understanding of love, claimed Bergmann (1980), requires illumination of falling in love as a special ego state, solving the problem of why a particular person is selected as a love object and explaining the capacity to maintain a sustained love relationship with one person over a long period of time, "with fidelity, maturity, and a preponderance of love over envy and aggression in the relationship" (p. 57). He interpreted falling or "being in love" as a temporary undoing of separation and individuation, and the finding of a way back to a state of bliss known before individuation—which he postulated to be the feeling state of the symbiotic stage.

This type of interpretation involves committing the genetic fallacy, explaining all facets of complex adult patterns of love as derivatives of impressions from the earliest infantile state and of universal fantasies. As an example, Gediman (1981) made the most careful analysis available of the various versions of the Tristan and Isolde myth with particular emphasis on the *liebestod* motif. Tristan and Isolde each form a selfobject for the other. She concluded,

> The "exquisite anguish" in the yielding swoon of the lovers casts its spell because it is evocative not only of sexual passion, but also of the early ego state of fusion and merging. . . . In this way, I find it useful to view the rhythms of parting and coming together, the theme of all courtly myths, as derivatives of the rapprochement rhythms of establishing distance between two people, both literally and intrapsychically. (p. 620)

What Do Lovers Seek?

The common oedipal interpretation involving Tristan, Isolde, and King Mark seems weak and contrived. The story is not primarily sexual or triadic, and sex here is manifestly just a vehicle of preoedipal union. Could it represent, as many commentators have said in agreement with some of the authors quoted earlier, a preoedipal union with the mother—a dyadic relationship? The libretto of Wagner's drama is dyadic and symbiotic over and over again. This is especially true of the second act, in which the language is almost unintelligible and "who is saying what" is so blurred together in the mystical union that only the music carries the message. It is clear that such longing is regressive when it appears and represents a turning of one's back on the frustrating world of Day. But Tristan is successful and well thought of by everyone; he is a worldly hero and a mature man. The only latent dynamite is that his needs have always been subordinated to his sense of duty throughout his adult life, even long before the opera opens.

Tristan and Isolde in one sense is a paean to the power of the instincts, but notice that *both* Tristan and Isolde seek the union and *both* are transfigured by death, which is idealized by Wagner alone. Bliss here represents the total sudden gratification of a primordial wish, but what is the wish? Clearly it is for everlasting union and an oceanic feeling that goes with it. Tristan seeks for the wound-healing mother with magical power. Isolde seeks for a lost part of herself, and in this sense Lacan's (1977) interpretation that the child's greatest and most basic desire is to seek to become what the mother most desires, which Lacan labels with the signifier "phallus," seems to fit. Yet all of this is surely inadequate to explain the gripping power of this overwhelming work of art and the universal appeal of many great works of art on the theme of longing and desire.

Another way to picture the situation is that the lovers have a passion to restore contact with Being, for falling away from Being represents daytime preoccupations (the realm of the Day)—what Heidegger (1962) labeled as an immersion in the "they." Their search in this sense is existential and represents the longing for an authentic life (Chessick, 1986), which can occur for the neurotic Wagner only in death. Indeed, that is the point Wagner was trying to make in the opera, but I believe he was carried by his artistic genius into a realm beyond his muddled quasi-Schopenhauerian philosophy. We are brought into a deeper philosophical preoccupation with the attempt to somehow make contact with Being—a preoccupation that Heidegger insisted has been the fundamental task of all metaphysics from even before the time of Plato and Aristotle.

The unanswered question is whether passion of this all-consuming power can be explained reductionistically on the basis of infantile longings alone or whether something transcendent is in it, such as Freud's Eros and Thanatos at work. Are we simply dealing with the explosion of long-repressed and unsatisfied needs? Or have lovers like Tristan and Isolde become gripped in cosmic forces unintelligible even to themselves?

Of course, the regressive element in love is found in both women and men. Fenichel (1945) wrote, "an archaic type of self-regard (or even of omnipotence) comes back again in an oceanic feeling of losing one's ego boundaries" (p. 86). He stressed the narcissistic gratification involved in fusing with a partner that contains the projected perfection and idealization. This explains the explosive "falling in love" that can occur during periods of chronic narcissistic wounding, as has been repeatedly described, for example, of the aging therapist carrying on many frustrating long-term cases and depressed in his personal life (Dahlberg, 1970) who "falls passionately in love" with a patient, illustrated and discussed in Chapters 16 and 17 of the present book.

Another explanatory approach to the oceanic feeling that follows fusion and loss of ego boundaries, one that utilizes the object relations channel, is to stress the role of being in love as reassurance against separation, anxiety, and death. Fenichel in his reference to the subject emphasized the narcissistic bliss in the oceanic feeling that such union brings. Ross (1968) postulated "the need for the sustained eternal existence of an immutable protective loving object" (p. 269) and "dread of object loss" as the basis for religious faith and other creative phenomena including those which, like the oceanic feeling, involve the loss of ego boundaries. He vaguely added that "there is a case of narcissism in all religious belief" (p. 274), but he did not seem to notice that the phenomena of "loss of ego boundaries accompanied by profound ecstasy" and "detachment from the external world" are common to *both* mystical religious experience and sexual fusion with a passionately loved person. He did realize that certain religious experiences like that of St. Teresa are "often imbued with erotic intensity" (p. 270).

It is a logical and philosophical error to attribute the oceanic feeling that Romain Rolland (Freud, 1930a) viewed as the core of religious experience or other mystical experiences of this sort simply to regression to early forms of narcissism or to conflict/defense formulations. This *may* be true in some cases but it is not *necessarily* true in all cases. This well-known reductionist fallacy runs throughout Freud's views of religion (Chessick, 1980); he dismisses the *Credo quia absurdum* of Tertullian in one page as believable only to those influenced by the "artifices of philosophy." Freud's (1927a) *The Future of an Illusion* contains *two* sets of illusions, those Freud attributes to religion and those of Freud himself in his religion of science, the latter already under attack by Nietzsche (to be described in Chapter 17), and it also contains a highly debatable philosophical a priori premise: "But an illusion it would be to suppose that what science can not give us we can get elsewhere" (Freud, 1927a, p. 56).

The paradox in this premise is immediately manifest when we open *Civilization and Its Discontents*. Freud (1930a) began it with a magnificent paragraph pregnant with value judgments about aims and ideals, which certainly cannot come from science. He then characterized both the oceanic feeling and the state of being in love as merely regression to a primary developmental state where ego boundaries are not yet established, "the restoration of limitless narcissism" (p. 72). Freud's only philosophical argument for this explanation is that he was "inclined" to trace these phenomena "back to an early phase of ego-feeling" (p. 72). There is no way to validate such an explanation either by philosophic argument or by science, since early preverbal experiences are never initially communicated, and verbal descriptions of them are contaminated extrapolations from later reports—contaminated both by psychic distortion and by later experiences and conflicts.

Harrison (1979) stressed Freud's ambivalence about the matter of transcendence and explored the roots of this ambivalence in Freud's relationship to his mother: "One might say that Rolland denied the preoedipal 'bad mother' in a lifelong embrace, via his mysticism, of a hallucinatory formless, divine mother who represented his lost primary narcissism; whereas Freud simply isolated the most traumatizing aspects of his early life with explicit aversion" (p. 414). How to establish the scientific validity of even such a plausible psychohistorical interpretation remains a very open question.

The term "oceanic feeling" used by Rolland (that Masson, 1980, claimed he could trace to Sanskrit sources) and "explained" by Freud is related to Kohut's (1978) concept of cosmic narcissism. The philosopher Gaston Bachelard (Jones, 1991) originally wrote about the "oceanic feeling" but Bachelard did not worship science and was much aware of the naive epistemological profile assumed by classical science, and of the significant creative aspects in all scientific and artistic endeavor. Bachelard insisted that the subject projects his or her dream upon things, and this is equally true in both art and science. Masson (1980) correctly stressed the dark side of the ocean metaphor, with its implications of suicide and annihilation. Kohut (1978) distinguished between the primordial "oceanic feeling," which is experienced passively, and the creative activity of an autonomous ego that produces "the acceptance of transience and the quasi-religious solemnity of a cosmic narcissism" (p. 456).

The explosive outbreak of a profound narcissistic need in a person like Barry, who always kept his nose to the grindstone and served by subordinating his personal needs to those of others, should not be confused with the historically and anthropologically evident universal longing of humankind for the fusion with "God" or some sort of transcendent experience. The former is a clinical phenomenon not rare in the treatment of aging narcissists in our time and explainable by concepts such as those of Kohut's (1971, 1977, 1978) self psychology. The latter represents a boundary beyond which science cannot pass. Explanations from religion are no less applicable to articulating this yearning for an oceanic feeling than such speculative conceptions as Freud's "death instinct." Reductionistic psychoanalytic hypotheses are clearly explanatory for such states when they appear in cases of psychopathology, as in the psychoses, but become open to much debate when applied to those individuals of obviously great psychological strength from all civilizations and all ages who have reported such experiences and even found in them new sources of strength and conviction. The explanation of this puzzle remains unresolved. As Freud (E. Freud, 1960) wrote in a letter to Romain Rolland, "Your letter of December 5, 1927, containing your remarks about a feeling you describe as 'oceanic' has left me no peace" (p. 388).

After a disturbance in the psychologial equilibrium of primary narcissim,

> the psyche saves a part of the lost experience of global narcissistic perfection by assigning it to an archaic, rudimentary (transitional) self-object, the idealized parent imago. Since all bliss and power now reside in the idealized object, the child feels empty and powerless when he is separated from it and he attempts, therefore, to maintain a continuous union with it. (Kohut, 1971, p. 37)

Under overburdening adult stress there is regression to early configurations, what I described in Chapter 1 as a sliding backwards on the ego axis; the true believer seeks mystical merger with God, while the nonbeliever is more prone to outbreaks of passionate longings. The power of this passion is explained on the self psychology channel by the need to maintain the vital bedrock of the personality, a cohesive sense of self, which is threatened with fragmentation under the pressure of severe narcissistic wounding. The very psychological existence of the person is at stake, and in this situation nothing else matters. For example, Prosen, Martin and Prosen (1972) pointed out how the "middle-age crisis" in men who must deny the aging process is a sufficiently noxious narcissistic wound in certain men to set off an obsessive search for an idealized woman, a search which can attain "hypomanic" intensity, and which is based on the hoped-for fusion with the vaguely remembered fantasized mother of childhood ... a woman he never finds. This approach will be very important as we try to understand Ezra Pound and Barry.

These situations, which can occur at any time in a person's life, have been labeled "boundary situations" by the psychiatrist-philosopher Karl Jaspers (1932b). They have not received sufficient clinical psychoanalytic exploration or metapsychological delineation. Phenomenologically, they are ultimate situations requiring one to face existential questions, and they also have ethical ramifications because they require crucial choices in a person's life; they represent crises in human existence in which conflict and its meaning become poignantly, tragically clear. Jaspers emphasized death, suffering, guilt, and struggle with the uncertainty of the world (Sartre's "contingency"), and two more general boundary situations, that of the particular historical determination of one's particular existence and the relativity of all that is real—its self-contradictory character of being always somehow what it is not.

Falling in love reflects the grappling with a boundary situation, as does creative endeavor that serves the function of psychological self-repair for the artist. Using the example of Sylvia Plath, Silverman and Will (1986) pointed out that when such efforts at self-repair fail, suicidal violence threatens to break out. A sweeping narcissistic regression may occur, with a longing for death as a release and ultimate bliss, a death that may be self-inflicted in one way or another as a violent expression of narcissistic rage. We are dealing here with a clinical matter of the utmost importance, a collapse of the ego, a fragmentation of the self.

This should help us empathize with patients like Barry and artists like Ezra Pound who are driven to pursue self-defeating activities at any cost in spite of our best psychoanalytic efforts at explanations and interpretations; with the tragic and puzzling suicide of wounded narcissistic poets so common in our time; and with what it is like to long for someone with your whole heart and soul, living in a state of continual agitation, ignoring the claims of the external world, and feeling that you must fuse with that person no matter what the cost to yourself, your career, or your very life.

8 RELATIONSHIPS MALE AND FEMALE

The eyes she had! . . . everything there, on this old muckball, all the light and dark and famine and feasting of . . . (hesitates) the ages! . . . The face she had! the eyes! like . . . chrysolite!

—*Samuel Beckett,* Krapp's Last Tape

To what extent did Ezra Pound and Barry escape enmeshment with their parents? Melanie Klein's early theory of artistic creation was that the creator wishes to rediscover the mother of his or her early days who has been lost. Klein (1929) reported her clinical experience of the tremendous anxiety of children over the child's sadistic desire to destroy the mother and rob the mother's body of its contents. She maintained that the dread of being alone, of the loss of love, and the loss of the love object mother is a basic infantile danger situation. In her theory the urge to create arises from the impulse to restore and repair the injured object after a fantasied destructive attack.

Pound and Women

Although Ezra Pound once or twice mentioned falling in love, there is no evidence from his behavior toward women that he ever did so with any passion. His attitude toward women did not fundamentally involve the usual romantic love or sexual desire. William Carlos Williams, "who had as close a knowledge of Ezra's early love affairs as anyone, observed: 'if he ever got under a gal's skirts it must have been mainly with his imagination'" (Carpenter, 1988, p. 57). He never seriously fell in love

109

with any woman; his relations with women centered around respect and intellectual exchange. When he became involved with women the relationship usually shaded off into a friendliness that he maintained by mail, sometimes over many years. For example, in his youthful flirtation with Hilda Doolittle a very intense relationship developed, but the intensity was motivated by having one's mind illuminated by new ideas "rather than that of a young man in love with a girl" (Carpenter, 1988, p. 63). Although he appeared to be in love with her and there were some kisses and caresses, his main interest seems to have been the narcissistic one of "educating" her, and the exchange of poetic ideas.

He displayed his typical consciously "artsy" personality and dress to a variety of girlfriends at once, as, for example, to Mary Moore, whom he never told about Hilda Doolittle. But it was clear that his interest in them, beyond a kiss on the forehead, was mainly to flirt and exaggerate the romantic aspects in writing and talking without committing himself. He preferred constructing a romantic ideal out of touch with reality and flirted better by correspondence with women when they were separated from him by many miles geographically. Of course, this did not satisfy the women, and eventually they would drift off and become attached to other men.

Another way of looking at Pound's attitude toward sex is illustrated in his arcane *Canto XXXIX* (Pound, 1950), which contains a depiction, at times vulgar, at times esoteric, of "the ingle of Circe" and girls saturated with sexuality and orgiastic pleasure. But this canto culminates in a fertility rite that leads to the conception of a god. The love cult of the troubadours, a kind of sexual-religious mysticism, had more appeal to Pound than an actual intimate relationship with a mortal woman.

He was much more interested in gathering around him "privileged" disciples whom he considered to be a small group of advanced thinkers in the arts. He would speak on many topics, jumping from subject to subject, descanting in a monologue while the disciples would listen with rapt attention. He considered himself an expert in many fields of knowledge, including political science and sociology as well as economics, art, and education. His main interest and quest seemed to be to become regarded as a celebrity, perhaps *au fond* to meet the narcissistic needs of his mother.

In that quest, when he arrived in London he began to hang around a bookshop that was known to attract contemporary *literati*. He was able to ingratiate himself to them and to others by his brilliant personality when he wished to display it. This networking eventually led to his introduction to Olivia Shakespear, a married woman 21 years older than he was, who was beautiful and charming. Carpenter (1988) wrote, "romantic friendship with such a woman was very much to Ezra's taste, far more than the notion of marriage to somebody nearer his own age" (p. 105). And so he began a relationship and eventual correspondence with Olivia Shakespear of the type described earlier.

His customary descanting monologue performance enacted at the home of the Shakespear family made an exciting impression on Olivia's daughter Dorothy, who was a year younger than Pound. She developed passionate romantic love as a reaction to his exhibitionism, perhaps out of the adolescent need to find an idealized self-object. It gradually dawned on Pound that she adored him, and he basked in the sunshine of her feverish admiration.

At this time the self-centered Pound published what would become one of Barry's favorite poems, to be found in the collection of Pound's (1949) *Selected Poems*, titled "Sestina: Altaforte." T. S. Eliot labeled this as one of Pound's best early poems. It is a loose rendition of a poem by the troubadour Bertran de Born, whom Pound had already impersonated in another striking poem titled "Na Audiart." The latter poem, more romantic, was another favorite of Barry's. These two poems in a sense sum up Pound's personality at the time; the latter is about the romantic construction of a perfect idealized woman and the former displays the troubadour's boasting aggressiveness and love of battle. A sestina is a form of rhymed or unrhymed poem with six stanzas of six lines and a final triplet, all stanzas having the same six words at the line-ends in six different sequences. Altaforte was Bertran de Born's castle. Audiart refers to Lady Audiart, who scorned Bertran de Born, so that in his poem he tried to find various parts of other women and put them together to make a woman that was her equal. The title "Na Audiart" is an allusion to Provençal Bertran de Born's poem "Lady Though You Care Not For Me."

Pound and Men

Pound seems to have done better with men, as, for example, in becoming a friend of the writer Ford Maddox Ford in London; he became an important supporter and also introduced Pound to significant members of the British literary establishment. Pound impressed them with his rebelliousness, cleverness, brilliant assertiveness, and impish and elfish behavior, as well as his poetic experiments, which seemed to enliven a rather dull poetic era in London. He was bored with the interests and enthusiasms of others and was not particularly interested in conversation; what he liked to do was to declaim about many topics to a group of admiring listeners. Within a year he had become a public figure in London on his road to celebrity status; he dressed like the stereotype of a Bohemian artist, like an actor preparing for a character role.

It should be kept in mind, however, that in spite of all this charlatanism and tomfoolery, Pound was writing some very impressive and innovative original poetry, such as "Dance Figure" in 1912, another of Barry's favorites in Pound's *Selected Poems*. During his first two years in London he applied for various teaching positions at universities in the United States and was rejected. He decided that he would nevertheless return to the United States after visiting Italy, and he planned to stop off in Paris briefly on his way to Italy. Leaving for Italy in March 1910, he carried with him a promise from Olivia Shakespear that she and her daughter Dorothy would try to join him there in a few weeks.

He really knew very little about England except for the city of London, but Pound's plausible view was that all great art emerges from major cities and that all civilization has developed from these cities and from little groups of advanced thinkers, such as those he gathered around him. He claimed that the United States had failed to produce great art because it lacked a magnificent capital city.

When Olivia and Dorothy Shakespear met Pound in Italy, it was a great shock to the mother to discover that Pound now was transferring his affections to her daughter. Olivia actually derogated her daughter to Pound in a fit of jealous rage. Of course, Pound enjoyed Dorothy's infatuation with him, but he did not consider that a reason to commit himself exclusively to her. He left them and returned to the United States in 1910, where it was already recognized by literary reviewers that he was hungry for publicity. He had nothing but contempt for most American poets and their poems, and he was at first unhappy in the city of New York, where he went hoping to make money in some business enterprise or other.

Pound's Return to Europe

He returned to London in less than a year. At the same time he did report interest in the brash aggressiveness of New York City life and begin to concern himself with helping contemporary struggling American poets in the self-appointed role of European critic and mentor. Pound felt conclusively that his home was going to be Europe, and he decided to travel about in Europe as a nomad for a while. His poetry slipped during that period and he gradually became aware of the fact that he was not going to be able to revive the poetry of the Provençal troubadours.

There was also a certain continuing cruelty in his behavior to the various women mentioned earlier; for example, when Mary Moore or Hilda Doolittle came from the United States to visit him, he insisted that Dorothy Shakespear invite them to tea. He had no inclination to get married and preferred to have a number of ladies interested in him but not to be committed to any of them. It is clear from his writing at the time that he was not in search of sexual gratification.

Hilda Doolittle was attracted to odd and lonely individuals and soon became a disciple rather than a romantic partner of Ezra Pound. Even as early as 1905, in *Hilda's Book,* comprising twenty-five rather amateurish poems he wrote for her, Pound indicated his detestation of Western social and religious organizations, basing his values on more ancient sources such as those of the early Greeks or Chinese. This is very important information toward understanding his creative work. It was Professor Doolittle, Hilda's father, who objected strenuously to Pound's relationship with his daughter and who first labeled Pound as "nothing but a nomad" (Tytell, 1987, p. 28).

During his first stay in London, Pound also managed to form a lasting friendship with the famous Irish poet William Butler Yeats. It should be noted that it was possible then, as it is not now, for a poet to eke out a sustenance by assorted writings published in little magazines, public lectures, and teaching assignments, and, if necessary, work as a translator. Pound had a great flair for self-publicity, a talent for interesting other intellectuals, a charm which he could put on when he wished to do so, and genuine ability as a poet. These things combined made him a very well-known individual at an early age, and opened doors to him wherein he might exert power and influence in the literary world of London. But Mullins (1961) related that for the next decade Pound was continually attempting to find little magazines and arrange short-run publications of his books of poetry as an outlet for his work; "He finally realized that it is easier to write an epic poem than to manage an intelligent periodical in the 20th century, and he retired to Italy to work on his *Cantos*" (p. 55). Even Yeats was much influenced in his poetic work by Pound, who also dominated Yeats's popular literary soirees.

In 1912, at the age of twenty-seven, Pound was already a well-known figure on the literary scene. He was sincerely trying to practice the dispassionate contemplation of beauty. I believe it would be an instance of Freudian reductionism to interpret this simply on the basis of pathological sexual repression and sublimation; Pound from the beginning had his eye on something transcendent, as was even recognized by his compatriots. With all his obvious narcissistic psychopathology, he clearly was obsessed with getting into contact with something greater than himself, something involving an emotional and intellectual contemplation of beauty, beginning with physical beauty as described by Plato in *The Symposium* and moving up the ladder to higher and higher levels. His great and enduring interest in Dante's poetry is consistent with this obsession. It would be amateurish to interpret all this merely as a series of defenses against Pound's sexual conflicts, his hidden feeling of sexual inadequacy, his unconscious homosexual proclivities, and his unresolved oedipal struggle as well as his narcissistic enmeshment with his mother. Certainly these factors were present and

Pound was a quite seriously disturbed individual, but a phenomenologic study of his early work impressively reveals the stirrings of true genius searching for a sense of Being, a search for aesthetic transcendence.

Barry's Orientation

At about the same age that Pound returned to London, Barry finished his formal training as a specialist in psychiatry. This required working for three years as a resident at a major teaching hospital, after which it was necessary to practice for two years before becoming eligible to receive specialty board certification, a requirement in those days. Barry was also carving out a minor reputation for himself as a teacher of psychiatry and an author of some scientific articles. In common with Ezra Pound, he had a certain capacity to gather students around him and to communicate clearly a number of psychiatric theories that were difficult to understand and murky, as well as the capacity to analyze the epistemologic assumptions behind these theories and to clearly display their strengths and their weaknesses. Under the tutelage of his uncle he also did some work on the chemistry of the nervous system, suggesting a new scientific approach to the study of the nervous system that involved a mapping of the brain by means of identifying the predominant chemical compounds present in the various anatomical sections of the brain. He dropped his interest in this after he finished his training; he was not cut out for laboratory research.

The publications and his teaching success brought him a certain amount of local renown but also considerable envy from his peers as well as from older established psychiatrists who felt threatened by his exposure of the tenuous roots behind their practices. For example, there was a wealthy neurologist who practiced psychiatry (these individuals call themselves "neuropsychiatrists") in the same building where Barry worked. His treatment of the psychoneuroses was to apply ultraviolet radiation to the patient's head. Techniques such as these rested on poor scientific foundations, and Barry was not reluctant to expose them. As a result he made some powerful enemies. Barry, perhaps playing the game (Berne, 1964) of "poor me," liked to think of himself as the protagonist in Greene's (1956) novel *The Last Angry Man*. Indeed, like that protagonist, he was seriously devoted to helping his patients, and he also died of a premature coronary occlusion.

At this point in his career, Barry managed to publish his first paper in a philosophy journal, a study integrating neurophysiology and philosophy. He identified certain nervous system circuits as definitive in determining, shaping, and forming our perceptions; this was a Kantian view. Always drawn by the magnetic attraction of metaphysics, he audited Charles Hartshorne's class on Whitehead's (1929b) *Process and Reality* at the University of Chicago. It was his first experience with professional philosophers, and a dismal one indeed. Hartshorne tended to autistically speculate and absent-mindedly philosophize in class, I suspect somewhat in the manner that Wittgenstein notoriously did, rather than to help much with the explication of Whitehead's very difficult text. Although Barry had read Whitehead's other and much more readable books, there are sections of *Process and Reality* that are simply so obscure he could not understand them. Some of Whitehead's concepts, such as "prehension," seemed to him both scientifically naive and lacking in common sense.

In spite of all this, the confrontation with Whitehead's metaphysical system enabled Barry to compare and contrast the prosaic, pragmatic clinical practice of medicine with the poetic and speculative thought of a philosophical genius. In this sense he was again getting a glimpse of the light that shone through the poetry of Ezra Pound, although in Whitehead's metaphysics it was coming from quite a different direction. Barry did not remain a disciple of Whitehead for very long, moving on to Plato, Kant, and eventually even toward Hegel in his later years, as we shall see.

Barry in Love

Barry's first love was clearly his mother. Although he was reticent in sexual matters, he was not as repressed as Ezra Pound and he was capable of developing intimate relationships with women. Because of his background, as I have described it in previous chapters, he was slow in receiving sexual initiation. His first girlfriend seduced him into an affectionate relationship during a summer season, but this did not develop past the same hugging and kissing Pound did with Hilda Doolittle. Pound was sixteen years old and Hilda was fifteen. Barry was fifteen and the girl was sixteen in this instance.

Barry promptly went on to form a serious steady relationship with a lovely girl, Paula, who was one year younger than he was, and he maintained this relationship for about two years on a very regular basis. He genuinely loved her. In the words of Saul Bellow (1997), "I had fallen in love with her when I was an adolescent schoolboy. This tremendous feeling came, as they say, 'we know not whence'. . . this love, direct, from nature, came over me" (pp. 70-71). Paula bore a striking resemblance to his mother, but she had a much better personality in that she was soft and loving and kind. They were both very young. Paula was under considerable pressure from her parents to become engaged to Barry, whom they imagined as a promising successful physician in the future. They deliberately left the couple in their home alone together for substantial periods of time on weekends, and of course this developed into sexual play. It almost culminated in sexual intercourse, and Paula was quite ready, but Barry stopped at the last moment. He knew that if he began a sexual relationship with Paula he would ask her to marry him and be permanently committed, because Barry was that kind of serious person and he loved Paula. After he moved to the University of Chicago he was so immersed in his studies that he had much less time to see her and the relationship lost its intensity. They drifted apart.

Barry never found out what happened to Paula, although he made repeated efforts to contact her later in life. She disappeared, to his great sorrow. In the fourth year of medical school he met Paula's mother briefly, and she was again very impressed by his appearance in a white laboratory coat with a stethoscope sticking out of the side pocket. All the medical students at this point were very interested in looking like doctors! As the costume of an artist was to Ezra Pound, so the costume of a doctor was to Barry, but to his credit, as he matured he tended to abandon this costume and dress in an ordinary but conservative style of clothing.

To Barry, Paula was always his lost beloved. She clearly represented a derivative image of the beautiful young woman who was the mother of his oedipal and preoedipal days, not the elderly mother whom he remembered as an adult (see Prosen et al., 1972). This "longing for the unknown beloved" remained with Barry until his death. So for Barry, the long-awaited woman would always be absent. "Come when you must," the fragment from *To The Long Awaited* by Rilke begins (Freedman, 1996, p. 353). In 1914, Rilke, at almost forty, separated from his wife, and in a state of almost suicidal despair, received an admiring letter from a woman he did not know, Magda von Hattingberg. Calling her Benvenuta (the Welcome One) he (Hattingberg, 1987) began a passionate correspondence that went on daily for a month (Prater, 1986). He poured his heart out to her and longed for her, but she rejected him. He knew from the start he could never find a selfobject in her. Hence, "You my beloved, lost in advance, you who never arrived" (Freedman, 1996, p. 377). A magnificent poetic fragment (Rilke, 1984b, p. 131) remains as a momento to this longing.

Immersed in premedical studies at the University of Chicago, Barry had little time for any social life. The women at the university for the most part were older than he was and were very marriage-oriented. Fortunately, during a summer in which he earned some money by manual labor, he met a lovely and charming young girl who was two years younger and who had as little sexual experience as he did. They got on extremely well together because she was a very tactful, resourceful, adaptable, and unusually pleasant individual. She represented for Barry a fountain of nutrition, well-being, and repose in the maelstrom of his competitive medical work. Her parents despised him, considering him a starving student (which he was) and worrying that he would try to take advantage of their daughter by making her work to put him through medical school. Successful and wealthy people, they were appalled by his naiveté, lack of good business social graces, and poor taste in clothes. One of their mottoes was "You are what you wear." If this is true, Barry was dilapidated indeed.

In spite of these obstacles and every repeated effort her parents made to destroy their relationship, Barry and Mary persisted, and eventually got married. He lived happily, or so he thought, in an intimate relationship with Mary for many years until their children left for college, after which Mary became preoccupied with interests of her own and decided to leave him.

Barry was a good father to his young children and was quite delighted with them until the children became adolescent and, to his surprise, began the usual rebellions and explosions. Barry was by that time aging and burning out in his psychiatric work, and the adolescence of all four children coming almost at once seemed to be more than he could handle without extreme stress. After their college years his children grew away from him and, although there was a superficially polite relationship, there was such a difference in interests that it made intimacy impossible.

His children were healthier than he was and much more prosaic and practically oriented, whereas Barry always had a kind of mystical seeking to his personality and an intellectual involvement in nonmaterialistic, quodlibetic issues. He was also politically an idealist, a democratic socialist by inclination, and much influenced by Freud and the early writings of Marx. His children were not interested in politics or economics at all and, as is so common in the current "me-first" generation of American citizens, they often did not even bother to vote or inform themselves on national or international issues and events.

Saul Bellow's novels again come to mind here, for his heroes, like Barry, often struggle between an unauthentic life in the real world that would immerse them in meaningless materialism and petty distraction, and the life of the mind, with its dangers of autism and narcissistic introspection. As Kakutani (1997) put it, "On one side, community with the threat of shallowness and vulgarity; on the other, self-reliance with the threat of solipsism" (p. 28).

After Barry's wife left him when he was middle-aged, Barry had only one more intimate relationship with a woman. This woman, a former patient of his, also had an eerie physical resemblance to his mother (his wife did not), and her personality was more like that of his mother, characterized by a hot temper. She was unhappily married and her relationship with Barry did not involve sexual intercourse but rather physical caressing. This seemed to have had an immensely soothing and nurturing effect on both of them, although it happened only occasionally. For the first time since his early adolescent experimentation with Paula, Barry experienced an ecstatic pleasure in simply leisurely gazing at a naked woman. He began to understand the preoccupation of many artists, such as the aging Degas or Bonnard, with painting the female nude in many natural positions. Of course Degas's nudes in the bath were somewhat more voyeuristic, realistic, and animal-like, whereas Bonnard's paintings of the aging Marthe are more ethereal, mystical, and iconic, but both painters understated the erotic aspect of their scenes (for details see Hyman, 1998). The American painter Thomas Eakins, roughly a contemporary of Degas, was perhaps more direct. In his extraordinary painting "William Rush and His Model," created in 1907-1908, he expressed the essence of his work and ideas. For him, as for Barry, artistic creativity was stimulated and inspired by the human figure, which to Eakins represented the fundamental basis of beauty. It is impossible to translate this transcendent experience into words, and only the genius of our artists can communicate it to us. At first Barry was seduced into this relationship by the woman, but once it began it became almost an obsession for him.

This obsession developed at the same time he was bitterly disappointed in the conduct of one of his daughters, who was unhappily married and committed adultery. In his fantasy life Barry made an effort to discover this young woman with her lover and put an end to her adulterous affair and, being at the time a burned-out and divorced individual, he wrote the story of his current life and how he imagined it to end in the form of a play. This unpublished play, his only humanistic work that is in a finished form, is reproduced in Chapter 16.

Barry's marital history illustrates the fact that the appropriate object choice of a person in the teens is not necessarily an appropriate object choice for a person in middle age. Barry's wife recognized that Barry had become increasingly needy. She was less and less inclined to slide into the common role of the nurturant mother that so many aging men desire and respond to late in their marriages. Now that her children were grown up, she wanted autonomy to fulfill her own desires and create her own project and an individuality of her own. Greatly to her credit, she gradually developed these things and matured. Her second marriage was quite different and much more self-enhancing. She lived happily with her second husband many years after Barry's death. She never visited his grave, nor did his children.

A similar problem occurred with his final girlfriend, the patient, who became tired of ministering to Barry's needs and gradually withdrew from him. This increased the pressure on Barry to turn inward and raised an impossible tension between his need to use creativity as a selfobject function and his lack of talent and of reinforcing recognition.

While Ezra Pound had many superficial acquaintances but no genuinely intimate ones, Barry had few superficial acquaintances but a number of very significant intimate ones. He was much more able to share in relationships and was less demanding of adoration than Pound. He also had less need to use people for his purposes, although he also had less to offer to scintillate, inspire, and provoke them. His sexual activity as a young man was somewhat diminished, but Barry's sexual performance on the whole was considerably closer to what we might label the normal than that of Ezra Pound.

Friends and Early Creative Efforts

Barry always had a few close male friends, but he was not a popular person who had much social life. He did not enjoy lecturing to disciples as Pound did, nor functioning as an educator or informer of his friends. There was genuine camaraderie between Barry and his male friends, who were usually peers of Barry, in the same position in life as he was. One of the most unfortunate developments in Barry's life was that as time progressed these friends either moved away or died. By the time he was well into middle age he had lost some of them and was engaged only in correspondence with the others; there were no close friends in his immediate vicinity to whom he could turn in order to share his experiences and his troubles involving his wife, children, and patients. Several times in his life he was able to make up for the loss of old friends by developing new intimate acquaintances, but it became harder and harder as he grew older. His parents died, his in-laws despised him, and his children were preoccupied with their own lives. Again he turned inward, attempting to create.

Barry left many volumes of handwritten notebooks with drafts or copies of his correspondence, at times containing the prototypes of papers that he wrote and published later, at times proposing drafts of and outlines for creative writing, and at times describing personal experiences. The quotations from Barry in the rest of the present book are from his unpublished notebooks and correspondence, since it[19] his creative efforts that interest us, not his published didactic writing summarizing the scientific work of other psychiatrists. In the latter, whatever literary skills he possessed were not devoted to artistic or creative endeavor, but were put in the service of practical gain to enhance his reputation as a teacher and bring him referral of patients.

The first entry in the first notebook occurred when Barry was still an intern. He wrote of the death of Mr. B of a sudden coronary occlusion. Mr. B was the professor who taught humanities at the University of Chicago in Barry's first year of college, and his death was felt as a shocking personal loss, which perhaps initiated the beginning of these notebooks. He wrote, "My only memory of him as I think back is in his explaining *Don Juan,* the tone poem by Richard Strauss. He demonstrated Strauss's unique idea of putting the richly melodious theme in suddenly after a number of atonal bars, by singing it loudly to the class with a graceful sweep of his hand. The class tittered. He was a gentleman."

The second entry is labeled, "After Two Months of Depression, While Listening to the St. Matthew Passion in Rockefeller Chapel." Here the young intern wrote that his philosophy is one of revolt:

> This is adolescent, yet I revolt on an expressive level against the mundane, greedy, and brutally vulgar society in which I am forced to live, and unconsciously against the demands of my ambitions that come from my parents who insisted on making me what I cannot be. This period of my life cannot be viewed as anything more than a state of dynamic equilibrium between my natural tendencies and rational beliefs on the one hand, and the mass of pressures that move me from without. It leaves one with, beside a depression, also a sort of feeling of suspension and a sense of awe at the power of the forces that toss one about in the world, like a cork bobbing on the ocean's surface.

There is a six-month gap in his correspondence because he was working on a manuscript that never was published; this manuscript was to be dedicated to his beloved uncle (mentioned in previous chapters), who at that point was seriously deteriorating from generalized arteriosclerosis. Barry explained, "I have to write because I feel this to be my major interest in life. . . . I will devote all my spare time to the manuscript, for it is the hub of my life around the periphery of which everything else is arranged. I feel possessed of an uncanny vital force only while I work on it— it is a genuine sublimation." There is already at this early date some mention of Ezra Pound in Barry's notebooks, who for Barry characterized a revolution in literature with attention to immersion in culture as the highest psychic aim of a human life and with focus on the criticism of language.

At the point Barry started his psychiatric training, he noted the death of his father's young brother (the high school basketball star mentioned in Chapter 2) from a myocardial infarction at a premature age, and from time to time there is mention of other male and female relatives who died from the same disease; his family clearly was predisposed to it. There are a few other brief excerpts from his correspondence written during his specialty training worthy of our attention. Barry insisted that there are certain needs and passions that are specifically human: the needs for relatedness, transcendence, and rootedness, the need for a sense of identity, and the need for a frame of orientation and devotion. He viewed mental health as characterized by the ability to love and create, by a sense of one's experience of self as the agent of one's powers and of emerging from infantile attachments, and by a clear grasp of reality both outside and inside of ourselves.

His inward turn is already manifest in an early entry about Beethoven, who composed the *Adagio* of the Rasoumowsky Quartet No. 2 (Opus 59, Number 2) from an inspiration that occurred to him on a placid, starry night. Barry wrote, "Let the contemplative, inward, expressive, almost religious mood of this choral structure set the theme of my conclusion: a mingling of the magnificence of the eternal with an inward perfection of the spirit."

Barry's first efforts at playwriting appear in an early volume of his notebooks, and were stimulated by his reading a biography of George Bernard Shaw. The outline of the play titled *Three Gen-*

erations contains three acts. The first setting is around 1910, in a lower middle-class home, with the sound of the tedious Hannon piano exercises being played softly in the background. "Grandmother" and "her daughter" and "precious son" (Barry's uncle on his mother's side) are present while "Grandfather," a plain working man, sits at the table and noisily slurps coffee out of a metal pot. This act consists of a long dialogue between the grandmother and her daughter (obviously Barry's mother) on how to make a fancy kind of soup, with the interposition of complaining by grandmother, her haranguing of Grandfather, and her making invidious comparisons of Grandfather with her precious son. The "other daughter" (Barry's mother's sister), comes in from having finished her piano exercises, and Grandmother describes at length her life and thwarted ambitions while supervising her daughters to set the table, finishing the preparation of the meal, and continuing to depreciate Grandfather.

In Act II the setting is now 1925, and it is more middle class. The precious son is studying postgraduate medicine and has a dignified looking mustache. Grandfather and Grandmother are there, as before. There is a new character who is twenty years older than Barry's mother's sister, very fastidious and impeccably dressed, a surgeon. He sits, smoking cigarettes out of a long holder, in a chair where he intermittently dozes and reads the newspapers. Once more Grandmother is haranguing Grandfather and complaining to her daughter (Barry's mother) about Grandfather's lack of taste and about Barry's mother marrying someone ordinary in contrast to this wonderful surgeon, whom mother's sister has married in obedience to Grandmother.

At the same time, mother's sister's daughter (Barry's brilliant cousin) sits at a table studying. There are voices of children playing and laughing outside. The young girl looks longingly out of the window once or twice, but says nothing. Grandmother's daughter (Barry's mother) tries to change the subject by asking for advice on how to cook another type of soup, as her cooking invariably has no spice and is flat and tasteless. But Grandmother is busy praising the little girl whom she considers to be a genius, just like her precious son from the first act.

The third act is left unfinished except that it contains the same characters, as well as one new little boy, who is studying and fat. This act is to contain the scene of Barry's mother having a tantrum in front of her mother when she refused the offered soup, as mentioned in Chapter 4. It focuses on the little boy and centers on the familial expectation that he must be a great man. In turn the little boy begins to explain some subject to his mother, who listens in transfixed ecstasy, happy with the child's exhibition of knowledge and so blinded by her wishes that she does not realize he is making it all up. Grandmother finishes the play proclaiming that this is the reasonable life and everyone is happy and healthy. All drink a toast except for Grandfather, who has fallen asleep.

Barry's primary interest in his psychiatric training was already in the creative process. For example, he studied ballet dancers and commented on their well known shibboleth, "You dance for yourself and those who watch." The ballet dancer uses her face and her body as an instrument on which she plays. Barry noted the taboo on sexual discussion among ballet dancers; even though the dancing is sexual and suggestive at times, this is not articulated among them. (The "autobiography" of that superb prima ballerina Maria Tallchief, 1997, seems to contradict this notion, but it is hard to tell how much her story has been distorted by the ghostwriter to increase the sale of the book.) Barry was also impressed with the dancers' idealization of the choreographer (as vividly demonstrated in Tallchief's [1997] "autobiography"). He suggested rather naively that the excitement before and the breathlessness after a performance carries a hint of the orgiastic nature of the whole thing, perhaps a silent repetition of the primal scene.

Even as a novice psychiatrist he attempted to look at the springs of creativity, which he considered to involve neurosis, anxiety, and narcissism. He tried to study the equivalence between the longing schizophrenic patients expressed as he grew to know and understand them (this was possible before the days of psychopharmacology and managed care made it impossible), and the longing expressed in the myth and music of *Tristan and Isolde*. He believed this equivalence demonstrated that Lewin's (1950) "oral triad" was found in the psychodynamics of creativity also.

With some of the youthful brashness displayed by Ezra Pound, Barry apparently sent a manuscript of his early meanderings to the famous psychoanalyst David Rappaport, who politely replied that he should pinpoint one problem, exhaust its psychodynamic implications, and avoid a mélange. This is something Barry was never able to do, which resulted in the same mélange of impaired writing that is demonstrated in Ezra Pound's *Cantos*. The difference, however, is that in Barry's writings there is little evidence of real literary genius or major creative originality, unlike Pound at his best.

These unpublished notebooks and copies of his correspondence or prototypes of his letters are the main substance of Barry's failed creative work. Most of the humanistic material does not find itself revealed in his actual publications, which were primarily scientific, medical, and psychiatric. One reason for this was that he could not find a publisher for his humanistic contributions and speculations. Therefore, his creative energies were poured into notebooks and correspondence, and he was able to publish only scientific articles. The required and publishable style of scientific writing greatly restricted the possibility of creative expression in an artistic fashion and required meticulous study and objectivity with considerable attribution to earlier publications by other authors. In contrast to this, artistic writing tends to speak more directly to the reader with less encumbrance of jargon and attribution. An extreme of this style is in Pound's poetry, which contains innumerable allusions to all sorts of literature in various humanistic disciplines such as politics, economics, sociology, psychology, and history, as well as the literary and visual arts. It requires an ancillary volume or two that scholars have produced in order to help the reader identify the allusions (see Edwards and Vasse, 1957).

This was the "modernist" style of poetry, but Pound carried it to an obscure extreme, assuming that the reader had a prodigious knowledge of esoteric sources. Barry, on the other hand, displayed his scientific writing by leaning heavily on carefully cited references and expressing his own views modestly and indirectly. This was perhaps a reflection of the difference in self-esteem between Ezra Pound and Barry; as Pound became more and more successful and well known his self-esteem evolved into a psychotic grandiosity, while Barry's repeated failures to publish direct creative artistic work represented a chronic narcissistic wounding and enfeeblement of himself. Kohut (1978), in one of his finest papers, described chronic narcissistic rage turned on the body as carrying a serious risk factor for coronary artery disease. In addition, it was already apparent that Barry was carrying a genetic proclivity for this disease, which eventually prematurely killed him.

9 FALLING IN LOVE AND CREATIVITY

For most, romantic love is the most moving of all lived events, the only experience capable of seizing the center of one's concern and ripping it out of the iron cage of the ego; of reversing the vectors of attention so that the reality of something outside oneself is at last, if only fleetingly, encountered. It is, for most, the only glimpse beyond. Did not Plato himself, in the incomparable Phaedrus, *identify the erotic as a divine disturbance? It is a kind of madness, he says there, the result of either genuine illness or perturbation sent by the gods. . . . In that urgent pull toward another, which wrenches us away from the dulling conventions, we are reminded of the Form of Beauty. . . [Plato wrote,] "The soul that has seen most of Being shall enter into the human babe that shall grow into a seeker after wisdom or beauty, a follower of the muses, and a lover."*
—*Rebecca Goldstein,* The Late-Summer Passion of a
Woman of Mind

De Rougemont (1983), in a much-quoted book written when he was thirty-two years old, claimed that the notion of passionate love reappeared in the twelfth century as a myth re-created by Gottfried of Strasbourg, and has now degenerated in the materialistic West. Nineteenth-century German romanticism tried to elevate it again in Wagner's opera *Tristan und Isolde,* the sublime music preserving the transcendental in that myth. But now everything is profane and just a semblance, he said, for people are immersed in a sexual flood. With the legend of Tristan and Isolde begins medieval humanism, wrote Gray (1985), a focus on the worth of the individual and on the fact that individuals uniquely develop and change. Wagner's opera idealizes death and shows how a sexualized passion can transcend everything and sweep away the rules and regulations of this world, as symbolized by the realm of Day. The music and the libretto are submerged in Schopenhauerian gloom and hopeless desire, and the opera at-

129

tempts to explore a mysterious realm of darkness beyond everyday reality. The power of longing produces an abnormally intense state, breaks loose, and destroys the bonds of civilized life. Where does this come from? Is this beyond the pleasure principle (Freud)? Is it beyond good and evil (Nietzsche)? Is death the ultimate end? Wagner's murky religion of death was clearly a failure and nobody followed it, but what is his art pointing to?

Drive Derivatives in Passionate Love

Freud (1930a) mused that human love is the only thing that may make sense out of the absurd condition of the existential world, yet for Freud, love was essentially a derivative of sex. According to Freud (1930a), "Normally, there is nothing of which we are more certain than the feeling of our self, of our own ego" (p. 65). In passionately falling in love, however, ego libido and object libido cannot be distinguished. Freud continued, "At the height of being in love the boundary between the ego and object threatens to melt away. Against all evidence of his senses, a man who is in love declares that 'I' and 'you' are one, and is prepared to behave as if it were a fact" (p. 66).

Can the libido theory really explain all there is about the phenomenology of falling in love? Viederman (1988) said, "One of the most powerful aspects of a new passionate relationship is the formation of a new sense of self" (p. 9). He went on to explain that the love experience helps us to understand what we can expect from our body and what we can expect our body to do. The unconscious illusion of at least some gratification of early infantile wishes occurring in requited passionate love allows an individual to approximate aspects of the ego ideal from childhood, an ego ideal that had its origin in the frustration of childhood narcissistic wishes.

Many authors, including Freud, agree that in the experience of passionate love there is a temporary intense gratification, or at least the illusion of potential gratification, of powerful archaic infantile desires that have long been frustrated and repressed. This leads to what Viederman called "a euphoric sense of fullness" (p. 10) or what other authors have described as the sense of power and extraordinary exaltation that goes along with achieving requited passionate love. Viederman also correctly emphasized passionate love as for a time enabling one to escape the constraints of reality, as one finds oneself in a passionate embrace.

Viederman stressed the illusion aspects of passionate love, but he did not wish to devalue it on this account, claiming that once it is experienced and reciprocated, it is the closest thing to what he called "ever-elusive happiness" (p. 10). This is close to the Freudian concept that the greatest happiness consists of the preferably sudden gratification of long dammed-up infantile wishes. To this Viederman added the importance of being able to be one's true self in the lover's presence and of having one's true self accepted by the lover. This intense mirroring obviously has a powerful effect on the cohesion of the self.

Narcissistic Sources

Benedek (1977) pointed out that the word "passion" comes from the Latin verb *patior*, which means to suffer, to be tolerant, or to forbear. Landauer's (1938) early paper already mentioned the narcissistic factors operative in passion, as reflected in an enhanced awareness of one's sexual being.

Gediman (1975) drew a parallel between the "twin narcissism" De Rougemont described of lovers like Tristan and Isolde, and the narcissistic elements in the core of the artist's fantasies, which are projected onto the image of an empathic, sometimes adoring audience. For her the narcissism of Tristan and Isolde is to be viewed in a manner less pejorative than De Rougemont's. Shifting back to the classical Freudian interpretation, she described twin narcissism as "a term for fusion of self and object which is evocative of an early ego state common both to lovers and some creative artists" (p. 411).

One unanswered question is whether falling in love and being in love can be explained metapsychologically as a compromise formation expressing the sexual drive along with contributions from the ego and superego. Certainly it is a complex experience, and definitely not just a pathological regression in order to achieve the "oceanic feeling" and a sense of blissful fusion with the mother of infancy. Contrary to Freud's (1914b) contention, being in love enhances rather than depletes the ego ideal and is a source of narcissistic gratification. As discussed in Chapter 7, a study of falling in love helps us to understand how the regressive breaking loose of archaic narcissistic structures, along with the concomitant longing, pain, suffering, and rage, can sweep everything before it and lead to the individual's psychological and even physical destruction.

As explained in Chapter 7, passionate love can be set in motion in the young by the state of flux and instability indigenous to that late adolescent phase, but, somewhat paradoxically, also in middle age by the relentless and leaden repetition of experience. For the middle-aged individual, wrote Viederman (1988), "It is easy to see how the search for change, the search for the new, the search for mystery can lead to a passionate experience that will act as a powerful antidote to frustration, disappointment, and repetition" (p. 12).

Looking at the matter from the point of view of self psychology, the search for a passionate love experience in middle age is better explained by the increased narcissistic wounding that inevitably takes place as the individual in the course of life realizes that he or she is not going to reach cherished goals and ideals. Passionate love can restore the damaged narcissistic equilibrium in these situations by achieving a fusion with the projected infantile ego ideal, even if it is an illusion and only temporary. As Kohut (1977) said, "There is no love relationship without mutual (self-esteem enhancing) mirroring and idealization" (p. 122n). I (Chessick, 1989, 1990, 1997a) believe this to be an important clue toward understanding the sad situation of the aging therapist "falling in love" with his or her patient, as the creative work of Barry illustrates in Chapter 16.

For Viederman (1988), passionate love must inevitably diminish but can be a growth experience. He described it as "an entirely personal and a subjective experience" (p. 13), unique, and one which depends on the individual's fantasies, wishes, and memories. Therefore, no accurate general definition of passionate love can be obtained; "when one experiences passion one is never sure of how much it approximates the experience of the partner" (p. 13). This has important clinical ramifications, since when a patient in the transference declares himself or herself to be "passionately in love" with the therapist, this may have an entirely different meaning than the therapist assumes it to have on the basis of the therapist's personal experience. This is also true in everyone's personal experience. Compare, for example, what Pound thought it was to be passionately in love, with the expectations it raised in Hilda Doolittle or Dorothy Shakespear, as described previously.

Phenomenologic Aspects

One of the most remarkable phenomenologic descriptions of the state of falling in love has been presented by the Italian sociologist Alberoni (1983). He pointed out the close relationship between the great collective movements of history and falling in love. The forces they liberate involve similar experiences of solidarity, joy and life, and renewal. There is the birth of a new collective "we" constructed out of two or more individuals, as when two people fall in love. In an existing social structure this may divide whoever was united and unite whoever was divided to form a new collective subject. "The forces that operate in both cases have the same violence and the same determination" (p. 6).

Alberoni emphasized the distinction between "ordinary sexuality" in our everyday life and the "extraordinary sexuality" which appears in the situation of passionate love. This distinction has not been sufficiently stressed in the literature. During the sexual activity of passionate lovers a new vital energy is often released, and there are new explorations of "the frontiers of the possible, the horizons of the imaginary and of nature" (p. 13). The human beings are in what Alberoni called a "nascent state," in which "eros overflows the structures and floods prohibited territories" (p. 23).

Alberoni, like many other authors, stressed the long preparation period before this occurs, which may be characterized by increasing depression and a slow deterioration in relations with previous love objects. He insisted that the experience of falling in love originates in an extreme depression, an inability to find something that has value in everyday life, the well-known existential malaise, "the profound sense of being worthless and of having nothing that is valuable and the shame of not having it" (p. 69). This can happen at any age and it is characterized by the "irreparable loss of something in the self, a feeling that we will inevitably become devoid of value or degraded, compared with what we have been" (p. 69). The experience of romantic love becomes one of liberation, fullness of life, and happiness, in which all alienation is temporarily extinguished. For example, when a creative person falls in love, he or she becomes more and more creative, and passionate love increases the capacity to enrich life with the fruits of imagination. Alberoni claimed that "artists, poets, and scientists live in the imaginary universe they have created, and when they fall in love, they tend to transport the person they love to this world of theirs" (p. 65).

Alberoni also regarded the outcome of falling in love as quite variable. He adopted Sartre's version of human intimacy; for Sartre, intimacy is doomed to end in some form of clash of individual plans and life projects. This may either result in a direct parting of ways or in the destruction of the individuality of one person by the other, at which point instead of the anticipated bliss there occurs the realization that the changed person is no longer valued as a limerent object (see Chapter 7). Sartre had problems with intimacy. In contrast, Bertrand Russell's (1929) view, expressed when he was 60 years old, for example, in his book *Marriage and Morals,* placed loneliness at the heart of the human condition and maintained that only passionate love can afford an escape from the indifferent universe. To this 60-year-old philosopher, passionate love was the most important thing in the world (Ryan, 1988).

Passionate Love and Death

As usual, our literary artists are far ahead of our psychoanalysts on this topic. García Márquez (1988) published a magnificent novel about a passionate love that arose in adolescence, was brushed aside by circumstance, and resurfaced with a happy ending in old age. Yet the love becomes associated with the symptoms of cholera and faces toward death. Again, *Dasein* (human being) is being-towards-death (Heidegger, 1962).

A pessimistic view of passionate love runs also through the sparkling prose of Ernest Hemingway, whose entire neurotic life and suicidal death were based on problems originating in twin-ship narcissism (see Lynn, 1987). For Hemingway, the normal human condition is loneliness and the fundamental human problem is coming to terms with it. The way of liberation from loneliness is love, but love, however intense, never endures. The Hemingway hero always loses his beloved, usually to death. This theme of redemption by love arose in nineteenth-century German romanticism, where also the link of passionate love with death rather than marriage repeatedly appeared, as discussed earlier.

Although it is true that the form of passionate love and perhaps even its duration are determined by the given culture and the historicity of humans, as well as by many specific indi-vidual factors, there still seems to be a long and consistent phe-nomenon found throughout various cultures in which passionate love and lust are related in various forms. Whether love is the highest human pleasure and beyond the pleasure principle, that is, beyond the libido theory to explain, as Gaylin and Person (1988) insisted, or whether it can be explained as a combination of heavy pressure for libidinal discharge along with ego and superego functioning leading to a compromise formation that then determines the form and object of the pas-sionate love remains an unanswered question. I believe it can be resolved, especially if the complementary factors of narcissistic disequilibrium and the restoration of the self are taken into ac-count.

The mystery of passionate love is that it is not linked to marriage, but, rather, historically speaking, is often associated with thoughts of death or at least the longing for death. Al-though passionate love may represent at some level the wish for union with incestuous objects and the overcoming of one's in-fantile sense of inferiority to the parental objects, there still seems to be an ultimate goal—permanent fusion in some eternal fashion in another world—consistently associated with it. This points to the deeper preoedipal roots of passionate love . . . or it can be equally effectively used as evidence of man's in-herent search for transcendence.

The "Mysterious Leap" and the Creative Process

Robert Louis Stevenson fell in love twice, each time with an older married woman. The second one divorced her husband and married him. Only after that marriage did he produce his great creative works. A century before Freud, Stevenson (1988) wrote:

> This simple accident of falling in love is as beneficial as it is astonishing. It arrests the petrifying influence of years, disproves coldblooded and cynical conclusions, and awakens dormant sensibilities. Hitherto the man had found it a good policy to disbelieve the existence of any enjoyment which was out of his reach; and thus he turned his back upon the strong sunny parts of nature, and accustomed himself to look exclusively on what was common and dull. . . . And now, all of a sudden, he is unhorsed, like St. Paul from his infidel affectation. His heart, which has been ticking accurate seconds for the last year, gives a bound and begins to beat high and irregularly in his breast. . . . The lover takes a perilous pleasure in privately displaying his weak points and having them, one after another, accepted and condoned. He wishes to be assured that he is not loved for this or that good quality, but for himself. (pp. 8-9)

The capacity for passionate love is inherent in human nature; both females and males seek to achieve this extraordinary state. Person (1988) devoted an entire book to the subject of passionate love, filled with anecdotes from literature and film along with psychoanalytic generalizations. Imaginative flashes of the possibility of a passionate love developing with this or that individual who crosses our path keep occurring to us, similar to flashes of sexual desire or fantasy. Passionate love is "a perpetual possibility waiting to be born" (p. 264), but these imaginative flashes are usually immediately "nipped in the bud" by the realistic situation in which there is not only no chance of reciprocation but usually the danger of a humiliating rejection. Unless there is some hope that one's love may encounter a less stringent response, the flashes suffer the same fate as fleeting sexual fantasies.

Following Freud, Person located the source of passionate love in our early lives, but she related it to the play of the imagination and in the springs of our creativity. She viewed it as potentially transforming and transcending the self, but opined that a mysterious leap is involved in falling in love, similar to a religious conversion. When this "leap" occurs, there is always a heightened drama and sense of self-awareness and, when the love is reciprocated, we experience a sense of intermittent transcendence and merger, with the "oceanic feeling" as a typical result.

When this happens, values and priorities may become reordered, new projects undertaken, new responsibilities assumed. This profound change in the self may last even after the passionate love affair has passed. Person emphasized the creative and positive potential of passionate love, a state which is discontinuous with the rest of our lives and can be a major agent of change even outside of the transference love of psychoanalytic experience. Some people manage to allow such love to flourish for a long period, especially if there are obstacles to its consummation, which permit the individual to experience intervals of merger and surrender while at the same time preserving autonomy. On the whole this approach to love views it as an ego function, an act of the creative imagination, in contrast to Freud's more id-related explanation involving a refinding of incestuous objects. But phenomenologically it remains a "mysterious leap."

This mysterious leap occurs when certain conditions are met. The first of these is the safety requirement of not having to anticipate the certainty of serious narcissistic wounding if one manifests one's love. The totally inappropriate appearance of passionate love suddenly in a situation that clearly indicates it will be rejected, and often cruelly and scornfully rejected, demonstrates very poor reality testing in the lover as, for example, in the autistic infatuation with a movie actor or actress seen in some cases of psychosis. At best such declared infatuation indicates a severe borderline (Chessick, 1997c) or masochistic disorder, and at worst it is not uncommon in schizophrenia or bipolar disorders.

The second condition is some association in the lover's mind of the beloved with either an incestuous love object or an object from childhood invested with healing and soothing power—a self-object—or both. At least there is the imaginative hope that the beloved will transform into such an object, given the proper persuasion and seduction. Arlow (1980) elaborated on this condition: "In every love relationship the individual acts out some form of complicated unconscious fantasy rooted in early vicissitudes of drive and object experience, a fantasy that ultimately determines, but only in part, the pattern of loving and the specific person or types of persons that will correspond to the object choice" (p. 127).

The third condition is that of the activity of the creative imagination. There has to be a problem situation that calls for creative imagination, such as a loss that must be ameliorated or a depletion of middle age that is becoming unbearable. The "leap," then, is one of the imagination, wherein the illusion is created that the beloved object will be able to perform all these roles, and passionately, so there will be a sudden release of dammed-up narcissistic and sexual tensions that have accumulated, sometimes for many years. This creative leap triggers the idealization and obsession with the beloved, and explains the exaltation and ecstasy when the love is reciprocated.

Certain people who fall passionately and romantically in love are also capable of enduring object love. Kohut's (1971) postulate of a separate narcissistic developmental line from that of object relatedness, in which narcissism is never outgrown but rather transformed, neatly helps to explain this fact. In addition, Kohut commented that for the average individual, idealization as a transitional point in the development of narcissistic libido survives only in the state of being in love, when one idealizes the love object. Kohut also said that the gifted individual idealizes and despairs about his or her creative work as well. So for the creator, the created work is a transitional object invested at least temporarily with narcissistic libido (Kohut, 1966, p. 261). In Kohut's later terminology it is a selfobject, performing a vital selfobject function for the creator. This is very important to keep in mind while trying to understand Ezra Pound and Barry.

Kohut (1978) also said, "People whose self is in need of sustenance, whether because of the energic drain and anxiety during a creative spell or for other reasons, will tend to establish narcissistic relationships to archaic selfobjects—whether in the form of one of the varieties of a mirror transference or through a merger with an idealized imago" (p. 813*n*). He claimed that in periods of intensive creativity an archaic selfobject transference occurs similar to those seen in the psychoanalytic situation—a "transference of creativity" (p. 814). It follows from this that creativity enhances the propensity for idealization required for falling in love, and that falling in love enables the actualization of one's potential for creativity since it lends strength to a self that would otherwise be enfeebled by the creative process.

This is not so mysterious, and can be depicted in metapsychological terms. Furthermore, the length of the passion can be understood as a function of the capacity of the lover to maintain the illusion in his or her creative imagination for an indefinite length of time, and of the degree of their proximity and time spent together. For some of us have a greater capacity to regress in the service of the ego than others, to maintain illusions and idealizations longer, and to engage in a play space in our fantasy lives. Freud said that with each sexual act the degree of idealization of the loved one diminishes—perhaps he was speaking from his own experience. Of course, familiarity makes it harder and harder to maintain idealization, whereas partings and obstacles fan the flames of illusion by keeping the reality of the beloved in a shadow and making it easier to project our wishes and fantasies onto him or her. That is why passionate love is often thought of as incompatible with marriage, and often (but not always) fades after the familiarity of marriage into either an enduring affection or a parting of ways. In Freud's terms the passionate or "lyrical" phase of love is replaced by a calmer, more rational, more durable "epic" phase.

Similarly, in the state of heightened creative imagination and expanded play space during passionate love there is an enhanced potential to create in other areas of one's life (Gediman, 1975). New values, projects, dreams, and even artistic compositions may abound. The increased cohesiveness of the self as a function of the mirroring from the beloved can also lead to better ego functioning, greater achievement, joy in life, and an enhanced sense of being alive. This transformation is no mystery and can be understood either in metapsychological terms stressing ego apparatuses, or in the concepts of self psychology.

But what of the longing for death at the moment of ecstatic union? Why is the long-awaited consummation often associated with death rather than life and companionship? Could this be due to guilt over breaking the incest barrier? Or would the final consummation of life secretly longed for be, indeed, the return to the inorganic? Was Freud right after all that the quest for nirvana is the fundamental human impulse and beyond the pleasure principle?

Falling in love cannot simply be explained as a refinding of incestuous parental objects, although this is always an important basic element in falling in love and in object-choice, as Freud said. What makes falling in love unique for each individual is the specific ego function involved in the act of creative imagination that each person uses, falling in love in his or her own way to solve specific intrapsychic difficulties. Falling in love represents a creative effort to find a solution for unbearable narcissistic and libidinal tensions, often in an emergency situation of object loss or narcissistic wounding. Depending on the nature of this effort, falling in love can be a constructive, helpful, and forward moving event, or it can lead to destruction and tragedy. But no generalizations can be made about the function of falling in love beyond the fact that it tends to occur when there is a serious problem to be solved. These problems of unbearable tension can range from the revived Oedipus conflict that occurs in normal adolescence or preoedipal pathology that suffers a resurgence in adolescence to the problems of old age, where loss, loneliness, and despair often predominate. Any variety of these problems are a challenge for solution by the ego; one of the solutions possible is the creative imaginative act of falling in love. Another is artistic endeavor.

Isolde was filled with rage, and she suffered from bouts of depression and even suicidal ideation. When certain women fall in love, it is possible that the repressed sadistic aspects of their preoedipal ambivalence toward the archaic love object, which falls across the image of the current love object, manifests itself in the wish for death of them both. The clinical exploration of the fate of the repressed hostility for the preoedipal love object in these situations of falling in love, when the finding is a refinding, remains a challenge before us. Perhaps the secret linking of passionate love with death rather than marriage lies in this direction, and would then be amenable to dynamic-genetic interpretation.

The phenomenology of falling in love only becomes intelligible when one views it as motivated by libidinal energies and narcissistic disequilibrium and molded into a compromise that is consistent with the historical and cultural horizons of the individual, so that it clearly incorporates the unique superego and ego functioning aspects of that individual. This is true even if one emphasizes the "oceanic feeling" or altered consciousness or "aberrant" experience in requited passionate love. Werman (1986) convincingly argued that such experiences in the adult cannot be simple replays of an infantile experience but instead represent "a complex phenomenon that derives from all aspects of the psyche, including the subject's value system and the influences of his culture" (p. 123).

Utilizing our self psychological understanding of the problems in maintaining narcissistic equilibrium, the extreme exaltation accompanying requited passionate love is no longer a mysterious or quasi-psychotic phenomenon but represents instead both Freud's concept of rapid gratification of long dammed-up infantile wishes, or at least the illusion of such gratification, and a powerful force toward the cohesion of the sense of self with the accompanying joyful experience that such improved cohesiveness of the self brings to the individual.

The mystery of falling in love lies only in the debate about the relationship between passionate love and death. If the pre-oedipal roots of falling in love are represented by the need to fuse with the mother of infancy in some eternal union, then we have an alternative and metapsychological explanation to the mystery of passionate love, which stands in contrast to viewing it as an aspect of the search for transcendence. The ultimate question behind all these transcendent experiences, whether manifested in falling in love, listening to Beethoven's *Emperor Concerto,* or experiencing some other incredible and indescribable sense of the sublime, is whether they represent phenomena that can be totally explained by internal dynamic forces striving to reach the highest possible equilibrium in the individual, or whether they are built into the nature of *Dasein* as a carrier of the expression of Being, which from time to time and sometimes in unexpected ways produces a lighting in the dark:

> She stood before me in immutable beauty
> smiling in effortless perfection
> and all longing, all mortal dreaming
> oh everything the spirit ever foretold
> of the regions of heaven in golden morning hours
> it was all fulfilled in this one still soul.

I found this in Barry's notebook, allegedly a translation from Hölderlin's *Hyperion*. Hölderlin (1965) also wrote, "What is all that men have done and thought over thousands of years, compared with one moment of love? But in all Nature, too, it is what is nearest to perfection, what is most divinely beautiful! Thither all stairs lead from the threshold of life. Thence we come, thither we go" (p. 68).

10 ARTISTIC ENDEAVORS

I do not claim that creative people are of necessity suffering from structural defects that drive them to seek archaic merger experiences. I suspect, however, that the psychic organization of some creative people is characterized by a fluidity of the basic narcissistic configurations, i.e., that periods of narcissistic equilibrium (stable self-esteem and securely idealized internal values: steady, persevering work characterized by attention to details) are followed by (precreative) periods of emptiness and restlessness (decathexis of values and low self esteem; addictive or perverse yearnings: no work), and that these, in turn, are followed by creative periods (the unattached narcissistic cathexies which had been withdrawn from the ideals and from the self are now employed in the service of the creative activity: original thought; intense, passionate work). Translating these metapsychological formulations into behavioral terms, one might say that a phase of frantic creativity (original thought) is followed by a phase of quiet work (the original ideas of the preceding phase are checked, ordered, and put into a communicative form, e.g., written down), and that this phase of quiet work is in turn interrupted by a fallow period of precreative narcissistic tension, which ushers in a phase of renewed creativity, and so on
— *Heinz Kohut,* The Search for the Self

What I have painfully learned in forty years of clinical experience and sixty-eight years of life is that the wonderful hope of the Enlightenment was ill-founded. This does not mean that the Enlightenment can be dismissed as representing the foolish prejudice of dead White males. It still remains the best project we have for eventually producing a world society fit for humans to develop their potentials and their aspirations. For this to happen, human rights must be defended everywhere and a springtime of diverse cultures must be encouraged to flourish. Hobsbawm

(1977) deplored the unfortunate loosening of restraints on human conduct in our time, and emphasized the pressing importance of restoring civility to contemporary human affairs. I will discuss the effect of all this on twentieth-century creative endeavors in the next chapter.

But the Enlightenment was wrong to postulate that man is a rational animal. Humans cannot live without myths that seem convincingly true to them but are obviously false to nonbelievers or to those who want objective evidence. It has always been one of the tasks of artists to create these myths or to rework the myths of the past into more contemporary form and make them pertinent, viable, and directly applicable to the particular culture or civilization of the artist's time. The destruction of these myths by science simply results in people searching for other myths or flatly denying the truths of science; hence, in our time, in the age of the scientific explosion that reveals many sacred scriptures of different religions to be simply wrong, we have a powerful movement in every country toward a mindless fundamentalism. This movement is extremely aggressive, hostile, and destructive of culture, and it expresses the rage that people experience when their myths are destroyed.

Since the days of the hand paintings in the caves of Lascaux, there is evidence of an irrepressible force that draws certain individuals to reach into them-selves in order to create and recreate these myths and to explore and produce various possible forms of art and sciences. Kohut (1978) claimed that when a creative person is led by his or her mind into lonely areas that have not previously been explored, "then a situation is brought about in which the genius feels a deep sense of isolation. These are frightening experiences, which repeat those overwhelmingly anxious moments of early life when the child felt alone, abandoned, unsupported" (p. 818).

Often individuals during a period of their most daring creativity "will choose a person in the environment whom they can see as all powerful, a figure with whom they can temporarily blend" (p. 819). Kohut tried to explain this as the wish of a self that has been enfeebled during a period of creativity "to retain its cohesion by expanding temporarily into the psychic structure of others . . . or to be confirmed by the admiration of others" (pp.

819-820), or attempting to obtain strength from an idealized self-object. He concluded, "relationships established during creative periods do not predominantly involve the revival of a figure from the (oedipal) past, which derives its transference significance primarily from the fact that it is still the target of the love and hate of the creative person's childhood" (p. 820). As in the case of the relationship between Freud and Fliess (see Gay, 1988), the idealizing transference of creativity became superfluous and ended when the creative work was done. During Freud's creative spell Fliess was the embodiment of idealized power but Freud did not need this kind of idealizing transference once he had completed his creative task.

Marcel Proust was an incredibly keen and perspicacious observer of humans and, like Kohut, he was sensitive to the vicissitudes of the self. One cannot read and reread Proust's (1981) *Remembrance of Things Past* sufficiently; it is in a class by itself for its perceptual depth of exploration of the secrets of the human psyche and its thrust against the style of Western civilization that characterizes our time. De Botton (1997) mentioned Proust's claim that every reader, while reading, is the reader of his or her own self: "The writer's work is merely a kind of optical instrument which he offers to the reader to enable him to discern what, without this book, he would perhaps never have experienced in himself" (pp. 24-25). Proust taught us that a novel helps us to articulate our perceptions and to recognize them as our own and formulate them in a better way. De Botton explained,

> Our mind will be like a radar newly attuned to pick up certain objects floating through consciousness; the effect will be like bringing a radio into a room that we had thought silent, and realizing that the silence only existed at a particular frequency and that all along we in fact shared the room with waves of sound coming in from a Ukrainian station or the night time chatter of a minicab firm . . . . The book will have *sensitized* us, stimulated our dormant antennae by evidence of its own developed sensitivity. (p. 29)

This is similar to the approach I advocated in Chapter 3, that of using several channels of psychoanalytic listening and understanding. A work of art, as Proust maintained, helps us to undo our habits, *"making us travel back in the direction from which we have come to the depths where what has really existed lies unknown within us"* (De Botton 1977, p. 103). Proust's magnificent novel incomparably demonstrates his contention.

I propose now to turn to the mature artistic endeavors of Ezra Pound and Barry in the light of these preliminary discussions of the creative process and of the importance of the kind of knowledge brought to us by the works of art. It must always be kept in mind that creative work is produced against the resistance of the practico-inert of the surrounding, more or less barbaric civilization in which the artist has to work. It is not possible to understand the phenomenology of the creative process and to accomplish a hermeneutic exegesis in Gadamer's style (see Chapter 20) of the knowledge provided by works of art without at the same time understanding the more or less thick resistance imposed on the artist by his or her place and time in history. An understanding of the creative process requires a psychoanalytic investigation using at least the five channels that I have previously described (see Chapter 3), as well as a phenomenologic study of the impact of the artist's work itself and an acquaintance with the historical and cultural milieu in which the artist was immersed. It is a multifaceted investigation; a purely psychodynamic interpretation of a work of art becomes reductionistic and neglects important phenomenologic and cultural factors. This is the disadvantage of Freud's interpretations of religion, mythology, philosophy, and art.

Pound as Wuz

Pound, now living more or less permanently in Europe, created and developed his mature method of artistic expression, which he sometimes called the "luminous detail method" or the "ideogramic method." He tried to choose some specific focus on a detail that might illuminate a work of art or a historical event rather than offering a multitude of material and details scattered in all directions. The detail he picked was typically related to whatever theme he was currently obsessed with and often included bizarre economic and political material, especially in *The*

Cantos. He tried to make his poetry correspond exactly to the shade of emotion he wished to express, and at times he was able to achieve this with amazing skill. He experimented a great deal with metrical schemes and *vers libre;* although he believed the latter could lead to "anarchy," at times that is exactly how his free verse sounds.

With Hilda Doolittle and others he launched *Les Imagistes,* a new movement in poetry, a school of images; he treated other members of this movement as "a couple of pet dogs" (Carpenter, 1988, p. 179). He took a leisurely walking tour of France and Italy, and spoke of his "damned mania for reforming things, due to my Presbyterian training" (p. 184), that would later include his innumerable grandiose and bizarre attempts to single-handedly reform the United States. The first vehicle of this reform, he decided, would be the new magazine *Poetry.* After receiving a request for money from Harriet Monroe, who had founded the magazine in the United States, his response was to appoint himself as its overseas editor. She was delighted. This launched Pound's energetic career of editing poems by even major poets such as Yeats and T. S. Eliot, and introduced his controversial poetry to American readers. It also unleashed his energies toward gathering contributions from other poets for *Poetry* magazine.

He felt he had an automatic right to edit everybody's poetry, published or unpublished, and most of his editing consisted of cutting parts of the poem out. "Yet though he had an acute ear for weak lines in other peoples' work, it is striking that he did not apply it to much of his own" (Carpenter, 1988, p. 193).

After he set himself up as the head of a poetic school and the self-appointed foreign editor and contributor to *Poetry,* Pound's grandiosity began to show itself in a more unpleasant form as he approached the age of thirty. He saw the public as a mass of dolts, denigrated the United States, and believed that the artist is a superman who will be the dictator of the future.

The imagist method was to write by means of unexplained and detached images rather than using similes, metaphors, or symbols, as in traditional previous European poetry. The images become the poetry and the reader of the poem "is left to do all the work of explanation, is expected to make all the effort necessary to establish a coherent narrative" (Carpenter, 1988, p.

194). The idea is that a specific image will present an intellectual and emotional complex in a brief moment of time, which, when experienced, instantaneously gives a sudden sense of liberation. This liberation is what we receive in the presence of the greatest works of art, a liberation from the prosaic material world, a sense of transcendence and beauty. Heidegger (Zimmerman, 1981) described this as the sudden illumination of Being in a time span equal to the blinking of an eye (*Augenblick*, a moment of vision), while present metaphorically as in a clearing in the forest. Of course, one has to be open to this experience, willing to be standing in the clearing, so to speak. The illuminative experience of a great work of art, the dramatic impact, the liberation, is almost impossible to articulate. This is an important source of didactic frustration and presents a major philosophical problem.

At this point, the acting out of Pound's grandiosity was confined to literary and artistic matters, and he tried hard to encourage other artists. He did not brag about his own work; his arrogance did not show itself in proclaiming the superiority of his poetry. Especially over the second and third decades of the twentieth century he "discovered" and encouraged major writers such as Robert Frost, D. H. Lawrence, and T. S. Eliot. He helped James Joyce and many other writers and poets of lesser ability. He championed Joyce not so much because he was impressed with the quality of his writing, but rather because Joyce was in an endless struggle with publishers who tried to censor his works. Pound at first (see Chapter 12) thought Joyce was a sort of ideal artist who had produced a master work and who was isolated and rejected by an uncaring world. He enabled Joyce to achieve publication by relentlessly bombarding various magazines and publishers with Joyce's manuscripts and letters from Pound recommending them.

Ezra Pound had two aspects to his genius. One of them appeared in his poetic experiments, which unfortunately became increasingly flawed by his mental illness, and the other was in his capacity to discover, promote, and encourage a number of the great writers of the twentieth century. He displayed a remarkable capacity for getting his own way and for networking and developing and maintaining contacts in continental Europe, England, and even the hated United States.

At the age of twenty-eight Pound married Dorothy Shakespear. Pound's marriage "was the first permanent relationship of his life, and it was to endure—albeit in a tenuous and melancholy form—until his death" (Ackroyd, 1987, p. 35). Further, this marriage enabled him to have an independent income from Dorothy's father that relieved him from the necessity of either earning a living or considering the reactions of an audience to his poetry. He was able from this point on to do whatever he wished and not to have to worry about publication and sales. He was a gentleman of leisure. This also fed into his grandiosity, because he was able to sneer at poets who had to worry about getting paid when their poems were accepted for publication. As he now viewed it, his work was of importance simply because it was there. Pound's parents were invited to the wedding only as a formality and were given very little information about Dorothy Shakespear or about the wedding itself.

The marriage was a cold one, and from all evidence Pound had little sexual interest in his wife, although "in his poetry he liked to give the impression of casual virility, with allusions to 'the dance of the phallus'" (Carpenter, 1988, p. 240). Dorothy Shakespear was helpful to him, took an interest in his work and in the poets he was encouraging, and in many ways seems to have functioned as a selfobject for him, as she had for her mother. Thus, Pound did not use an idealized selfobject, but rather a reflecting or mirroring selfobject, an auxiliary ego found in his wife, as was the case between Eugene O'Neill and Carlotta, his third wife who, "for many years completely fulfilled his needs for an empathic selfobject" (Kohut, 1991, p. 575).

Pound coined the term "vorticism" as the name of yet another new movement in poetry he supported. It emphasized primary forms of expression even in painting and music, and it expressed "the inexorable haste of his own mind, which, whirlpool-like, was constantly hungry for matter to suck up and expel" (Carpenter, 1988, p. 247). He was not the leader of this movement, but he enjoyed the battle to get it established; the leader was Wyndham Lewis, and the publication that launched the movement was a "little magazine" called BLAST, appearing in 1914. It was soon followed by Pound's introduction to T. S. Eliot, the superb poet and critic, who was more impressed by

Pound's energy as expressed in his poetry than by Pound's poetry itself. Pound promoted Eliot everywhere and was instrumental in the publication of his first famous poem, "The Love Song of J. Alfred Prufrock." The advent of World War I during this period seemed largely ignored by Pound, although Mullins (1961), in contrast to Carpenter, claimed that "Pound also was deeply shocked by the war. Never again would he be content to be merely an artist" (p. 102).

Pound became interested in Fenollosa's translations of Chinese poetry (which were not very accurate), and he began to use Chinese ideograms in poetry in a highly idiosyncratic manner. Previously he had been enchanted by the Japanese "Noh" plays, but the Chinese poems appealed to him more because they seemed thoroughly imagist. His putative "translation" of Chinese poems under the title of *Cathay*, although inaccurate and inadequate as translation, was filled with energy and set a pattern for modern verse that was followed by many poets. Unfortunately, the success of *Cathay*, or at least the enormous controversy it provoked, convinced Pound that he was now an expert in Chinese. Actually, the best he could do was painfully spell out some of the Chinese ideograms with the aid of a dictionary, but he convinced himself that he had an intuitive understanding of the Chinese characters. His belief that all he had to do was look at the Chinese ideograms to instinctively spot mistakes or inadequacies in the translation without even using a dictionary strikes me as the first definitive slippage in his reality testing.

The Fenollosa style of translation appealed greatly to Ezra Pound because it emphasized the nonrational habits of mind, what today some psychologists would call those aspects of mental processes that are mediated by the right brain. Pound's ideogramic method "consisted of doing away with abstract argument, or any other obviously rational process, and instead, 'presenting first one facet and then another' for the reader to contemplate and meditate on—lining up ideas or images side by side, but not linking them by any stated theory" (Carpenter, 1988, p. 273). Carpenter (1988) concluded, "while at its best the Ideogramic Method could genuinely illuminate—as in, for example, the finest passages in the Pisan Cantos, where the juxtaposition of apparently disparate memories and notions

produces a feeling of enlightenment and intuitive understanding of the world—at other times the result was just a
muddle" (pp. 273-274). This muddle in Pound's hands began to
resemble the loose and disturbed associations as well as the idiosyncratic speech habits characteristic of schizophrenia. Combined with the hypomanic quality of his behavior and the
scattered flight of his ideas, one might consider the possibility
of a developing *DSM-IV* schizoaffective disorder of the bipolar
type (his muteness in late life had a severe depressive or possibly
even catatonic quality).

It was in this furious state of mind that he began work on *The
Cantos* in 1915. He described it as an endless poem of no known
category, and it was supposed to deal quite literally with everything of importance in human experience that in his judgment
had not been adequately expressed elsewhere. At the same time,
paranoid thoughts were occasionally now overtly expressed, for
example, in a note he appended to *Cathay* claiming that he was
personally hated by many, and in a letter to the *Boston Evening
Transcript* accusing the newspaper of malice and insisting that the
staff of the newspaper detested him. He became an increasingly
angry person, and this anger began to affect his judgment. By
1917, the suburban culture anti-Semitism from his childhood
reemerged as an obsessively virulent theme in his writing and in
his published poetry. He developed a kind of backwoodsman dialect in his correspondence, with errors of typing and spelling
that seemed weird and that few regarded as funny.

At the same time, he made a considerable technical advance
in the rhythm of his poetry when he published "Homage to
Sextus Propertius," a very erotic poem that demonstrated he was
still being quite successful in his artistic endeavors. Whether this
poem suggests that Pound had become sexually active and
promiscuous in his behavior or whether it represents simply a
shift in his fantasy life is not as important to the purpose of the
present book as is the well-known clinical fact that the onset of
fragmentation of the self is often heralded by an outbreak of
sexual promiscuity in a person who has up to that time been
rather chaste, reserved, and repressed in his or her sexual life.
This has been noted on a variety of listening channels by several
psychoanalysts. For example, R. D. Laing (1969) described the

outbreak of sexual activity as a last ditch effort to counteract the person's ontological insecurity when it increases to the point where a schizophrenic explosion threatens.

Shortly after World War I ended, Pound gradually became aware that he had lost supremacy in the literary circles of London intellectual life to T. S. Eliot. He was enraged by the discovery among academics that he had mistranslated the poetry of Propertius because of his inadequate knowledge of Latin, leading to his further public narcissistic wounding. In this ambience he applied the ideogramic method in writing Canto IV. On the theme of seduction and slaughter as the result of sexual entanglements, "Its technique is to place before the reader first one and then immediately another image of this, from classical or medieval literature, superimposed or set in montage without any connective tissue" (Carpenter, 1988, p. 347). There are also images from his private memories that one could not possibly understand without knowing a lot about Pound's personal history, producing a nearly incomprehensible poem that seems to be presented using a stream of consciousness technique. Cantos V, VI, and VII appeared increasingly opaque and incomprehensible.

By the age of thirty-five Pound became obsessed with an economic "social credit" theory that was generally regarded by professional economists as a crackpot idea, and he also developed a major acceleration of his anti-Semitism. I would regard this as a paranoid crystallization secondary to the repeated narcissistic woundings he had to endure and to his gradual realization that T. S. Eliot and other poets were becoming famous while he was becoming unknown and obsolete. Even T. S. Eliot was worried about his future, although Pound continued to write poetry and published *Hugh Selwyn Mauberley*, containing some of his most poignant retrospective reflections on the disaster of World War I. Although not as incomprehensible as Cantos V, VI, and VII, this poem is also obscure (Espey, 1974, devoted an entire book to the elucidation of it), but it again presents innovative and important verse technique. One is not surprised to learn that at this point Pound decided to leave London and move to Paris. I believe this was his attempt to contain his narcissistic rage by trying over again to become a celebrity in a different environment.

Heymann (1976) regarded *Hugh Selwyn Mauberley* as "almost certainly the high point of Pound's literary career" (p. 40). It is his most definitive pre-Canto work. Heymann was more charitable toward Pound's preoccupation with crackpot economic theories and usury. He thought it developed because Pound was distressed about the war and disillusioned with "botched" civilization, as well as disappointed with his own role as a poet. He emphasized Pound's conflicts with the publishing industry in the United States and England, "which over the years had catered to commercial interests at the expense of the more creative forces of contemporary arts and letters" (pp. 33-34), and also Pound's concern with finances. Since Pound felt that artists were the antennae of the race, this mistreatment of contemporary artists struck him as a degeneration of the cultural level of our civilization. The Douglas economic theory that Pound embraced sought to restore civilization and make a place for the arts, literature, and the amenities in a system of economics. Heymann continued, "For the poet-turned-economist, this idea became, at length, an obsession. Then came the long downward slope to rabid anti-Semitism, fascism, and paranoia" (p. 35).

Tytell (1987) maintained that "Pound's efforts during the war years on behalf of others were the expression of a private war, an unequal contest between the forces of art clamoring for recognition and the bourgeois community that wanted only security and bread" (p. 131); Pound's name in England stood for "dangerously different." Pound's talk was described as full of strange sounds and cries and he created "the picture of an antagonist for the arts flailing the Philistines and finally reviling them" (p. 131). One of the most remarkable and unfortunate features of such poets as Pound, T. S. Eliot, Yeats, and others was their extreme right-wing conservatism, "a belief in the enlightened firm hand of a noble despot and a rigidly controlled economy. They all shared the fear that democracy would gradually erode all cultural standards" (p. 139). Harrison (1967) studied this in detail. He reviewed the work of the "anti-democratic intelligentsia," as he called it, including Pound, W. B. Yeats, Wyndham Lewis, T. S. Eliot, and D. H. Lawrence, illustrating their longing for stability in society at any political cost and their conviction that culture has been sacrificed to democracy. He pointed out that "Eliot and

Pound, in particular, sometimes claim to write only for a small group, mainly consisting of other poets, because they despair of finding any public of sufficient intelligence to understand them, or with enough discrimination to appreciate their poetry" (p. 204). He also mentioned their tendency to think of the artist as a superman who deserves political power, and he emphasized their search for absolute certainty and transcendence in beauty and mythology or religion.

In that vein, Tytell (1987) wrote that for Pound the core of *The Cantos* would especially be "his beliefs about the ritual value of archaic worship of divine forces" (p. 142), with emphasis on the old gods and divine principles that existed before the Judeo-Christian myth. Pound hoped to use a kaleidoscopic approach, presenting a variety of incidents rather than relying on one central story, and presenting many shifting points of view in order to suggest the flux of reality. The trouble is that the fragmenting effect of each kaleidoscopic shift of action or place or persona runs the risk of losing the reader, and it often does.

Pound struck back fiercely at the mountains of criticisms that were heaped on him by the London literary establishment. Curiously, the more he was criticized, "the more assiduously he seemed to provoke criticism" (Ackroyd, 1987, p. 41). I believe he was unconsciously trying to actualize the sense of alienation he always had about himself, and provoke an ambience that would justify his emerging paranoia, as so often happens in this disorder.

Unfortunately, Pound turned from his energetic encouragement and support of many artists and the arts to the bizarre Douglas social credit theory. It appealed to "Pound's naive and dogmatic populism, which considered the woes of mankind to be the product of some shadowy system conspiring against the individual—a system likely to be manipulated by financiers and Jews" (Ackroyd, 1987, p. 52). This corresponded exactly to Pound's growing paranoia. In 1922 he wrote the *Hell Cantos* (XIV and XV), "a sustained and vicious attack upon English culture" (Ackroyd, 1987, p. 52). Cantos XIV and XV picture important contemporary London citizens (not named but easily identified) as condemned to be mired in excrement. Pound seemed obsessed by defecation and its physiology and, as T. S. Eliot said, Pound's hell consisted of other people. How remarkable that such pathological and scatological material should emerge just after Canto XIII, which contains some of Pound's most beautiful renditions of Confucian thought! Perhaps having recognized, like Confucius, who also considered himself a failure, that he would not be able to reform English culture, Pound shifted from haranguing to reviling the English. But Confucius gradually withdrew into studies in order to avoid further narcissistic wounding, whereas Pound became paranoid and thrashed about in a rage, attributing his wounding to malevolent enemies. Nothing Pound did was now praised and it is not hard to see that he was receiving one narcissistic wound after another and watching himself, often through his own provocation, being relegated to the literary dustbin.

Mullins quoted the picture offered by Iris Barry of Pound in London in 1916: "Pound talks like no one else. His is almost a wholly original accent, the base of American mingled with a dozen assorted 'English society' and Cockney accents inserted in mockery, French, Spanish, and Greek exclamations, strange cries and catcalls, the whole very oddly inflected, with dramatic pauses and diminuendos" (p. 105).

I believe that, seething with narcissistic rage, Pound underwent what Harry Stack Sullivan called a paranoid crystallization around the time he left London, where he had lived for twelve years, for Paris. Sullivan (1953), using the interpersonal channel of psychoanalytic listening (see Chapter 3), speaks of the "paranoid transformation" (p. 347) of the personality:

> At the beginning of this transformation, the only impression one has is of a person in the grip of horror, of uncanny devastation which makes everyone threatening beyond belief. But if the person is not utterly crushed by the process, he can begin rather rapidly to elaborate personifications of evil creatures. . . . as the process goes on, he begins to wash his hands of all those real and fancied unfortunate aspects of his own personality which he has suffered for up to this time . . . the beginning phase of the paranoid state has a curious relationship with what I call moments of "illumination". . . the transfer of blame—in which the person suddenly "sees it all." The beginning of this process comes literally as a sudden insight into some suspicion and it comes with a blaze of horror. (pp. 361-362)

Thus, in psychopathology there can also be an "illumination," often in a sudden moment. The normal human capacity to spontaneously and sometimes in a sudden moment respond to a work of art with a sense of transcendence is here distorted and utilized not to go beyond one's self but to implode one's self into an involuted, private, and isolated delusional world.

Sullivan's (1953) concept of "malevolent transformation" is quite valuable in understanding this development in Pound's personality. It basically represents a miscarriage of the need for tenderness, in which a child discovers that manifesting the need for tenderness toward the potent figures around it leads basically to anxiety rather than relief. Under these circumstances the child learns that it is highly disadvantageous to show any need for tender cooperation from authority, in which case,

> he shows something else; and that something else is the basic malevolent attitude, the attitude that one really lives among enemies—that is about what it amounts to. And on that basis, there comes about remarkable developments which are seen later in life, when the juvenile makes it practically impossible for anyone to feel tenderly for him or to treat him kindly; he beats them to it so to speak, by the display of his attitude. And this is the development of the earlier discovery that the manifestation of any need for tenderness, and so on, would bring anxiety or pain. . . . this distortion, this malevolence, as it is encountered in life, runs something like this: Once upon a time everything was lovely, but that was before I had to deal with people. (pp. 214-216)

As Pound entered middle age, this paranoid transformation of his personality became increasingly apparent and, like many patients with this disorder, the manifestations of it became an obsession with him that destroyed what he had proposed to make his major artistic work, *The Cantos*. I believe that the roots of his paranoid transformation came from his unresolved narcissistic grandiosity, which at first had been fueled by his early successes in London. However, as is so often the case with narcissistic characters, he blazed up, burned out, and was surpassed by more meticulous workers, then becoming more and more desperate to maintain a position of eminence. As his reality testing deteriorated, he proposed more and more grandiose and simplistic schemes for reforming the entire world. We can trace his slipping farther and farther back on the ego axis (see chapter 1).

Pound had very little capacity for psychological introspection in spite of his great artistic sensitivity. Although Barry had a great capacity for introspection, he was unable to transform it into any successful artistic endeavors. He had to be content to channel his energies into mundane scientific expositions. So, like Pound, Barry had two manifestations of his project: On the one hand there was the secret life of artistic creativity which was unrecognized and unappreciated, in contrast to Pound's poetry which at first *was* appreciated, and on the other hand there was the energetic production of scientific papers which did bring him recognition, just as Pound received recognition for his realistic energetic attempts to help other artists and poets.

Barry As He Was

Foucault's tragic and premature death unfortunately cut short the development of new and fertile ideas that force us to rethink our most fundamental premises of discourse and practice in the human sciences. Foucault delineated three kinds of intellectuals. The "universal intellectual" speaks for the conscience of the collectivity. Sartre was the last of this group, said Foucault. The "specific intellectual," a type that emerged since World War II, is an "expert" in a specific field. Foucault said the first of these was Oppenheimer. A third, rare type is the "social thinker," such as Marx and Freud. These, Foucault (1984) explained, are "founders of discursivity" (p. 114) and work only in the human sciences. One returns repeatedly to their texts even if the texts contain errors, and each reexamination of these texts modifies their field of endeavor. These authors have "established an endless possibility of discourse" (p. 114). I believe that Foucault, in spite of his exaggerations and rhetoric, deserves to be a member of this third, rare group of intellectuals.

Barry was much influenced by both Marx and Freud. Marxists believe that the intellectual should generate and catalyse the development of working-class (proletarian) consciousness and lead the praxis of the masses as the proletarian class actualizes its destiny to establish communism (not to be confused with the Soviet tyranny). Those intellectuals who do so from the inside, as members of the proletarian class, are what Gramsci (1985) called "organic intellectuals," and those who lead it from the outside are representatives of Lenin's "vanguard party intellectuals." In sharp contrast stands the traditional bourgeois intellectual, the self-proclaimed detached thinker, or, in Sartre's term, the "classic intellectual."

Foucault's "universal intellectual" is similar to Sartre's "new intellectual." This type of intellectual unites with the masses and stands for humanity and universal values, in contrast to the "classic intellectual," who stands only for the values and interests of the bourgeoisie and not for that of humanity in general. Sartre insisted, however, that all apparently original and individual thought of intellectuals must be understood as situated within the context of historical development.

The "mad" artists and poets, such as Goya, Nietzsche, Van Gogh, Rilke, Artaud, de Sade, and Hölderlin, create outside the discourse of "normal" people and herald a new *epistème*, claimed Foucault (see Chessick, 1992b). The insights of these artists force the world to question itself. Even traditional psychoanalysis cannot comprehend such creativity in ordinary psychodynamic terms, as Freud (1928) said: "Before the problem of the creative artist analysis must, alas, lay down its arms" (p. 177). Hence, the artist has a role as an "intellectual" also, an extremely important function that is often overlooked in our age of technology.

Much influenced by the early writings of Marx and by the genius of Freud in this prepsychopharmacology era of psychiatry, Barry established his career from about the age of twenty-four to thirty-five, the same age range described in this chapter for Ezra Pound. After finishing his training he took advantage of his growing reputation as a teacher to evade military service. At the time he was in training he was deferred from the Korean War under legislation that required him to take an Army Reserve commission and then enter active Army duty immediately after finishing training. However, shortly before he finished his training he wrote a letter of resignation from the Army and at the same time enlisted in the United States Public Health Service, where he was much wanted to take charge of their psychiatric residency training program. Due to an error at the Pentagon his resignation from the Army was accepted, and he was automatically commissioned in the U.S. Public Health Service. The discovery of this error later caused a great deal of difficult interservice debate in the Pentagon, and Barry was warned that if he ever found himself in the Army again he would be treated with great severity. Fortunately for him, that never happened.

He was stationed at the federal prison for drug addicts in Lexington, Kentucky, for two years. His main memory of that place involved the one-star general who was in charge. This officer had an air-conditioned office, although no other facilities at the prison were air-conditioned. He required all the officers of the U.S. Public Health Service on the station to wear full winter uniforms even in the hot Kentucky summer, and even after a previous memo had instructed officers to purchase summer uniforms (which Barry dutifully obeyed, using his own money, as required). When Barry complained, he was told, "That's discipline, Doctor." His other memory of this general involved office space. Barry's first office assignment was a converted bathroom where he could hear toilets flushing from the plumbing of other bathrooms throughout the day. On his first day of duty the general appeared in his office, sat in Barry's chair, and put his feet on Barry's desk to remind Barry who was the boss on this station. About a year later Barry was transferred to an office in the basement that was infested with red ants. The general was no friend of Marx or Freud.

The advantage of this transfer, however, was that Barry could avoid everyday activities in the prison, since he was in an isolated office. This allowed him to study and prepare for board specialization and to read a great deal. During this year he worked his way slowly through James Joyce's *Ulysses* and came to realize what a masterpiece it was. Pound had used good judgment in championing Joyce, and his influence on Joyce was obvious. They both worked with Homer's universal story of Odysseus (Ulysses), which also opens and appears intermittently in Pound's *Cantos*. The study of *Ulysses* was the high point of Barry's military service, probably the only time in his life when he had enough leisure to study in detail a book of this scope and depth.

Returning to Chicago from his military service, Barry applied to take his examination for the American Board of Neurology and Psychiatry. This was scheduled to take place in New York City in December of that year. After careful study in the usual preparatory courses, he packed his suitcase and carried it, along with his little doctor bag containing neurological instruments, to the airport. At the ticket counter where he checked in to get a boarding pass, he was informed that all flights to the East coast were canceled. Barry had prepared rigorously for two years for this examination. He told the airline clerk that he was a brain surgeon who needed to be in New York to do surgery the next day on an emergency basis. The clerk could find only one flight left for the East coast, but it was going to Boston. Barry took the plane and landed in Boston that evening. He then rode the commuter train from Boston to New York, sitting up all night and watching the snow pile up in a terrific snowstorm.

When dawn broke, not Homer's "rosy fingered dawn" over the Mediterranean sea but a gray gloomy curtain of falling snow, some commuters got on the train and, fortunately for Barry, one of them sat next to him and asked him where he was going. When he said he was going to the Columbia University College of Physicians and Surgeons, the commuter advised him not to go all the way into downtown New York but to get off at the station around 155th street. Barry did this, wading into a snowstorm and looking for a taxi, but none were to be seen. Finally one taxi came along, and he piled into it along with several other people going in different directions. The taxi driver took him within walking distance of the hospital, and Barry trudged through the snow, arriving two hours late for the eight-hour examination. When he arrived, he was told that he was too late to take the examination.

Fortunately for Barry, one of the proctors of the examination was a former teacher of his who took pity on Barry after he explained what happened and offered him a chance to take the examination at his own risk. What he would have to do would be to work at a much faster pace and eliminate any rest periods. Barry went up to one of the wards in the hospital and coaxed the nurse to give him ten milligrams of Dexedrine; he then returned and took the examination and successfully passed it. He spent that night on the slow train coming back from New York to Chicago because all the planes were grounded.

Barry began his career by applying to be on the staff of one of the major psychiatric hospitals in the city. In order to do this he had to submit to an interview with the head of the department of psychiatry, who was a famous psychiatrist with a reputation of being very nasty to the junior staff. During this interview Barry smoked a pipe, again using poor social judgment. He had to light the pipe repeatedly because it kept going out while he was talking, and he placed the matches in an ashtray on the desk of the chairman of the department. About halfway into the interview, a fire flared up in the ashtray from all the partly used matches. Barry and the chairman of the department sat and watched the fire. It was another serious humiliation for Barry and marked him permanently with one of the most influential psychiatrists in the city as being of no account and as a person that no one should pay any attention to or take seriously.

He began visiting various doctors to urge them to refer patients to him. Soon he ran into the tremendous prejudice in general medicine and dentistry against psychiatrists. For example, Barry's friendly dentist enthusiastically encouraged him to ask the dentist's brother, a gynecologist, to send Barry patients in need of psychiatric help. A meeting was arranged. When Barry, an innocent young man at this time, entered his office, the first thing the gynecologist said was, "Well, how is the psychiatry racket?" Barry tactfully defended himself and disclaimed any participation as a racketeer, but, of course, he never received a referral from this man.

Barry then began a general hospital psychiatric practice, and one patient made a special impression on him that he could never forget. This unfortunate individual was an elderly musician in the Chicago Symphony Orchestra who had suffered a stroke. As a result of the stroke the fingers on one of his hands were clumsy and had lost the dexterity necessary for the musician to play his instrument. His wife could not accept the fact that he could no longer be a professional musician and had to retire; she subjected him to repeated attempts to build prostheses to support the fingers, prostheses which were painful and unsuccessful. Gradually the old gentleman sank into a greater and greater depression, which was why Barry was called upon to help treat him. He had to be placed in the hospital, and his wife was extremely angry at Barry because she saw no reason for this depression and attributed it to chemical causes. In those days there were very few medications for depression and Barry attempted to do psychotherapy, but it did not succeed because the gentleman's problem was an interactive one with his wife. It was only when Barry confronted the wife about her denial of what had happened that any progress was made in the treatment; as the old gentleman was relieved of his prostheses his depression improved, but his wife removed him from the hospital as soon as possible and dismissed Barry as the therapist. Barry was gradually learning about the phenomenology of both the performing arts and of marital relations in their pathological aspects.

Because of his reputation as a good teacher, Barry was able to obtain a teaching position at one of the major universities in the area. He did very well as a teacher, but he soon ran into difficulties with the individual who was listed as the codirector of the psychiatric residency training program. This individual was one of the most powerful individuals in American psychiatry, and he was thoroughly corrupt. At the time when Barry collided with him, he was forcing the residents to enter psychoanalysis with him and exploiting them by assigning them to various places where they could work for him at the same time. When Barry complained about this he made a permanent evil enemy of a very powerful individual, who, for the rest of his life, disparaged Barry to everyone he met. He seriously damaged Barry's reputation, because for many years it was not recognized that he was a corrupt and degenerate individual. Later he was successfully sued by a group of women whom he had assaulted in his office after injecting them with hypnotic drugs, and he was forced to retire from practice. But that was too late to help Barry.

During this period of extreme stress in dealing with such a dangerous enemy, Barry was raising a family with no apparent difficulties. It was at this time, however, that he showed the first evidences of fragmentation, because he got involved sexually with a colleague who subsequently moved away from the state in order to be free of him. This involvement was largely one of pregenital play and was not consummated by sexual intercourse, and it related mostly to Barry's intense and increasing need for pleasurable stimulation as a soothing vehicle for the discomfort and stress he was enduring. Not long afterward, he discovered that his blood pressure was elevated and his cholesterol was too high.

By the time he was thirty-five, Barry began his lifelong battle with cardiac risk factors. He attempted to bring down his blood pressure using a low-salt diet and attempted to reduce his cholesterol by introducing a low-cholesterol, low-fat diet. These techniques enabled him to bring down the readings to a borderline range, one which these days would be considered too high by present standards. He also began an exercise program, but it was not a cardiac exercise program, only light exercise without attention to raising the pulse rate to a properly prolonged level. At this point his life was fairly stultified into a routine full-time practice. His main tool of treatment was psychotherapy, since psychopharmacology had not yet crowded out everything else in psychiatry, as it has today. That is where his career remained until his death.

Like Pound, Barry continued in two directions at once. In his public direction he was teaching, practicing, and publishing papers in psychiatry. These publications consisted mainly of introducing the work of others and presenting their work in the best possible and understandable form to audiences and students, enhancing Barry's reputation as a teacher. But in his private persona Barry was endeavoring to think and create in a literary fashion. Lacking Pound's good fortune and genius, he never published any of this, and his artistic endeavors were contained mainly in his unpublished written notebooks and copies of his correspondence, all given to me after he died by his ex-wife, who was glad to be rid of the clutter.

His private creative thinking and writing was more philosophical and less imagistic than that of Pound; he was unapologetically more of a left-brain person. For example, he cited Thurber's saying, "All men should strive to know before they die, what they are running from, and to, and why" as the basic model of his intellectual life. There was a strong bent in private toward the pursuit of knowledge for its own sake, and again he was aware of the division of energies in his life. On the one hand he enjoyed doing good for other human beings, which was object-related, clinical, and very valuable but, as he wrote, "less satisfactory to intellectual thirst and hard to do in an age so materialistic and with so little regard for the suffering of others." On the other hand he felt that the pursuit of knowledge and removal of false beliefs, although it was more egocentric, was perhaps more suited, as Aristotle said, to the nature and function of humans.

As quotations from his notebooks and correspondence show, Barry had considerable insight into his dilemma during the period of his life covered in this chapter:

> At this time I seem to be very paradoxical. It is the emotional zenith of my life, with all one could ask for materially, wife, children. They are marvelous. Yet intellectually I am at the very low point. Perhaps the conclusion should be that if one does not develop animal faith as Santayana called it during the first years of life as a consequence of a successful mother-child symbiosis, then one is doomed to an empty wandering at least in some sense, for the rest of one's life.

This could have been written as well as by Pound, "the nomad," as by Barry! Barry continued,

> There is always the period of feeling it is not enough, a certain core that cries out for a special identity, for a central theme. Is this central theme or core, this need for meaningful structure to my intellectual existence nothing but a stifled cry to be back with my mother? If it is, then my whole life is a farce and a failure.

Ezra Pound in his final years probably asked the same question about his whole life. But Barry went on,

> What if there is something more to what I am looking for? Schopenhauer's pessimism points to art and aesthetics. He retreats to mysticism, a loaded word. There is something to aesthetics, both the endeavor and the contemplation that is separate and different from the joy of material things and of object relations. Is this simply communion with mother? It doesn't matter if it is looking at or painting a picture, memorizing a language, music, or mathematics. It must be done *for its own sake;* that is the one requirement. Here is my central theme. Leisure is the basis of culture (author's note: Barry must have been reading Pieper, 1952). Leisure, the basis of making life meaningful through creative activity.

Very difficult. Without it life degenerates into the animal and one is totally at the mercy of the everyday ups and downs, of the cruel blows dealt us all the time by pitiless unfeeling nature. I must put some leisure time away for contemplation and creation, or I am really lost. I must go my own lonely way to grapple in the dark with what may well turn out to be nothing but the wish to restore a phantom of the past.

Paradoxically, one of the most striking aspects of Barry's life was that it offered him little leisure. Much time was spent trying to keep his weight down, his blood pressure down, and his cholesterol down in a constant battle with these coronary artery disease risk factors. He was overworked, with two full-time jobs that raised his tension to an almost unbearable level. He was very aware of his emptiness, his chronic narcissistic rage, and of a deep early fear of being penetrated and destroyed in his relationship with his mother (see Chessick, 1993b, 1996d). He could never balance his needs for soothing, for material success and the support of a family, and for leisure for his artistic endeavors; there was a continual tension among these factors until the end of his life. He felt his situation was unnatural, ahistorical, acultural, and irrational. He was tormented by the thought that he was betraying himself and his best judgments and impulses.

Although he enjoyed the practice of psychotherapy, he was always frustrated by the weakness of the method and the inadequacies of it to deal with the serious psychopathology that he was constantly combating in his office. Many patients needed to be seen several times weekly but could not afford it, a problem that has since become a very serious calamity in our current era of "mismanaged" care. He wrote, "Others have reached crises in their lives and the capable have consolidated their identities and come out the better. I am afraid I will just drift on the road of least resistance . . . pursuit of truth for its own sake: Are there hierarchies of truth? Some more worth pursuing?" He experienced considerable anxiety and insomnia at times, and he began to feel that he was increasingly crippled by his neurosis.

With the advent of psychopharmacology, Barry began to sense the ominous shift that was threatening to materialize and distort the whole practice of psychiatry. Here is a fragmentary draft of one of his undelivered, unpublished lectures, somewhat in the style of Pound's frustrated flailing at the Philistines:

> Ladies and gentlemen: I believe work in biochemistry and physiology in psychiatry is done mainly due to pressure from other medical disciplines that we should be a "science," and by people who are either unaware of the deep and explosive powers of human fantasy or who by reasons of personality are unable to relentlessly pursue an understanding of such powers. Such basic science research is carried out by people who have never sat down more than five minutes to listen to a patient, and by the castoffs who have never been able to grasp what psychiatry is all about and who want to prove it is all chemistry anyway.
>
> If we want to help psychiatric patients we must quit being "scientists" and learn to be men of leisure. This brings me to De Grazia's book: Here is the proper attitude to enable one to tune in to the fantasy life; to be able to free associate one must be at leisure, one must be on "slow time."
>
> Mental illness precipitates out of pathological interpersonal relations imposed on a constitutional and genetic makeup. To understand human process is essential to treat mental illness. Drug treatment is purely symptomatic . . .

Barry went on to outline the work of De Grazia (1962) in his notebook, and he became increasingly concerned, as was De Grazia, about the pressures in our culture against the achievement of free time and leisure, such as the lack of a tradition of leisure, the vast wasteland of television, and the heavy emphasis on shopping and lunching and networking. De Grazia wrote, "Design on the world fractionizes your view. Not only that, it unsettles the mind. The crowding of desires, one upon the other, can shake a man's head until it rattles" (p. 420).

Like Pound at this time of his life, Barry felt an increasing sense of being a "loner." This was even pointed out by Barry's wife, who was beginning to be dissatisfied with his preoccupation and scribbling in notebooks. He developed a certain suspiciousness of people, anxiously expecting hassle and trouble from them, but not nearly to the extent manifested by Pound. When patients raged at him he became anxious due to memories of his raging mother. Yet he did good basic psychiatric work, and his reality testing remained intact. As he slipped slightly backwards on the ego axis, his laboring ego began to smoke and sputter in the form of free-floating anxiety and a mild dysthymia.

While his notebooks filled with incidents of disappointment and humiliation, he began writing a series of essays on his contemporary culture. None of these was ever finished. He noted that writing a creative description of some incident that took place would have a self-soothing function for him, somehow enabling him to stand away from the pain of the incident and master the trauma involved. It then became his habit to write either letters to friends or notebook entries or both describing these incidents, so that his correspondence and notebooks increasingly became quite clearly a selfobject for him, almost an imaginary companion. There was a "twinship narcissism" at the root of this behavior, as described in Chapter 7. In his loneliness, especially since his wife was so preoccupied with raising their children, he needed something to restore his narcissistic equilibrium.

His aims at the age of thirty-five were listed as the wish to discover his own nature and place in nature, to achieve in the arts, and to make his good intentions effective in the world: "Now we will see who I am and what I believe." Barry never achieved these aims and his written entries went tediously over the same ground again and again over the years and never developed any closure or sense of resolution. In that sense the volumes of his notebooks and correspondence resemble Pound's *Cantos,* an endless epic leading nowhere. Barry gradually realized that he was at a dead end, a realization that came to Pound only much later in life.

As he entered middle age, Barry wrote,

> Chronic depression is the price one pays for loyalty and faithfulness to one's wife and children. As Somerset Maugham pointed out, loving kindness often does not bring happiness although it is an affirmation of our will and independence. To escape from the idea of death and the death of God is why there is all this family breakup in middle age.

Barry began turning more and more to the enjoyment of the ballet, music, the visual arts, and literature, which he also found to be an escape from his chronic depression and anger. He tried to strike a balance between work and aesthetic activities, even though it meant a reduced income. At the same time he thought of reading and writing as a way to move away from "science" and toward understanding people, but he never found a unifying theme to his work. He also maintained an interest in pure mathematics, metaphysics, languages, and chess—abstract intellectual exercises that he thought represented an escape from the world of material reality, just as that offered by the arts. At this point he was anti-Hegelian, but he admitted that life at rock-bottom is a mystery and a tragedy: "Only through loving kindness can we alleviate it a bit." He believed that art, which is able to take us outside of ourselves temporarily, is "beautiful," but that there are no other eternal criteria for beauty; the sense of the beautiful varies from era to era. Nevertheless, he thought art was extremely important for human living.

Like Pound, he became interested in Chinese thinking, especially *The Analects of Confucius* (1997), which he read in translation. Both Pound and Barry intuitively recognized that like themselves, Confucius was also a witness to the collapse of civilization in his time. Barry wrote,

> The tranquility, objectivity, and direct honesty of Confucius's epigrammatic style affects the mood of the therapist. It enables him to maintain balance and perspective in the face of the chaos of the patient's defenses, and to penetrate in an empathic way to a feeling identification with the patient. It is not so much the individual wisdom of any saying, but the life style of Confucius as reflected in *The Analects* that influences the psychic field of the therapist. It enhances his tranquil capacity not to be thrown by confrontation with the patient's passions, which, if psychotherapy is to be successful, must happen; his optimism in the outcome is due to his good faith and good faith in the basic virtue of the patient, which given a chance in the proper atmosphere, will express itself.

At the age of thirty-five Barry wrote,

> How still it is at midnight! I am a scholar in exile, unaccepted by anybody, anywhere, alone, going in an opposite direction from psychiatry. I'm finally beginning to find myself while

looking frankly with horror at my mother. I should have done this at age 18 but now it is too late. Now I can only go through the motions and become increasingly uncomfortable around people. They nauseate me. Sartre said hell is other people. I try to make a living and do a decent job of work and to be a good husband and father, and I am all right at all this. But I am also searching and searching for a center that I cannot find. In the television series entitled "Civilization" I thought I spotted it; it's almost a fantasy life about being civilized that clashes with the money-making mentality in our culture. "Civilization," the TV series, was another cipher, as Jaspers would call it, toward transcendence.

Even an atheistic human must either strive toward some idealistic goal or live in a totally hedonistic and materialistic way as most people do. There is no way to say what is best, and perhaps nobody chooses their way. Every way represents an ego solution, and then we die, and soon we are forgotten. It really is a dismal abyss! Nietzsche said that if one looks upon monsters, one must take care that one does not become one, oneself. He warned us that if you gaze down into the abyss, the abyss may enter into you. This is from *Beyond Good and Evil* (author's note: see Nietzsche, 1886).

Ezra Pound could have easily written something like this quotation, if he would have been capable of introspection. Alas, he was not, until it was too late.

11 OUR CIVILIZATION

Leisure and idleness. — There is something of the American Indians, something of the ferocity peculiar to the Indian blood, in the American lust for gold; and the breathless haste with which they work—the distinctive vice of the new world—is already beginning to infect old Europe with its ferocity and is spreading a lack of spirituality like a blanket. Even now one is ashamed of resting, and prolonged reflection almost gives people a bad conscience. One thinks with a watch in one's hand, even as one eats one's midday meal while reading the latest news of the stock market; one lives as if one always "might miss out on something," "Rather do anything than nothing": this principle, too, is merely a string to throttle all culture and good taste.

— *Nietzsche,* The Gay Science

The great literary artist Leo Tolstoy (1947) centered one of his major novels on the problem of evil. Humans, who are evil, try to correct evil but by their nature they cannot. What then, is the solution? We know that fish are more aggressive among themselves than most species of animals. Humans are more like fish. Aggression is basically species- or life-preserving, and among most animals inhibitors are built in, such as submission rituals and an instinctual prohibition against killing one's own species. Humans did not need this in evolution because they are not so physically powerful as many predators, but suddenly, with the explosion in technology, as any Hollywood movie today nauseatingly and vulgarly demonstrates, they can kill multitudes of their fellow humans very quickly. There are no submission gestures built in humans by evolution to provide inhibition against intraspecies aggression (Lorenz, 1966).

The famous ethologist Konrad Lorenz (1987) mourned the imminent destruction of the environment and perhaps the ex-

171

tinction of the human species. He described the decline of all the attributes that uniquely constitute humanity. He complained about our reckless pursuit of power and our neurotic and insatiable greed, as manifested in the development of our technocratic system. Kohut (1978) depicted the tragedy of humans suffocating in an increasingly inhuman environment that humans themselves continue to create. Sartre (1963) maintained it is need and scarcity that impel our inhumanity to each other. As mentioned in previous chapters, Sartre defined the practico-inert as the material environment and everything else in our finitude, including our human bureaucratic structures and social arrangements. There is a constant tension between the human as a product of the means of production and the socioeconomic structures built on the means of production. The practico-inert works against the human who is a historical agent trying to actualize his or her basic project.

Academic philosophy has been of little help on these problems. Jacoby (1987) pointed out that the last generation of intellectuals wrote for educated readers but they have been replaced now by the "high tech" narrowly specialized intellectual in academia. The nonacademic or "public" intellectual who is widely read and politically concerned has become an endangered species. Similarly, positivism as an intellectual philosophy, said McCarthy (1982), conceals a commitment to technological ("high tech") rationality devoid of concern for humans behind the facade of value freedom, and it cannot justify itself.

A jaundiced attitude toward traditional intellectuals is maintained by historians to the present day. Pipes (1990) described the Russian intelligentsia as simply intellectuals who wanted power. The concept of an intelligentsia began with the Enlightenment. Before that, human nature or "essence" was thought to be unchangeable. It was the Enlightenment thinker Helvetius who introduced the idea that humans can be made over through politics. The sciences of human affairs, attempting to use "reason" to construct humans and society, replaced spontaneity by "consciousness" and socialism. The Enlightenment was the era when the notion of the intellectual became important, a notion that began in the sixteenth century with the rise of science; by the seventeenth century it was definitely believed that human nature could be changed through science. For example, the physician and philosopher Locke maintained that there were no innate ideas. Pipes was very hostile to intellectuals who, he said, claimed to know "things in general," and he insisted that the ideology of the Russian intelligentsia was materialism, utilitarianism, and positivism, all of which are in disrepute today.

Cheerful rationalists still exist. For example, Durant and Durant (1968) offered an optimistic paean to progress. They maintained, after publishing many popular volumes of history, that revolutions produce chaos and that the only true revolution is the enlightenment of the mind and the improvement of character. They referred to the term πλεονεξία *(pleonexia)*, a classical Greek concept indicating the appetite for more and more of everything, the character and conduct of a πλεονέκτης, one who arrogantly claims more than his or her due. They believed civilizations decline because their leaders fail to meet the challenges of change, but I think this is a very superficial explanation. The recent history of Western philosophy consists of the breakdown of the crucial Enlightenment assumptions of the Age of Reason (Jones, 1969), founded on a belief in the existence of a rational order of eternal truths, truths that humans could discover, understand, and could act upon. In our era the quest for certainty is even considered by some as a manifestation of neurosis, or at least of philosophical naiveté.

The Great War

World War I was the pivotal event leading to a changing consciousness in the modern age. This can only be understood when one studies the documents and photographs of what the years of stalemated trench warfare were like at that time on the Western front (and on ancillary fronts, such as in the ill-fated British attack on the Dardanelles), and what this war did to an entire generation (Eksteins, 1989). One of my (Chessick, 1996a) most influential teachers, the pioneer psychoanalyst Franz Alexander, produced a curiously neglected book (Alexander, 1960) describing what his life was like before World War I and then between the two world wars in his European formative years. He

(Alexander, 1951) concluded that human relations are dominated by irrational forces and humans are losing faith that their lot can be improved through technical advances alone. The natural sciences have become a curse rather than a blessing in the hands of men and women ignorant of interpersonal relations, and he hoped that the solution would be a more scientific enlightenment about humans, a hope that was shared by Freud (1930a).

Alexander called attention to the coexistence of regressive and progressive forces in human life, vividly demonstrated here in the stories of Ezra Pound and Barry as these forces shifted them back and forth on the ego axis. An adult neurosis consists of a conflict between mature attitudes and regressive tendencies aroused by frustration or narcissistic wounding. The neurotic tries to uphold adult ambitions for a sexually and socially productive existence, but at the same time he or she is drawn by the magic attraction of the past, when gratification was experienced under the protection and care of the parents. These parents remain as ghosts or "introjects," and individuals with psychopathology such as Ezra Pound and Barry may spend and ruin their entire lives either serving or rebelling against these ghosts. I have seen this in my clinical work over and over again; the purpose of it is to cling to the fantasy that one still has one's parents with (within) them as bad as the parents might be, so that one is not alone like a small child lost in a busy department store.

A great many thinkers were deeply affected by the Great War and subsequently by World War II (which was simply a continuance of the Great War). For example, Husserl attempted to defend reason against the irrationality of Europe, so manifest in these devastating self-destructive wars. Natansan (1973) explained how Husserl searched for a universal certain foundation that would be prior even to the objective sciences. Husserl (1913, 1970) felt that focus on what he called the life world was a way to establish this, using his phenomenologic method, as described in Chapter 1. Unfortunately, Husserl was a very obscure, unclear writer, often changing his concepts obsessively, and locked in a dangerously solipsistic approach from which he was unable to wriggle out. So his quest failed, although it influenced many important thinkers after him.

World War I was when the age of θάνατος *(thanatos,* death) began, wrote the philosopher-novelist Percy (1987). He asked, "Why does it take two years of prison for a man to be able to sit still, listen, notice his kids, watch the sunlight on the ceiling?" (p. 43). Another way to phrase this complaint is to call attention to the stifling of the spirit in our era. Taylor (1989) insisted that there is an absolute necessity for moral ideas to be embedded in cultural practices and religious faith, and that this need is not an illusion. I believe his complaint embodies the recognition that humans are not rational animals, in spite of Plato's moral theory assuming they are. To whatever extent we abandon the notion that through science and reason alone human life and human civilization can be perfected, we will return, as in the golden years of ancient China and classical Greek culture, to respecting the role of myths, art, religion, and philosophy for being crucial in lifting human spirits, reinstilling a sense of transcendence, and reorienting the goals of everyday life. This is the centerpiece of Ezra Pound's poetry. Barry's recognition of this, as he gained psychiatric and medical experience of the misery and suffering of humanity in spite of the technological miracles of our age, gradually moved him to a quasi-Hegelian view in which art, religion, and philosophy were the highest and irresistible manifestations of Truth and Beauty.

If this sounds far-fetched to the modern reader, imagine the difficulty Barry would have had in trying to present this idea to the twentieth-century scientific community—it was an unpublishable idea. But Barry was a teacher; one should not forget Russell's (1969) description of teachers as "more than any other class, the guardians of civilization. They should be intimately aware of what civilization is, and desirous of imparting a civilized attitude to their pupils" (p. 117). For Russell, "Civilization, in the more important sense, is a thing of the mind, not of material adjuncts to the physical side of living. It is a matter partly of knowledge, partly of emotion" (p. 117). Russell (1969) described the details of this view in his "unpopular essay" on the functions of a teacher:

> So far as knowledge is concerned, a man should be aware of
> the minuteness of himself and his immediate environment

in relation to the world in time and space. He should see his own country not *only* as home, but as one among the countries of the world, all with an equal right to live and think and feel. He should see his own age in relation to the past and the future, and be aware that its own controversies will seem as strange to future ages as those of the past seem to us now. . . . On the side of the emotions, a very similar enlargement from the purely personal is needed if a man is to be truly civilized. . . . The civilized man, where he cannot admire, will aim rather at understanding than at reprobating. He will seek rather to discover and remove the impersonal causes of evil than to hate the men who are in its grip. All this should be in the mind and heart of the teacher, and if it is in his mind and heart he will convey it in his teaching to the young who are in his care. (pp. 117-188)

There is no doubt that the production of a civilization, as Clark (1969) suggested, requires confidence in society and human mental powers, energy and will, a sense of permanence, a margin of wealth, humaneness, and a balance of sorts between established religions and aggressive nomads like Ezra Pound.

Corruption

Both cultures and individuals have to continually oppose a tendency to become corrupt, a tendency to fall away from their youthful ideals as time passes, under the vicissitudes of life. Corruption does not happen to everybody, but due to the inevitable pressures of life there is a continued force that must be resisted throughout life; those with a strong sense of self are able to maintain their ideals into old age, while those with narcissistic pathology like Ezra Pound and Barry are least able to do so. Erikson (1959) described everyone's life as ending either in integrity or in despair and disgust.

I will discuss corruption in terms from two or three of the channels or theoretical standpoints I use, based on the writing of Freud and Kohut (as described in Chapter 3) that some have rejected. The ego ideal is usually defined as a set of functions within the structure of the superego. It contains representations of the image of an admired, idealized object, of the self I ought or want to be, and of actions "that either ought to be done or ought to be avoided" (Moore and Fine, 1990, p. 640). Although there is disagreement on the details, it seems clear that out of the experiences and identifications early in life each of us sets up an internal notion of the kind of person we wish to be and how we wish others to be affected by us.

Technically speaking, what I am describing here has not been much discussed in the literature before. In Freud's metapsychology, which I still consider to be a valuable "heuristic viewpoint" (Fölsing, 1997, p. 136), it represents the vicissitudes of the progressive withdrawal of narcissistic libido from cathexis of the ego ideal and back to a cathexis of the ego itself, analogous to Freud's (1914b) concept of secondary narcissism, in which narcissistic libido is withdrawn from objects and returned to the ego. The cause of this withdrawal, as in the situation of Freud's secondary narcissism, is progressive narcissistic wounding arising from many inevitable disappointments encountered in the vicissitudes of life and its goal is the attempt to prevent further pain. So the ego ideal tends to shrivel up under the impact of reality, which punishes all but the most talented or lucky individuals for their attempts to live up to it, because each failure constitutes narcissistic wounding and results in a withdrawal of libidinal investment of the ego ideal and reinvestment in the ego, which is both restitutive and a safer situation. In the extreme case of libidinal investment in the ego we observe psychotic grandiosity, as in Napoleonic or Hitlerian psychopathology.

A similar phenomenon accounts for the decline of "Cultures" into "Civilizations" and then into chaos and barbarism, as described by Spengler (1926, 1928, 1962). In a distinction usually not made today and which can be confusing, Spengler differentiated "Culture" from "Civilization" as one might differentiate the seasons of spring and summer from autumn and early winter. For any social organization, he said, there is a springlike phase of vigor and development, a blossoming from the energies and ideals of the founders of the organization, which is then followed in time by a rigidification, bureaucratization, and decay, and a falling away from the ideals of the society until the final collapse. The early phase Spengler called "Culture" and the later phase he called "Civilization," in a pessimistic theory that condemned all social organizations sooner or later either to inevitable stagnation or collapse. The most dramatic example of this in our time is in the history of Russia (Pipes, 1990) from the time of a revolution characterized by the highest hopes and ideals about the intrinsic social nature of humans, which then evolved through Stalinism, corruption, and decadent bureaucracy, until the final implosion of the entire system, which happened so suddenly it surprised everybody. Philosophers and psychiatrists were and still occasionally are deeply influenced by Spengler's theory; even Heidegger's most fundamental concept of "being-towards-death," which led to Sartre's existentialism, was taken from Spengler.

The ego ideal of a culture is set by founders such as Confucius, the early Greeks, the American colonists, or even Marx, Engels, and Lenin. Spengler, who was not aware of the profound significance of narcissistic wounding although he had a number of his own narcissistic difficulties, attributed the decline of cultures to an inherent botanical organicity, borrowing from the romantic philosophy of Goethe.

The educator Robert Hutchins, who was not psychoanalytically oriented, described the corruption of the individual in moralistic and Aristotelian terminology. He worked with an unusual type of college student (see Chapter 5) those attracted by the "Hutchins Plan" at the University of Chicago that reflected Hutchins's high idealism. To these young students in the springtime of their lives and much influenced by Hutchins (who was in turn influenced by the Aristotelian philosopher Adler), the disinterested pursuit of truth was the highest ideal, one not far from Freud's claim that psychoanalysis requires of both the patient and the analyst devotion to such a pursuit regardless of the pain or consequences involved. But individuals and cultures share the common problem that when the ego ideal is divested of its narcissistic libido there is consequently less and less motivation to live up to it, since there is less and less gratification when an identification with the ego ideal has been achieved.

Spengler

Spengler, the charismatic German thinker, developed the Italian philosopher Vico's (1744) original notion of the inevitable decline of societies. His writings, appearing just after Germany lost World War I, became immensely popular. Claiming that "man is a beast of prey, I shall say it again and again" (Spengler, 1962, p. x), he died in 1936 after first colliding with and then reconciling with the Nazi ideology in Germany. Spengler (1962) considered the "megapolis" as the worst feature of what he called "Civilization," a decadent phase of each "Culture." He forecast larger and larger cities, which he conceived of as being laid out for 20 million inhabitants, and covering vast areas of the countryside. Cairo, Tokyo, Los Angeles, Mexico City, and Bangkok are good approximations of this prediction today. He offered many examples of the development of megapolises in history, and concluded that the end of all these cities is inevitably the same. After the city, beginning as a primitive barter center, develops to its zenith as a Culture city (which for Spengler is the ideal city), a line of inevitable corruption begins. Gradually it balloons into a world city or megapolis, which then undergoes an inevitable decline and ends with a handful of nomads camping in the ruins.

Spengler prophesied that (White male) Western Europe would lose its world hegemony and that Western Culture, like all other cultures, would decline. The trend toward separatist ethnic groups and sprawling megapolises that he predicted to occur as a Culture becomes a Civilization is already apparent in the United States. For Spengler, each Culture has its own new possibilities of self-expression which arise, ripen, decay, and never return. These Cultures grow with the same superb aimlessness as the flowers of the field, a romantic concept that Spengler borrowed from Goethe, who, in his holistic or organic ideal of "nature," described plants and animals developing in the same fashion.

As Spengler (1962) put it, the problem of the "Decline of the West" is the problem of Civilization. There is an organic succession in which Civilization is the inevitable destiny of each Culture: "Civilizations are the most external and artificial states of which a species of developed humanity is capable" (p. 24). As

an example of the change from Culture to Civilization he chose
the shift from the Greeks to the Romans: "The Romans were barbarians who did not *precede* but *closed* a great development" (p.
24). Spengler continued, "Unspiritual, unphilosophical, devoid
of art, clannish to the point of brutality, aiming relentlessly at tangible successes, they stand between the Hellenic Culture and
nothingness" (p. 24). He attempted to demonstrate an inevitable
line of development in human groups culminating in Civilization, in which "appears this type of strong-minded, completely
non-metaphysical man" (p. 25). This kind of individual represents "Civilization," a late phase of the decline of every Culture,
and it should be kept in mind these are the persons who formed
the surround of Ezra Pound and Barry.

Spengler wrote chiefly about what he called the Greco-
Roman or "Apollinian" Culture and the Western or "Faustian"
Culture; more briefly he discussed the Culture of the Mediterranean, which he called "Magian." The Apollinian Culture is that
of the Greek city-states and static geometry; the Faustian Culture
is characterized by our era of expansion into limitless space, the
art of the fugue, dynamics, and introspection; the Magian Culture is reflected in algebra, astrology, and alchemy. The Magian
Culture combines Judaism, Byzantium, and Islam, whose propo-
nents, he said, dwell in a magic world of mysterious presences.
Contemporary problems in trying to deal rationally with fundamentalism in the Middle East can be traced to this mindset. In art
the dome symbolizes the Magian, the free-standing temple or
nude statue symbolizes the Apollinian, and the soaring vaults and
spires of the Gothic cathedral symbolize our Faustian Culture, a
culture characterized by exploration and exploitation. Spengler
insisted that the art forms of the West are now over, and our
Western or Faustian culture is now in the Civilization phase.

More generally, Spengler (1962) maintained that "the energy of culture-man is directed inwards, that of civilization-man
outwards" (p. 28), so there is an expansive tendency, "a doom,
something daemonic and immense, which grips, forces into service, and uses up the late mankind of the world-city stage, willy-
nilly, aware or unaware" (p. 28). There has been a line of
development in the Western world which leaves us as a "civilized,"
not a Gothic or Rococo people: "We have to reckon with the hard

cold facts of a *late* life, to which the parallel is to be found not in Pericles' Athens but in Caesar's Rome" (p. 31).

Spengler claimed that the transition from Culture to Civilization occurred in the Western world in the nineteenth century, just as it occurred for the classical Greek world in the fourth century. When this happens, "In place of a type-true people, born of and grown on the soil, there is a new sort of nomad, cohering unstably in fluid masses, the parasitical city dweller, traditionless, utterly matter-of-fact, religionless, clever, unfruitful, deeply contemptuous of the countryman. . . . The world-city means cosmopolitanism in place of 'home.' . . . To the world-city belongs not a folk but a mob" (p. 25).

Heidegger (1962) later took up this concept of "home" when he drew the distinction between the planet on which we dwell as an ancient landscape and background providing a context for authentic everyday life, and as the site of an inauthentic existence marked by "turbulence" and exerting a whirlpool effect, pulling individuals in the world city into a frenzy of what one of my affluent Chicago North Shore patients called "shopping and lunching" (and, I would add, compulsively "networking," even on the golf course or during intermissions at a play or concert). For Heidegger, the big city embodies the basic feature of our epoch, homelessness (Petzet, 1993). As Spengler (1962) put it, in the megapolis there is "the reappearance of *panem et circenses* in the form of wage-disputes and sports stadia—all these things betoken the definite closing down of the Culture and the opening of a quite new phase of human existence" (p. 26). The hallmark of Civilization today, Spengler insisted, in contrast to the Culture of yesterday, is the way in which rhetoric and journalism serve money, which represents the power of Civilization. "It is the money-spirit which penetrates unremarked the historical forms of the people's existence" (pp. 26-27) in a Civilization.

In this shift from Culture to Civilization, said Spengler (1926), cosmopolitanism replaces home, cold matters of fact replace reverence for tradition and age, scientific irreligion replaces the old religion of the heart, society replaces the state, and natural rights replace hard-earned rights. In short, "any high ideal of life becomes largely a question of money" (p. 33). Johnson (1991) published an extremely detailed description of the period from 1815 to 1830 in which the so-called modern age began, an age of technology that Spengler would define as the Civilization phase of Western culture. Spengler concluded his first volume by predicting that a spiritual crisis will involve Europe and America, a prediction that certainly has come true.

Spengler noted that some Civilizations do not disappear; certain ones like India and China, he thought, may last indefinitely in their decadent form. Spengler also conceded that cultures can perish through external assault rather than through the inherent corruption process he described, as when the Spaniards invaded the Western hemisphere and destroyed the Old Mexican world. Or, in his concept of "pseudomorphosis," a culture too close to a stronger culture can perish by what he called "spiritual damage." For example, Russian Culture was deformed by the intrusions of West European Faustian Culture, first in Peter the Great's reforms and again in the Bolshevik revolution. Whereas Russian Culture is what Spengler called a "flat plane culture," characterized by low-lying buildings and calls for nondiscriminating brotherhood, as in the novels of Dostoevsky, the ancient Egyptian Culture is a one-dimensional world, its architecture predominantly a corridor enclosed in masonry, and moving down a narrow and inexorably prescribed life path.

Spengler depicted a similar line of corruption in the development of philosophy, correctly forecasting the current trend away from Platonic idealism and toward Rorty's (1979, 1982) pragmatics, neo-Marxist criticism, and hermeneutics (Chessick, 1992b). Like Hegel (1821), Spengler (1926) insisted that each philosophy expresses only its own time. He explained that Kant's "necessary forms of thought" are only forms of Western thought. Spengler, not Heidegger, introduced the importance of longing and dread, a "trickling-away" (p. 78) that we feel in the present as our dread of mortality; death as a frontier, inexorable and irreversible. Spengler contended that this *"enigma of time"* (p. 79) runs through all creativity and philosophy, a theme later made famous without attribution by Heidegger (1962). Spengler (1962) concluded that we cannot help it "if we are born as men of the early winter of a full Civilization, instead of on the golden summit of a ripe Culture, in a Phidias or a Mozart time. Everything depends on our seeing our own position, our *destiny*, clearly, on our realizing that though we may lie to ourselves about it, we cannot evade it" (p. 34). Both Ezra Pound and Barry were trapped in this reality.

Hutchins

Hutchins (1968) struggled with a similar and perhaps more familiar line, that of decline and corruption of the individual. This was a reflection of his own life-long internal struggle; he considered himself to be a failure at the end of his career (Ashmore, 1989). In a lecture to college graduates from the University of Chicago, he claimed that the least corrupted individual was the college student. He worried endlessly about what would happen to the graduates of colleges as they went out in the so-called "real world" characterized in our era, as Spengler said, by the money spirit. Hutchins (1935) explained,

> I am not worried about your economic future. I am worried about your morals. My experience and observation lead me to warn you that the greatest, the most insidious, the most paralyzing danger you will face is the danger of corruption. Time will corrupt you. Your friends, your wives or husbands, your business or professional associates will corrupt you; your social, political, and financial ambitions will corrupt you. The worst thing about life is that it is demoralizing. (p. 1)

Hutchins concluded with an exhortation to the graduates of the university not to let "practical" people tell them they should surrender their ideals because they are impractical. He begged them, "Do not be reconciled to dishonesty, indecency, and brutality because gentlemanly ways have been discovered of being dishonest, indecent, and brutal" (p. 4), and he urged them to take a stand now when they are graduating, before time corrupts them. In his moving and rarely quoted speech, Hutchins warned of the dangerous decline of one's idealism from its peak in one's traditionally idealistic college days, which parallels the decline of the Culture phase of a society, to the Civilization phase, a decline characterized by the bored, retired valetudinarian who spends his or her life infected by the money spirit in the broker's office.

Hutchins's claim that college students are not corrupt may seem strange to those who work with contemporary college students. Allan Bloom (1987) pointed out how American college students today enter college barely able to read and write, are utterly bewildered by the ideas in the "great books," and are further confused by arguments among academics about "political correctness." They may end up disappointed and demoralized, with a sense that nothing seems to be valuable in our society except "plastics" and to be a "big green pleasure machine," as depicted in the movie *The Graduate*. But students and teachers like Bloom still exist, even in the most humble colleges, and they offer impressive services to society through the ideals they represent to their students and as models of cultured gentility like Barry's Mr. B (see chapter 8), even if they do not receive the financial or social rewards of a professional basketball player or a corporate CEO. This same sense of highly energized ideals was generated by Freud among his students and pioneers, and Freud attracted those who fearlessly wished to explore the human psyche and were willing to sacrifice for this exploration, regardless of their various motives for doing so.

In his final publication, Bloom (1993) wrote:

Tolstoy's two great novels, *War and Peace* and *Anna Karenina,* were the introduction to high literary taste and Continental thought for a large segment of American college students when I was young. This was one of the last moments of immediate and natural literary influence on the daily life of the more or less educated. The graciousness of life, the incisive presentation of conflicting passions, and the direct presentation of great ideas seemed to be the royal road to an education and the cultivation of civilized sensibilities. The problems of modernity, particularly justice in the organization of the social and the economic order, were addressed directly in Tolstoy and in that other great Russian source, Dostoyevsky, and Russia itself appeared to be the place where the drama of justice would have its denouement. Psychological depth expressing itself in sentimental and unrestrained relations, strange compulsions, triumphs, and especially humiliations appeared to illustrate our Freud, whose victory was still fresh and inspiring. (p. 231)

How Corruption Develops

The explication of the forces producing a decline in cultures and in individuals is more sophisticated now, drawing upon concepts from psychodynamic depth psychology than it was in the days of Spengler, Heidegger, and Hutchins. The problem of life lies in the necessity to withstand the inevitable narcissistic wounding which occurs, both as a function of the vicissitudes of every person's existence and of the struggle for existence of a Culture as it endeavors to manifest itself and blossom in a surrounding world of barbaric, unempathic, and hostile expansionist Civilizations (Kohut, 1978). As wounding through disappointment in people occurs, there may be a shriveling of the soul as I have described it similar to what Freud (1914b) called secondary narcissism, a tendency of the libidinal investment in objects to be withdrawn into the self. This takes place not only as a consequence of inevitable narcissistic wounding but even as the consequence of the anticipation of narcissistic wounding, as when recognizing our necessary physical decline and death, which brings scorn and indifference in our youth-oriented Civilization. Hence, we observe the common phenomenon of elderly people who, in their manifestations of disgust and despair, lose interest in the problems of others and become extremely preoccupied with themselves, their finances, and their innumerable physical complaints.

This may progress to a major withdrawal of libidinal investment in the ego ideal, so that in the final stage of our typically corrupted individual we observe also a cynicism, rage, and a Scrooge-like mentality, what Erikson (1959) called despair rather than integrity: "Such a despair is often hidden behind a show of disgust, a misanthropy, or a chronic contemptuous displeasure with particular institutions and particular people—disgust and displeasure which . . . only signify the individual's contempt of himself" (p. 98). In my experience, people vary in their capacity to withstand the forces that propel one toward this corruption process, as a function of their ego capacity to withstand narcissistic wounding or, as Kohut would put it, as a function of the basic cohesiveness of their nuclear selves.

Similarly, in a Civilization we observe the development of the big city dweller described by Spengler, who has withdrawn libidinal investment from neighboring people as well as from any sort of humanistic, philosophical, spiritual, or religious ideals. As this individual steps nonchalantly around the homeless street beggars, he or she marks what is usually described as the Alexandrian phase of a society (what Spengler would call a Civilization), named after that ultimate representative of corrupt and disintegrating Hellenic culture, the so-called Alexander the Great. In this form of Civilization, art becomes gigantic, morals become flexible, and religious observances perfunctory. Cosmopolitan tastes, populist standards, and esoteric cults predominate. High and low fashions or fads come and go with amazing rapidity, and extremes of feminism appear, including hatred of men and confusion in gender roles to the point of denying even biologically obvious differences (for example, extreme feminists demanding urinals instead of toilets in women's bathrooms).

Massie (1991) described in great detail certain crucial and representative individuals as well as the general populace of the British and German Civilizations of the twenty-five or thirty years before the actual outbreak of World War I. His work demonstrated the theses of both Spengler and Hutchins quite dramatically, although it is reportorial history with no philosophical intent. The unfortunate link between the decline of individuals and the decline of Cultures is that individuals with power in Civilizations are already in the stage of the personal decline of their ideals, and therefore are more likely to accept and even foster rather than resist the corruption and disintegration taking place of the springtime values of the Culture and of the individual. Hence, the public elects banal amoral mediocrities again and again who symbolize the corrupt status of the group ego-ideal and who hasten rather than oppose further decline.

I agree with Spengler's (1962) idea that cultural cities and Cultures have the tendency to become megapolis-centered Civilizations, although I would not call it inevitable. Civilization is characterized by the practical, prosaic nonmetaphysical human. The money spirit prevails, and because of this Civilizations have an expansive tendency, as we observe today in the era of rampant capitalism and as was manifested in the rampant colonialism of the nineteenth century. The turning point for Western Culture to become a Civilization was 1800, said

Spengler, a time that was characterized by the extinction of inner religiousness. From this point on in the present book I will maintain Spengler's distinction between Culture, a springtime phase of creativity, art, and human aspiration, and the later phase of Civilization as just described.

Contemporary Civilization

The philosopher Herder maintained that history reveals the spirit of nations (Appleby, Hunt, and Jacob, 1994). For Hegel (1821), history reveals truth, including philosophical truth, and nations are the carriers of such truth. This implies a certain relativism, for the status of truth in Hegel's view depends on historical circumstances. An offshoot of this kind of thinking is the current collection of viewpoints loosely labeled as postmodernism, discussed in Chapter 5. As mentioned there, many narratives of legitimation have lost credibility in postmodern civilization due to the blossoming of technology, the horrible wars, and the decline of confidence in any permanent values; hence Nietzsche's announcement of the death of God, with the implication of nihilism. This leads to pessimism and loss of the role of philosophy as a metadiscourse to legitimize science or anything else, so we are left with the problem of legitimation of knowledge (Lyotard, 1984). Callinicos (1990) observed that an intelligentsia that is politically disillusioned, materialistic, and aspiring to a consumer lifestyle generates the discourse labeled as postmodernism. He argued, as did Bloom (1987) (see Chapter 5), that postmodernism is a symptom that arose originally from the writings of Nietzsche. Callinicos turned to Marx, whom he thought had a deeper historical understanding of the transient nature of social structures and offered more optimism for the improvement of the human condition.

Clearly there is a crisis regarding the contemporary human condition, the practico-inert against which Ezra Pound and Barry had to press to achieve their creative endeavors. For example, Eagleton (1993) asked, "How *could* the humanities not be in crisis in social orders where it is perfectly clear, whatever their own protestations to the contrary, that the only supremely valuable activity is one of turning a fast buck?" (p. 29). More recently, Bellow (1997) in his old age acidly described contemporary "commonplace persons" as,

> run-of-the-mill products of our mass democracy with no distinctive contribution to make to the history of the species, satisfied to pile up money or seduce women, to copulate, . . . the men and women alike, on threadbare ideas, without beauty, without virtue, without the slightest independence of spirit—privileged in the way of money and goods, the beneficiaries of man's conquest of nature as the Enlightenment foresaw it and of the high-tech achievements that have transformed the material world. (pp. 42-43)

More generally, there has been a loss of the traditions of civility and of the liberal democratic way of life as described almost fifty years ago by Lippman (1953) and in great detail in Riesman's (1955) popular classic that distinguished between inner-directed and other-directed persons. This has been followed by an increased general meanspiritedness, less and less regard for the sick and the poor and the mad, and a decreasing support for and even a fear of contemporary art and artists.

A society with high growth potential, what I would call a Culture, at first, while a barter center (Spengler), consists of persons directed by tradition and myth. It gradually shades over into a society with a transitional population consisting of inner-directed people. When the society becomes a Civilization, it is constituted by other-directed persons. Riesman explained that tradition-directed persons have no thought of themselves as individuals and exist in an unchanging social order where the culture minutely and rigidly controls behavior. When there is a transitional stage the society engages in exploration and then colonialization and expansion; the inner direction for the individual in that society is implanted by the parents early in life. There is a forced childhood and a constant expectation of more accomplishments. This shift was briefly illustrated in Barry's outline for a play (see Chapter 8).

Civilization, a society characterized by incipient decline, manifests increased centralization and bureaucracy. In this sort of a society other people, not so much the material environment, become the problem. The mass media is used for guidance, and being popular, well-liked, and conformist or "well-rounded" are the chief sources of direction in life. Freud's culture was a transitional Culture and the modern United States is a Civilization, one in which there is a legitimation crisis (Habermas, 1975) in the political system and a motivational crisis in the sociocultural system. A legitimation crisis occurs when the system cannot maintain a requisite level of mass loyalty; a motivational crisis arises from changes or corruption in the political system. As Taylor (1985) put it, modern capitalism has a legitimation crisis built into it. ⸺

There is not an exact overlap between Riesman's description of the kinds of free societies and Spengler's distinction between Culture and Civilization, but there is enough of a general overlap to at least approximately fit the picture of decline from an early, tight-knit, highly energetic group of individuals who are spiritually excited by some myth or another and produce great developments in the arts, religion (e.g., the early Christians), and philosophy, to a gradual transition and deterioration into a materialistic, exploitative Civilization, characterized finally by the money spirit, political corruption, and an overall descent into vulgar barbarism and general incivility.

What characterizes a Civilization in decline, such as the one that Barry and Ezra Pound were immersed in? Galbraith (1958) described the "affluent society" where "wants are increasingly created by the process by which they are satisfied" (p. 128), and "we are single-mindedly devoted to getting more" (p. 144). These are artificial and media-created urgent wants. A lack of balance develops between goods and public services; there are more and more of material goods and less and less quality public services. An extreme view of this was presented by Baudrillard (1988), who even became apocalyptic in his later writings. Baudrillard sees in the affluent or consumer society "a fundamental mutation in the ecology of the human species" (p. 29). In this society humans are indoctrinated into consumption, whereas previously they were just made to work. This consumption is not related to use or need but to gradations of social status reinforced by advertising. Galbraith suggested that instead of struggling to maximize one's income, one should seek instead to maximize the rewards of all the hours of the days. The response of contemporary conventional wisdom to this is to consider it foolishly impractical as well as fuzzy- or muddle-headed, although it represents insight as ancient as Confucius.

The dark side of rampant global capitalism has been pointed out again and again in similar terms by many authors. For example, Fromm (1941) described how hostility and resentment develops in the middle class as the drive for relentless work and efficiency increases and emotional and sensual expression is thwarted. People endure an increased sense of aloneness and powerlessness. The problem of modern man, said Fromm, is that he goes after cultural goals not his own and "life runs through his hands like sand" (p. 255), as illustrated in Barry's situation. The hedonism of the counterculture and the instant pleasure orientation so rampant today in the so-called "me-first generation" of impulsive, self-indulgent ideal consumers is simply a caricature of middle-class traditional capitalist values in the affluent society (Erenreich, 1989).

More precisely, Oscar Wilde (1982) already acerbically recognized that in a capitalist society, "We live in the age of the overworked, and the undereducated; the age in which people are so industrious that they become absolutely stupid" (p. 365). This situation, argued Barry, results from the lack of opportunity for genuine leisure. Linder (1970) distinguished four kinds of time: work time, personal affairs time, consumption time for using goods earned by work, and cultural time. The latter he labeled "idleness," and he distinguished it from the true idleness of unemployment and poverty. As we saw in the previous chapter, Barry was already aware of the contemporary problem of finding leisure in his era. To put it another way, Jacoby (1994) explained that "thinking, reading, and art require a cultural space, a zone free from the angst of money making and practicality" (p. 15). Without a certain sense of repose or leisure, a liberal education shrivels. He thought the current arguments over multiculturalism and political correctness distracted from serious social concerns in the United States.

Bloom (1993) labeled isolation and the sense of a lack of profound contact with others as the disease of our time. He also lamented that the activity of solitary reading with its need for leisure and calm has diminished to the vanishing point. One of his heroes, as it was also for Barry, was Jane Austen. For Bloom she represented reason and leisure in human affairs. Contrast the need for reason and leisure in human affairs, for example, with the results of the failure of the United States government to provide universal health insurance, the only advanced industrial nation to do so. Instead, for-profit corporations, sensing large amounts of money to be made, quickly form. They hire from the glut of doctors, reduce the number of specialists, destroy medical research by drying up the funds for it, set standards of work and retirement, and place the making of profits above the health needs of any individual. Already many horror stories involving the meanness and lack of care of remote bureaucratic managers for seriously ill patients requiring expensive treatment have appeared in the newspapers. Health care planning and marketing become a corporate health care services industry, a medical-industrial complex for profit, leaving out the indigent strata of society entirely (Starr, 1982).

The existence of what he called a culture industry was already recognized and criticized by Adorno (Cook, 1996). Assailed by powerful social and economic forces beyond its control, the family's ability to foster ego autonomy and spontaneity has collapsed. The reification of cultural life led to what Adorno labeled the culture industry of late capitalism. (I prefer to call this the Civilization industry of rampant capitalism.) Adorno believed that modern art gets through to people to change their political attitudes, whereas the culture industry, especially television, reinforces regressive behavior. The media as a vehicle of politics stress conformity and are controlled by huge multinational corporations. Clearly, this undermines participatory democracy, and it represents one of the most serious corruptions in Western society. Postman (1985) described how on television public discourse becomes nonsense and "entertainment" becomes the supra-ideology of all discourse; even "news" is fun and should not be taken seriously. In what is currently called "infotainment," news programs exchange images instead of ideas. The media disseminate misinformation, or misleading information that creates the illusion of knowing something while actually leading one away from knowing, or misplaced, irrelevant, or superficial information. The philosophy of the commercial (and of modern psychiatry under the thumb of the pharmacology industry and mismanaged care) is that all problems are solvable, solvable fast, and solvable through the inventions of technology and chemistry. Complex arguments are avoided because they lead to intolerable uncertainty, and the "sound bites" are so brief and fragmented that contradictions are allowed in this manner to disappear. Clearly, a population distracted by trivia and a Civilization redefined as entertainment carries a tremendous political danger for democracy. Currently, elections, for example, generate a barrage of distorted, brief, and repulsive "negative commercials" that actually seem to influence the electorate. Although there was no significant television in the formative and earlier creative years of Barry and Ezra Pound, radio served the same function at that time; hence, Pound turned, as we shall see, to radio broadcasts in fascist Italy as part of his grandiose attempt to singlehandedly reform the United States.

What Is to Be Done?

Fromm (1955) expressed a horror of modern television, which he called a *folie à millions,* a socially patterned defect. In opposition to the "infotainment," sex, and violence preoccupation of the media, he maintained that a spiritual life is a human necessity and must be based on the common ideas of all the great teachers, but this seems to me to be a rather vague prescription. Fromm hoped to develop humans with a productive orientation and a loving relation to the world, and so he deplored the state of humans in a capitalist society and argued instead for communitarian socialism where, allegedly, every worker is responsible and interested. But so far, all the experiments in this direction have failed.

Voltaire argued that we should fully accept life's realities and social responsibilities. He was a humanist trying to improve the lot of people by reason and by fighting fanaticism and superstition, a hero of the intellectually curious (Torrey, 1938). Skinner (1948) tried to design a society based on materialist behaviorism. Not only is behaviorism not scientifically correct, it goes deeply against our ingrained notions of freedom, democracy, and the family as a fundamental unit. People produced by a Skinnerian organized society cannot create and are vulnerable to dictatorship. A school of thought on the mind-brain problem that attempts to eliminate the mind entirely and describe everything in behaviorist terms embraces discredited positivism and turns a blind eye to the vital spiritual side of humans.

The sociologist Max Weber worried that bureaucracy envelops us in all systems, even in the democratic socialist system, forming an iron cage around us. This is another version of Sartre's practico-inert, but expressed in even more dramatic language. Weber worried that the earning of money, more and more of it, too often becomes the end of life. He fretted about the absence of transcendent values, an absence that implies history has to be understood by a study of social behavior and not, as Marx and Hegel thought, as an inevitable unfolding. For Weber history is meaningless, an absurd succession of events (Diggins, 1996). There is no unambiguous hierarchy of values, he asserted, and in his (Weber, 1930) most famous book, *The Protestant Ethic and the Spirit of Capitalism*, he suggested that capitalism is a product of the Protestant ethic. For Weber (Macrae, 1974) capitalism *is* the Civilization of the Western world, not just an economic form. It is a manifestation of a spirit, a historical movement based on actions of certain men, and is the unintended consequence of the Protestant ethic. Technology prevails and the world loses its savor. Poetry, faith, and myth disappear and an oppressive calculating mechanical crushing order prevails.

Rorty (1989) tried to approach the disintegration of Culture into the Civilization described by Weber by introducing the ironist, an individual who faces up to the contingency of his or her central beliefs and recognizes that they are historicist and nominalist. The liberal ironist maintains that among these ungrounded desires are the wishes that human suffering will be diminished and the humiliation of humans by other humans will stop, although these desires do not rest on any external value hierarchy or metaphysics. Today, he said, we worship nothing, and everything is seen as a product of time and chance. Everything is contingent, and among the liberal society's heroes are the alienated poet and revolutionary—like Ezra Pound in his early years. But Rorty, unlike Ezra Pound, did not become grandiose or fascist. He remained, and is today, a liberal ironist. He (Rorty, 1997) asked, for example, in reviewing Wilson's (1996) outstanding book on the new urban poor (remember Spengler's megapolis), "why millions of American children are leading utterly miserable lives in the ghettos, and what can be done about it" (p. 11). He failed to ask more stridently, however, why perfectly sensible remedies already proposed have either failed to be voted upon by Congress or defeated when they come up for a vote, such as proposed legislation establishing health care for rich and poor alike. What has happened to our political system and what should be done about it?

Both Rorty and Heidegger labeled the metaphysician as a person who thinks there is an essence to terms like justice, beauty, truth, and so on. Rorty maintained that the gap between intellectuals and the public is widening because many intellectuals today insist there is no center to the self and there is no natural order or starting point, as claimed to exist by Habermas and metaphysicians (I discussed this debate in Chapter 5). But when ironists deconstruct these metaphysical starting points, their opponents call them irresponsible, and stress the ease of transition of Rorty's liberal ironism into nihilism and even a regression to fundamentalism or neo-Nazi mythology. As I previously mentioned (see Chapter 10), humans must have a cultural and spiritual life based on myths, and if we deconstruct the grounds of the commonly accepted mythological, religious, and philosophical premises of society they will regress to an obstinate, violently defended (*jihad*) mindless fundamentalism.

Huntington (1996) advocated a mutual accommodation between "different civilizations," rather than fostering the continuing Western belief in the universality of Western Civilization, a belief which he regarded as false, immoral, and dangerous. It is not possible at the present time to decide whether Huntington is correct, or whether, as others (Fukuyama, 1992) have maintained, there will eventually be a global Western-style capitalistic system, in which all countries will be capitalist democracies and history has come to an end. At the time of Barry and Ezra Pound there was a greater belief in the ultimate universality of Western Civilization than there is today, but they both had grave reservations about the fundamental assumptions of this Civilization and were searching continuously for something beyond it. They were aware that their contemporary Civilization was in a crisis, a crisis constituted by the deterioration of what was previously believed to be accurate knowledge both of the self and of the right relationship between the individual and society.

Trilling (1955) maintained that there was an affinity between Freud's approach and the tradition of literary humanism, in that both paid attention primarily to the individual's self. For Trilling also, the deterioration of what was previously believed to be accurate knowledge of the self and of the right relationship between the self and our Civilization constitutes a crisis. According to Trilling, Freud believed there was some point at which it was possible to stand beyond the reach of Civilization, that Civilization was not all-powerful, and that there does exist a residue of human quality that Civilization cannot control. Trilling claimed the emphasis by Freud on biology is a liberating idea and supports the resistance to the pressures of one's contemporary Civilization. Freud assumed that somewhere in the adult is a hard, irreducible biological core that reserves the right to sooner or later judge, resist, and revise the Civilization; hence Freud's argument that more than parental actions form the child's personality, a view generally accepted today. Trilling emphasized Freud's description of a standing quarrel between the Civilization and the individual, since the self is not wholly continuous with its surrounding Civilization nor is it created solely by it. This same quarrel, claimed Trilling, has been a particular concern of literature over the past two centuries.

Creative work in the twentieth century has had to take account of the ongoing debate about whether there is any essence to humans. Marx said that humans are to a large extent formed by the practices of their life and that capitalist society generates the wish to have and to use as the most dominant desires that humans experience. Fromm (1962) stressed the importance of the development of the productive human, who is genuinely interested in the world and responds to it, the very opposite of what the mass media in the United States have fostered today. He hoped that under socialism, without the profit motive, what humans are and not what they have would become the crucial measure of a person. He believed the human is crippled under capitalism and cannot live up to his or her full potential; the human is alienated, a common argument by those who have been influenced by Marx. But what has become clear in the twentieth century is just how powerful, enduring, and productive capitalism is compared to other systems. Even Marx recognized this (Silver, 1994). Capitalism could not be eliminated from the top down by fiat; if it is to disappear it would have to slowly fall and be replaced by democratic socialism over many generations. Marx and Engels did not think far ahead about what socialism would be like. Marx said that humans make history, but they do not make it just as they please because there are circumstances to be encountered, and what is given to us and transmitted from the past also shapes what we do.

The collapse of socialism in the Soviet Union does not mean that democratic socialism is ended as a historical force. There are many arguments that support it as an alternative to rampant capitalism (Cohen, 1997). The debate remains unresolved at the end of the twentieth century as to whether rampant capitalism represents the end of history, or whether democratic socialism with its egalitarian ideals will eventually replace it and result in a corresponding transformation in the nature of human desire. If that should occur, the problem raised by Tolstoy will be solved. On the other hand, if it should not occur, we may be in the position described in Kafka's (Hiller, 1979) famous parable "The Building of the Great Wall," about endless senseless human endeavor, or we would have to agree, as Sartre (1973) put it, that man is a useless passion.

Let us not forget Heidegger's (1962, 1977, 1994) contention that each epoch or culture has a basic conception of Being that determines to the inhabitants of that epoch what it is that fundamentally matters. Our epoch, and also the time of Ezra Pound and Barry earlier in this century, produced devastation of the earth as the condition for a promised high standard of living and happiness for all, the darkening of the world, the flight of the gods, and the transformation of humans into a mass with a hatred and suspicion of everything free and creative and into devotees of speed and time-saving devices who paradoxically seem to have no time. Even the arts become just for pleasant diversion and entertainment, not for the expression of truths about ourselves and our world (Wood, 1995).

We are cut off from nature like fish out of water. Those who seek and attain ever-increasing wealth and power treat us and impel us to treat each other as objects to be used in pursuit of these goals. The movers and shakers of our global capitalist world pursue profit without any more concern about human needs or the human body than they have for our natural resources, the relics and even burial grounds of our ancestors, the places and properties that constitute our heritage, or the magnificent products of centuries of the arts—all are treated indifferently as inanimate manufactured objects for the purpose of manipulation and control. Ezra Pound and Barry were attempting to combat the false consciousness foisted on the public by the powerful, corporate-controlled media, that pictures consumerism and drugs as the solution to all human problems and the possession of material goods as the way to happiness and meaning in life.

12 CREATIVE FLOWERING

After all, that is, everybody who writes is interested in living inside them-
selves in order to tell what is inside themselves. That is why writers have
to have two countries, the one where they belong and the one in which
they live really. The second one is romantic, it is separate from themselves,
it is not real, but it is really there.

— *Gertrude Stein,* Paris France

The great speculative system of Hegel, revealing the ultimate forms of Absolute Spirit in art, religion, and philosophy, stipulated that

> In the Greek world the artist was the "maker of gods." It was through Art that the Gods (and their worshipers) became truly *humane.* One cannot say that Art *created* the Gods, for the "natural religions" existed before Homer or any other recognizably self-conscious poet. But Art created the divinely human (or humanly divine) *consciousness* of the Gods, and that function is over and done. (Harris, 1995, p. 105)

Try to keep in mind this function of art, and the question of whether in our time it is over and done with, when evaluating the creative flowering of Ezra Pound and Barry. Also remember Hegel's (1921) famous statement, "Whatever happens, every individual is a child of his time; so philosophy too is its own time apprehended in thoughts. It is just as absurd to fancy that a philosophy can transcend its contemporary world as it is to fancy that an individual can overleap his own age, jump over Rhodes" (p. 11).

199

Art as an Expression of Its Era

At the age of sixty-eight, Adrienne Rich turned down the 1997 National Medal for the Arts in the United States. This poet, who published more than fifteen volumes of poetry and viewed poetry as an instrument of change, has been criticized because there is a political aspect to her writing (for example, see Rich, 1995, her volume *Dark Fields of the Republic: Poems 1991-1995*). She argued that art should not be decorative and she claimed that her art was incompatible with the cynical politics of the Clinton administration. She also complained of the continually widening gap between the people in our country who have wealth and power, and the urban poor and others who do not, a problem already mentioned in my discussion of Rorty in Chapter 11.

T. S. Eliot was another poet obsessed by the collapse of civilization (Spender, 1976). He was a reactionary who preferred his monarchist idea of the Europe of the Middle Ages, in which there was a unity of belief and shared values throughout the whole society, to the modern Western civilization of fragmented aims and values. Ackroyd (1984) wrote that the central theme in Eliot's work was the failure of Western civilization without God and the emergence instead of efficiency and technology. He claimed Eliot's famous poem *The Wasteland* stresses the futility of all poetic styles and the absence of absolute truth, and he maintained that the plangent rhythm of the last section of the poem reads like it was written in a trance, while the early sections were written during Eliot's well-known miserable experiences in his marriage.

Eliot's great poem *The Love Song of J. Alfred Prufrock*, written in 1915 and published through the efforts of Ezra Pound, used everyday life and laconic language to demonstrate how life can be a feeble round of sterile habit and social conformity. While people are chattering aimlessly about art amid cocktails, Prufrock feels the impulse to remove himself from this milieu. Life becomes a waking dream in the deadly trap of convention; the speaker asks himself why it becomes this way and muses that even the life of a blind deep sea creature seems better. Questions stumble, falter, and end up lamely confused.

In his poems *Portrait of a Lady* and *Mr. Appollinax*, the modern living room is shown to conceal brutal lusts under hysterical conventions, painting a nasty picture of human relationships. Then Eliot wrote a series of poems in terse, acrid language about "Sweeney," who like Prufrock struggles to save himself from the blight that has withered his soul. Humanity is seen as the "red-eyed scavenger," the age of the hero is dead, and the age of rats and maggots is here. In the poem *Gerontion* we have an old impotent Sweeney; life is dry and sterile and rain has ceased to fall. Humans become estranged from that source of life, passion and spirit. The first seven years of Eliot's poetry presented this grim picture along with a notorious "genteel" anti-Semitism, in contrast to Pound's vulgar ravings.

Bazarov, a central figure in Turgenev's (1948) *Fathers and Sons* with whom Barry sometimes identified, as well as some of the characters in Dostoevsky's novels, prophesied the situation portrayed in Eliot's *The Wasteland*. Humans, masters of the physical universe, end by destroying themselves because they have destroyed their sense of faith. The terrible impersonality of the cosmos becomes unendurable and the decadence of society as described by Proust and Mann becomes a crucial problem. Humans are dispossessed of ancient dignity and grope in the darkness of their own making. Eliot's reactionary religious preoccupations in the poems constituting *Four Quartets* represent his solution. Only through humility can the human paradox be resolved, a paradox caused by the fact that humans have conquered physical nature but not their own nature. *Four Quartets* begins with two sentences from Heraclitus and introduces a meditation on time. It ends by reflecting on eternity and echoes Proust's (1981) contention that life as it flows in time is wasted and nothing can be recovered except what is timeless in art.

Perkins (1987) maintained that the *Pisan Cantos*, written in 1948, was Pound's response to Eliot's *Four Quartets*. (I discuss the *Pisan Cantos* in Chapter 14.) Perkins (1976) also claimed that for Ezra Pound poetry was not an amateur hobby and that in *The Cantos* he attempted to search for what is permanently valuable. So, as I have already suggested, there is a metaphysical purpose to *The Cantos* (see Chapter 18), and Pound failed in this purpose.

For Pound (1954), poetry is a composition of words set to music, and the whole of great art is a struggle for communication. Pound's critical writings were in effect a long war against mediocrity in art, but the chink in his armor was an egregious lack of humility in his critical temper. The subject of art for Pound is humankind and he attempted the infusion of ethical values in promulgating his doctrine of art for art's sake. He had great technical skill but his work was destroyed in meaning because of his naivete (I would call it poor reality testing) and paranoia. Russell (1950) offered the same criticism and claimed Pound's greatness lies in his influence on others and in a few marvelous poems such as *Hugh Selwyn Mauberley*, but not in *The Cantos*, which suffer from a lack of construction and a lack of matter. Pound's poetry is like the legendary little girl with the curl in the middle of her forehead. When he is good he is very very good, but when he is bad he is horrid. Pound himself eventually recognized that his *Cantos* represented an egregious failure.

Pound's Middle Years

This period of Ezra Pound's life and work covers the time span beginning with his move from London to Paris in 1921 up to the publication of *Cantos LII-LXXI* at the outbreak of World War II, in January 1940. Settling in Paris, Pound attempted to compose an opera, but when he got down to technical matters it was apparent that he was completely ignorant of musical theory. He also admitted that he was virtually tone deaf! Yet he constantly heard music in his head, to which the words of his poems were set (he would hum and sing to himself while composing poetry). He was very interested in the relationship between music and poetry, spending a great deal of time studying the original melodies of the Troubadours.

Pound's anti-Semitic hatred of Freud isolated him from the mainstream thrust of his contemporary modern artists. In Paris, "he soon became a familiar figure striding the streets, his head thrown back, beard thrust out. There were touches of grey in the beard now, hints at thirty-six of middle age" (Carpenter, 1988, p. 398). In this mode he met Gertrude Stein in Paris and also a variety of other artists. He and his wife lived essentially on her inherited income, and they lived quite simply. He became increasingly jealous of the success of James Joyce in Paris just as he had become jealous of T. S. Eliot in London. Eliot showed Pound a draft of *The Wasteland* when he went through Paris briefly on the way to a rest cure, and Pound subsequently made some extremely important editorial changes in the poem that ensured its survival and publication (for details see Eliot, 1971; Trosman, 1974). Eliot was much more successful in achieving what Pound always desired, a literary magazine (*The Criterion*) on a firm financial footing; out of jealousy Pound initially refused to contribute to *The Criterion*, but eventually he did. *The Wasteland* was a better poem than anything Pound had achieved, and perhaps this is why when he finished helping Eliot with it he returned to writing *The Cantos.*

With the publication of *A Draft of XVI Cantos* in 1925, Pound ceased to write any other serious poetry except other cantos. A reviewer of the first sixteen cantos complained that there seemed to be no structure, plan, or purpose among them. *The Cantos* clearly are a compilation of Pound's various ideas on innumerable subjects; one of the early reviewers pointed out (I think correctly) that at least in places "the rhythm is breathless and breath-takingly beautiful" (Carpenter, 1988, p. 422). At the same time his energetic efforts on behalf of other writers continued, and he gave an initial boost to Ernest Hemingway.

In Paris he began to see a great deal of the violinist Olga Rudge. This lady was a very determined and assertive individual, in contrast to Dorothy Shakespear, who was rather quiet and withdrawn, and who did not seem to fit very well into the Parisian scene. In autumn 1924 Olga Rudge became pregnant by Pound. He and Dorothy Shakespear moved to Rapallo, Italy, in 1925; Pound was forty. Pound became a familiar figure in Rapallo, substituting a wide-brimmed sombrero for his Latin quarter beret, and wearing a swirling cape and great yellow scarf with the usual Malacca cane. As he did in London and Paris, Pound fit well into Rapallo society, soon becoming familiar with the language, but Dorothy remained aloof and never became fluent in Italian.

On July 9, 1925, Rudge gave birth in the Italian Tyrol to Pound's baby daughter, named Maria. Pound did not announce the birth to more than a few friends and he was considerably reluctant to talk about her. Shortly after Pound's fortieth birthday, Dorothy left for a holiday in Egypt by herself and Olga Rudge moved in with Pound. Subsequently, Dorothy Shakespear became pregnant by Pound and on September 10, 1926, gave birth to a boy named Omar. Pound sent only confusing messages about their new grandchildren to his parents when he said anything about it at all. Dorothy took the baby to England and stayed there for a year. Omar remained in England and did not see his father until he was twelve years old. Olga returned to Venice and Pound continued to visit her there.

By 1924 Pound already began a falling out, due to envy as might be predicted, with James Joyce, who later remarked that Pound either made brilliant discoveries or howling blunders. Pound eventually even began attacking James Joyce openly in print, claiming Joyce had no common sense or intelligence (see Carpenter, 1988, pp. 441–443).

Although Yeats admonished Pound not to be so involved in political matters, Pound continued to do so and again began forming a group of disciples around him in Rapallo. There were many visitors such as Yeats, including other poets, writers, artists, and sculptors. Pound considered himself a one-man university. He gradually began to pose as "Old Ez," advising younger artists about everything.

His father retired and his parents thought they would come to Rapallo as their permanent retirement home. Homer Pound easily made friends in Rapallo but, as might be predicted, Isabel Pound remained aloof and snobbish. Ezra took Homer to the Tyrol, where Homer first had a chance to meet his granddaughter Maria, even though they could not understand a word of each other's language. Near the end of the 1920s Olga Rudge's American father bought her a small house in Venice, and Ezra began to spend late summer and early autumn with her there each year.

In 1926 Pound published a collection of his previous poems entitled *Personae*, which remained in print during his lifetime; Eliot made a slightly different selection of Pound's poems and published it as *Selected Poems* in 1928. By 1925 Pound had typed up most of seven more cantos, including *Canto XVII*, which contains some excellent examples of Pound's *logopoeia*, *melopoeia*, and *phanopoeia* (see Chapter 6). Yeats thought so highly of this canto he selected it for his *Oxford Book of Modern Verse*. The rest of the seven cantos wander all over the place, from economic theory, to references to *The Odyssey* and the Medicis, to a sudden appearance of a letter from Thomas Jefferson; "these and other items from Ezra's personal store flicker on the poem's screen with no sense of luminosity" (Carpenter, 1988, p. 445).

Acerbic critic F. R. Leavis began attacking Pound's obscurity as manifested in *The Cantos.* Pound responded that everything would become clear when the entire cantos were completed and even suggested that he would write notes into the text, but the last seven cantos in his *Draft of XXX Cantos* published in 1930 were of no help to readers trying to understand the earlier parts of the poem. Critics were invariably frustrated when they tried to find some evidence of structure or overall purpose in the *Draft of XXX Cantos.* Pound seems to have put in just anything that he was interested in at any time or that he thought might excite curiosity. Pound was forty-five years old in 1930, when these cantos were published, fully in middle age and regarded as out of date by the younger generation of artists. T. S. Eliot pointed out how both in the cantos as a whole and in the frequent passages on economics that are scattered in them Pound assumed that the reader should already know what he is describing, and that Pound seemed to refuse out of irritation to enlighten the reader. This to my mind again brings up issues involving grandiosity and impaired reality testing. He continued to produce cantos in the same style, peppered, for example, with prose fragments from the letters of Thomas Jefferson and the diaries of John Quincy Adams as well as prose quotations from a number of books on government and society. All this seemed to be arbitrarily selected.

In April 1932 Pound began making efforts to get in touch with Mussolini in person. They met on January 30, 1933, in Rome. This was a crucial event in Pound's life, and he seems to have formed an immediate idealizing transference to Mussolini, even though it was clear that Mussolini did not have the least understanding of what any of the cantos were all about; he called them "amusing." Pound "swiftly developed a world view in which the Fascist leader played a central part, and was portrayed as the ideal ruler, but where Social Credit rather than Italian Fascism was the political dogma. . . . Mussolini was at the centre of his world view because Ezra now hero-worshiped him as a man" (Carpenter, 1988, p. 492). Pound's literary interest had become extinguished due to the narcissistic injuries he endured when other poets, some younger, surpassed him in talent and fame. He was experiencing a middle age crisis and the familiar situation of middle age burnout. Mussolini and politics gave him something new to fuel the fire: "He began a period of frenetic activity, in which he set himself up as a prophet of salvation through right economics, an interpreter of history who could save the world from its errors, a scourge of government who could unmask international conspiracies" (Carpenter, 1988, p. 493).

Around this time Pound found a small apartment for Olga Rudge near Rapallo where she could live more cheaply than Venice and sublease her house in Venice during the tourist season. The triangle of Pound, Dorothy Shakespear, and Olga Rudge continued without any variation during the 1930s and generated considerable gossip.

Pound began writing dozens of letters every week to various public figures, politicians, and economists, generating an enormous amount of return mail and postal costs. He decided to embrace the Gesell economic theory, one that proposed the entire abandonment of the existing currency system of coins and bank notes and replacing it by "Free-Money," a currency that must be used quickly to buy something or it will go out of date like a newspaper and cannot be hoarded. This would prevent the rich from hoarding money and accumulating interest.

From 1934 to 1940 Pound produced more cantos; these were usually intended to be instruction in economics, sociology, or government. They were published as *Eleven New Cantos: XXXI-XLI* in 1934 in New York and *A Draft of Cantos XXXI-XLI* in 1935 in England. In this melange, *Cantos XXXVI* and *XXXIX* still stand out as fine poetry, but the beautiful passages are lost in Pound's scattered ragbag of ideas. *Canto XXXVI* translates Cavalcanti's canzone *Donna mi prega* in which a lady asks about how love operates. Pound/Cavalcanti's answer is that "love is not a rational process, but the passive experience of pure form. . . . Platonism —the perception of perfect forms" (Carpenter, 1988, pp. 511-512). Even though Pound probably misunderstood Cavalcanti, this answer is consistent with my discussion of ecstatic love in Chapters 7 and 9. Pound's characteristic theme of sexual love as an experience of sacred intellectual illumination was repeated in

Canto XXXIX, which describes Odysseus' men at the house of Circe. I have referred to this canto and its statement of a sexual-religious mythology in Chapter 8, and I will have more to say about the gropings of Ezra Pound and Barry toward an expression of ineffable Absolute Spirit or Being in subsequent chapters.

In his (1938) *Guide to Kulchur* Pound wrote, "Plato periodically caused enthusiasm among his disciples. And the Platonists after him have caused man after man to be suddenly conscious of the reality of the *nous,* of mind, apart from any man's individual mind, of the sea crystalline and enduring, of the bright as it were molten glass that envelops us, full of light" (p. 44). He became obsessed with "mysteries" such as the Eleusinian mysteries that were supposed to be the origin of the love cult of the troubadours, and in *Guide to Kulchur* he complained that rational thought and logical argument banished these mysteries: "His obsession with the Mysteries was therefore an oblique contribution to his growing irrationality and loss of judgment as the 1930s advanced," notes Carpenter (1988, p. 513), who correctly regarded *Guide to Kulchur* as "not a guide to anything except the labyrinths of his own preoccupations, nor a book about culture, a concept that did not greatly interest him" (p. 542). In this book appeared an increasing obsession with usury as the cause of all human problems, leading Pound to a more and more overt anti-Semitism.

The next ten cantos were published in 1937 and contain *Canto XLV,* one of the most beautiful sections of poetry Pound ever wrote, a litany against "Usura"; "it would be a magnificent, perhaps unflawed piece of work, were it not for the uncomfortable fact that it is a hymn to an obsession" (Carpenter, 1988, p. 547). This highly emotional canto combines in the most remarkable way Pound's poetic genius, his obsessive craziness, and his simplistic paranoid interpretation of the world's ills. The 1937 group contains some beautiful shorter passages in *Canto XLVII* and *Canto XLIX,* the former depicting women as predatory beasts who are interested only in sexual satisfaction and the latter offering a brief glimpse of an earthly paradise set in the distant past in China.

At the same time Pound began communicating with fascists such as Oswald Mosley in England and accepting their brutal anti-Semitism. He was obsessed by the bizarre idea that the personality of Jewish people was influenced by circumcision, and his private writing became filled with anti-Semitic slurs. He blamed the Jews for their persecution by the Nazis.

In 1938 Olivia Shakespear died, leaving Dorothy a large sum of money and ending Pound's financial concerns. Because of this he sailed to the United States in 1939. His central hope was to visit President Roosevelt but he was not allowed to do so. He was enthusiastic about Father Charles Coughlin, a notorious anti-Semite in the United States who published a newspaper and gave radio broadcasts containing Nazi propaganda. This seems to have been his model when he began to broadcast from Italy in 1941. His brain was immersed in a fog of fascism, as his American friends sadly noted.

His American visit failed, and he returned to Rapallo in 1939. Hitler and Mussolini formed a full-fledged military and political alliance and World War II began with Hitler's invasion of Poland. After his forty-sixth birthday Pound began dating his letters according to the fascist calendar, which began with the year of the march on Rome. Tytell (1987) reported, "Pound's letters had turned rancid and some of his friends told him so" (p. 226). By 1934 Pound had become aware of the amount of time and energy he was giving to what he called his "hysterical crusade on economics" (Tytell, 1987, p. 233), including the publication of over a hundred letters in periodicals in 1934 alone on economic matters. Pound's one-man crusade in 1935 led to the contribution of 150 articles and letters to periodicals, including a regular series of letters to Mussolini. He was becoming to his friends "an irritant whose anger surged without substantial insight" (Tytell, 1987, p. 239). Tytell sadly concluded,

> Before the first war, he had been the finest scout for literary talent in English, and that had led to his association with Yeats, Ford, Joyce, Hemingway and others. But these friendships had failed to help him become a literary power, a writer who set taste and helped determine what would get published in his own day. Pound had just never been taken seriously enough by the general public for that to occur. Rather than becoming a literary kingpin, he became seduced by the Confucian notion of the writer as political advisor to a ruler. (p. 234)

Apparently in his isolation and neglect in Rapallo he chose a more and more extreme path as a way to get notice, regardless of whether or not it was favorable notice, because he had such a tremendous need to repeat his initial success in London. "Pound had become an ardent supporter of Mussolini and had lost the ability to see the facts as they existed" (Tytell, 1987, p. 242), clearly demonstrating an area of Pound's impaired reality testing. He became increasingly abrasive, cantankerous, and mean-spirited, intensifying his anti-Jewish remarks. Heymann (1976) explained that the reason for Pound's virulent anti-Semitic lucubrations was because he had taken on too much, wasting himself in the process and scattering himself beyond human limitations: "It was as though he had badly misinterpreted the tone of some important aesthetic occasion, and in the agonized and agonizing yatter [sic] which emanated daily from Via Marsala 12-5, his friends and acquaintances noticed the error of tone more often now—the tone, many surmised, of a man no longer in touch" (p. 75).

At this point, as Ackroyd (1987) claimed, "His paranoia was the same as that which, in more powerful and determined men, led to the construction of Auschwitz and Dachau" and, "for all his attempts to keep at the centre of events, in fact, he had retreated into a private world of fantasy from which he never fully escaped" (pp. 77-78).

Although Mullins (1961) tried to defend *The Cantos* as a new poetic form representing a conversation presented by a truly international poet, I think the best objective assessment of *The Cantos* was presented by Stock (1970). The trouble with Pound's epic is that it was born of the wish to write a masterwork,

> rather than of a particular living knowledge which demanded to be embodied in art. At no stage was he clear about what he was trying to do. . . . Although he had no intellectual grasp of the work to be made he was determined nevertheless to write it. . . . the whole project . . . went on piecing together an endless row of fragments. Some cantos and some fragments contain high poetry and there is much that is humorous or otherwise interesting; but insofar as the work asks to be taken as a whole it verges on bluff. (p. 291)

It is clear that at the onset of World War II Pound was isolated in a number of ways. He was living within the Axis powers and defending the German and Italian point of view. "He was also isolated in the sense that he was imprisoned in a world of his own—a man with a mission to change the world both culturally and economically" (Stock, 1970, p. 371). Vanity!

Barry in Middle Age

I turn now to approximately the same period in Barry's life, from about the age of thirty-six to the age of fifty-four. That entire period was unremarkable in that he remained in the same city practicing psychiatry and writing copiously in his notebooks and in his exchange of letters. He raised his children, who in turn grew up and married, and he endured the gradual disintegration of his own marriage. He traveled. Barry mused, " 'nowhere' is to be on the train from Weimar to Berlin, when it is dark outside and cold and a full moon is glowing in the sky. If we have no enemy within us, no enemy without us can do us harm." At one point he wrote that one should not forget Lacan's concept of *objet petit a,* that part of the Other which is not there and we wish were there. Like Pound, he was immersed in the Homeric classics, and in thinking about his fantasies and his future he often referred to *The Odyssey,* Book 24, lines 11-15:

> He led them down dank ways,
> over grey Ocean tides, the Snowy Rock,
> past shores of Dream and narrows of the sunset,
> in swift flight to where the Dead inhabit
> wastes of asphodel at the world's end.
> (Fitzgerald, 1961, p. 457)

Beginning in his late thirties, Barry was also looking for an ineffable something that he called "high points." He remembered that the Dutch historian Huizinga (1924) observed there are three ways to escape from the afflictions of this life: The first is to believe in a better world beyond the grave, the second is to take active steps to better the world we live in, and the third is to weave oneself into a world of fairy tales. The preoccupations mentioned in Chapter 10 continued throughout Barry's notebooks and correspondence. He worried about the breaking loose of sexual fire in middle age, as exemplified by Bertrand Russell's (1945) complaint about Aristotle's *Ethics:* What does Aristotle have to offer to a man possessed by the devil? Barry thought of three unacceptable (to him) answers to give such a person: The first was salvation through deep religious faith, the second was repression by the superego with an inevitable subsequent depression, and the third was acting out, characterized by exciting affairs and cheating. In his insomnia, he endlessly asked what solution would be right for him, but he found none. Like Pound, he was generally irritated with everybody, although he hid it with much greater skill, and his rage was not nearly of the magnitude and chronicity that Pound manifested. Unlike Pound, he recognized that his irritation with human relations was his own problem.

On Barry's first trip to London he registered the sunrise on Portman Square, the Elgin Marbles, and Leonardo's *Madonna of the Rocks* all to be "high points" as he called them, ciphers that gave him a sense of transcendence. For him, "the real greatness of London lies in its block-to-block architecture." In the Tate Gallery he sat entranced among a group of Turner paintings and let them place Beauty and Truth into him, enjoying Turner's brilliantly expressed emotionality in his use of color and empathically sensing his (unfortunately misplaced) excitement about the forthcoming Industrial Revolution. As a midwestern American he found London and its galleries, offering many and variegated aesthetic sensations, to be humbling even more than humanizing. He felt closer to death and impressed with the brevity of life as he became immersed in English history, standing, for example, in Westminster Abbey at the grave of Newton, with that of Darwin and Herschel just off to his left: "One shrinks into greater and greater insignificance beside the tomb of an abbot buried in 1037."

Although his first impression of Paris was not as exciting as that of London, he grew to love Paris and visited it several times, spending many hours in the Louvre. "When it rains in Paris the cobblestones glisten as the sun subsequently comes out; the brilliant sunlight on the Paris-grey stone of these gigantic buildings;

the mixture of colors from dark grey to bright blue in the sky over the gables of the roofs; an artist's dream as Paris grows on a person, with a unique beauty all its own. It must be experienced passively, not actively as London."

Chartres filled Barry not with religious awe but with existential sadness. He felt it was a tragedy that men put forth so much effort to reach out to the spiritual, to find something transcendent, and yet these efforts ended in cold, dark, damp crumbling stone surrounded by bibulous peasants and tourists with cameras that annoy them: "I took many pictures of the rather melancholy statues at the portal of Chartres, with their eyes truly expressing a civilized hope and something spiritual, trying to find something worthwhile about this life even if it is only the hope of a better next life." He experienced Spengler's Faustian Civilization (see Chapter 11), the enormous outpouring of energy represented by the great modern cities of Athens, Rome, Paris, and London, "always reaching and never finding inner peace except in delusions, or temporary aesthetic joy." Experiencing the same excitement over the beauty of the city of Venice that Pound recorded in his cantos, Barry wrote, "Venice today contains the faded remains of what once must have been a magnificent civilization with a mixture of Roman and Byzantine influences. It still possesses a unique natural beauty of its own—the sun on the sea —and an architecture that without a doubt delights the eye. Ezra Pound was right to settle here; he is faded the same way" (Pound was still alive, living in Venice in his old age at the time). But Barry noted the pollution, corruption, and stupidity that are still destroying Venice as the barge, for example, replaces the gondola.

From a restaurant at the top of a hotel he watched dawn break over the Duomo in Florence. It was clear why Mark Twain thought the sight of this city was the fairest picture on our planet, the most enchanting to look upon, and the most satisfying to the eye and spirit. Barry's notebooks are filled with descriptions of paintings and statues from all over Europe that he studied with great care and responded to in a very personal fashion: "How many famous figures have achieved their supreme ambition of burial in a great European church, only to have their stone epitaph worn away by thousands of people over the centuries walking over their head?" He stood for hours in the ruins of the Roman Forum, even in the rain. He viewed the place where Keats died in 1821 at the foot of the Spanish Steps, and walked up to the top, where he attempted to enter the Hotel Hassler—but he walked around in the massive revolving glass entrance door of the hotel and went too far, ending up by walking into the glass wall. He was definitely not one of the "beautiful people," or the snappy international set.

He tarried a long time in front of the Moses of Michelangelo, wondering how Freud (1914a) really felt when he wrote about it. He found the proportions to be massive and the statue different from every angle: "Whether the tablets are falling or just resting depends on the angle from which you look at the statue. Also, whether Moses looks angry or with a far-away vision also depends on the angle from which one looks at it, so one can either see Moses enraged and dropping the tablets or visionary while resting the tablets; most likely anger is correct, but my nature inclined me to the other interpretation. One could sit for hours in front of this statue and that of Rachel and Leah—the one on the viewer's left—which is sublime and otherworldly in appearance." But he ended his tour of Europe again standing in the Roman Forum in the rain taking shelter under the archway of the old vestal virgin home "which rather by chance looked directly up at the ruin of the temple of Castor and Pollux." Returning home to reality, he found that his house had been burglarized and his stamp collection decimated and parts of it stolen.

Throughout his middle years Barry had a goal that he could never reach, to stretch out on the old couch in his front room and read for hours on a rainy afternoon, warm and comfortable and imaginatively drifting into the world of the book, for example, the world of that master novelist of all English novelists, Jane Austen. In the earlier part of middle age, an experienced psychiatrist, he found himself uninterested in social and community psychiatry and remaining preoccupied with individual psychotherapy, seeking to understand his patients thoroughly. The next fashionable move, from social psychiatry to psychopharmacology, was in an even more extreme opposition to Barry's orientation and left him feeling increasingly alone and professionally alienated, as Pound was in Rapallo. His income diminished more and more over the years as fewer patients appeared seeking medical psychotherapy, and when managed care and the huge insurance corporations took over the field of medicine there were almost no new patients available who could afford without insurance what Barry did the best.

By his forty-first birthday he awoke to the sexual fantasy of running off to Florida with a pretty girl. This occurred at a time when his children were in late adolescence and becoming increasingly estranged from him, a separation that had to occur but left him with nothing as a replacement. He noted the old Japanese saying: The longer one lives, the more shame one has to experience. The problem of controlling his weight was constantly a struggle and he suffered from an intellectual malaise, a sense of growing hopelessness and entrapment. Although he wrote obsessively again about many plans to resolve the situation, nothing ever changed.

Barry believed there were two stages of human growth. The first of these is self-authentication, the development of a secure sense of identity and resultant falling away of dependence on others for self-esteem. The second stage is transcendence, the development of a sense of Being somehow over and above one's self. This involves a perspective on life, nature, and the universe in which we feel fused with this cosmic order and can accept aging and death. Again and again he asked himself what he regarded as the crucial question of philosophy, whether the search for transcendence, regardless of the ciphers chosen to represent it, is possibly (as Freud would say) simply a search for the good mother in blissful reunion and/or simply an opiate for the horror of knowing that one will die. He felt one could never know the answer and that the search for transcendence was an act of faith: "We must live with this uncertainty and never know if it is all a delusion, just as solipsism can never be *proven* wrong."

He spent much time (while most of his colleagues were watching and enjoying football on TV) studying *Philosophy*, the masterwork of the psychiatrist and philosopher Karl Jaspers (1932a,b,c). In the third volume of his *Philosophy*, Jaspers (1932c) attempted to use what he called ciphers to "overcome the intellect" (Vol. 3, p. 122). There are a variety of experiences that give us an immediate feeling that cannot be described by the intellect, a hint that "reality" is more than what is empirically presented to the senses. These experiences differ for different people. Jaspers called them "ciphers." So transcendence, the world of Absolute Spirit or Being, cannot either be proven or clearly articulated, only hinted at by ciphers. If this "transcendentally related communication defaults" and we do not experience any ciphers, then we end with existential desolation (Vol. 3, p. 137). Jaspers argued that if we do not have philosophical faith in ciphers the only alternative is an empty not knowing, a radical despair that leaves us nothing but the void. But Barry asked whether this "leap from fear to serenity" described by Jaspers (Vol. 3, p. 206) is simply an opiate in the form of a mystical self-delusion, like the religions of the East. Barry wrote, "the fact that we relentlessly want something to exist or spend an eternity searching for it does not make it exist; it may just be a function of gross unhappiness and the inefficiency of our minds. Faith brings serenity but so do opiates." He agreed with the novelist John Barth that there is no ultimate reason for valuing anything, but he also insisted, along with the philosopher T. E. Moore, that personal affection and aesthetic experiences constituted the good, and he was sure that if one could not experience these one was sick. But again and again Barry asked himself why he could accomplish nothing in the direction of changing his situation, why he felt trapped.

As time passed and he received no recognition, Barry began to lose respect for himself because he could not live up to his original narcissistic goals. He recognized that he was an unsuccessful narcissist and was constantly overdriven to somehow accomplish aims that his talents did not permit. He continued to be concerned about transcendence and experienced a cipher in a planetarium when the lecturer showed the constellations of the zodiac on the ceiling and demonstrated their rising at the time of the Egyptians. The lecturer explained the "Age of Aquarius"; about 2300 A.D. the constellation Aquarius will either rise first or be the constellation in which the sun rises on the first day of spring. This shift is caused by the earth's precession. The lecturer pointed out that we are living in the dawning of the Age of Aquarius, a dawn that Barry of course had no hope of ever living to see.

He read with great jealousy how the philosopher Peirce was able to devote two hours a day to the study of Kant's *Critique of Pure Reason* for more than three years until he almost knew the whole book by heart and had critically examined every section of it (Körner, 1970). He wondered if the "natural disposition" to metaphysics postulated by Copleston (1964) was also a cipher, a natural tendency of the human mind to seek unconditional principles of unity or transcendental ideas. For Kant this is a regulative function of reason, but is that the entire picture? After all, mused Barry, Kant's wonder about the existence of the starry skies above and the moral law within as being unanswerable by science represent his indirect admission that the universe is ultimately a mystery. Today's astrophysical mystery is represented by the so-called "singularity," a concept that has rattled the brains of our best physicists (see Hawking, 1993). He became increasingly interested in the work of Hegel and subsequently of Heidegger, as much as he could understand these tortuous and obscure authors without professional instruction. The mystery of the moral law within he sometimes regarded as solved by Freud and modern anthropology, and at other times he remained unconvinced of a relativistic cultural origin to all morality. Were there no moral universals? Freud thought they were self-evident.

Barry had enough insight to recognize that he was in the throes of a harmful personal conflict that he could not resolve because of his unconscious childhood subjection to the demands and prohibitions of his parents. He was trapped, with an unconscious image of an internalized bad mother attacking him and acting like a severe illogical and punishing conscience. As he entered the fifth decade of his life his parents died, but he continued the struggle with them internally: "I awoke early, angry and swearing, feeling left out and alone. Yes, I am isolated and alone and I do not belong anywhere or to any group and there is not much I can do about it. It is hard to hide my depression and sense of the futility of it all." At this point Barry began to have thoughts of his mortality. He noticed the more he wrote in his notebooks and correspondence the more tired and drained out he felt, as if somehow he was investing all his energies or, as Freud would put it, narcissistic libido, in his written work while at the same time being mired in terrible frustration because there was no recognition or mirroring of his creativity. There is a certain similarity to the life of Franz Kafka, who worked in an insurance office during the day and produced his creative stories and diaries at night, but Kafka was a genius and Barry was not.

On November 2, 1972, Barry noted that Ezra Pound died at the age of 87, and he asked himself, "How could anyone so brilliant and with such poetic ability have been such a skunk? Nobody except maybe T. S. Eliot in my era had such an ear for the musical aspects of poetry." He inserted a clipping in his notebook of the photograph of a black gondola decorated with six wreaths carrying the coffin of Ezra Pound in Venice to the island cemetery of San Michele. He wrote, "I studied Heidegger this morning and some of Einstein's essays in the afternoon. Both were looking for the same thing, each in their own way, something above, behind, and beyond the dreariness of everyday material life. This is not so unlike the drug addict or the seeker after a romance, or even Don Quixote! This is why I cling to my reading and writing and to my friends in correspondence, and study an eternal dialogue of which I am not even a footnote, but even being present at it is something. How fortunate are those few who can devote their lives to it or even contribute to it and be recognized for their contribution!"

More ominously he continued, "As my narcissistic blossom dreams fail to blossom, then the sexual fantasies press up, perhaps as a substitute for the more remotely available passive lying-in-the-sun fantasies. The deep oral longings behind it all are a defect, make it hard to tolerate long-run frustration. For the first time I am beginning to believe in Freud's death instinct and it really frightens me. At times I feel I would prefer death to life. I never felt like that before, no matter how unhappy I was."

He was photographed in front of the Propylaea, about to enter the Acropolis in Athens. On the same trip, in Ephesus, he remembered how philosophical questioning began with Heraclitus, who lived where everything and everyone in the city were mixed together in great flux. No religion appeared as the only one and the sacred one, so the natural tendency in the face of so much nonsense was to disbelieve in all of them. The inevitable fluxing and changing of so many people in this bustling trade center led to a search for what was permanent: "The idea of the laws of change or the formula of change being what is permanent came from the genius of Heraclitus, who walked the streets of this big bustling metropolis in the heat and in disgust with himself and everybody else."

An antidote to this was the magnificent sunshine and the view from the Acropolis of Rhodes. After visiting the Greek islands he wrote, "I have come halfway around the world to discover the secret of the origin of civilized man and all I have discovered is that I cannot discover the secret." He noted sharp contrasts in Greece, for example, "cruising the Aegean sea in the warm sun looking out over the blue water, an indescribable blue, and smelling the stink of the antiquated cruise boat," or "the silent classic temples on the Acropolis stand in sharp contrast to the hellish noise and pall of pollution that envelop modern Athens."

Traveling in a boat on the Öslo Fjord he concluded that the life of the honest psychotherapist is characterized by the continuous agonizing reappraisal of countertransference, which he seems to have mixed up with his personal intrapsychic conflicts. He remembered O'Neill's comment in *A Moon for the Misbegotten*, that there is no present and no future; only the past lived over and over again.

In Copenhagen he visited the grave of Kierkegaard and spent a lot of time in the Tivoli gardens, enjoying the remarkable juxtaposition of the sublime to the ridiculous, the serene to the tawdry, valuable natural beauty and a cheap Las Vegas all jumbled up together, "even gourmet restaurants mixed with hotdog stands. . . . Kierkegaard and Copenhagen reflect each other." He began another unfinished, unpublished lecture:

Europe in the Twentieth Century

In the past year and a half or so I have had occasion for a variety of reasons to visit many of the major cities of Europe. What is happening? Where are humans going? At this time we are at the nadir of the dilemma. The magnificent cities of the Old World are becoming inundated by a swarm of locust-like little cars, breeding traffic congestion and industrial fumes and covering over the magnificent ancient and classic architecture like lava over Pompeii. The traditions and gentility, the civilizing effect of these great cities, have disappeared as everyone grabs for tourist money, with Americans, Germans, and Japanese heading the list of sheep to be shorn.

Centers of culture and learning and the great repositories of art are surrounded by barefoot hippies and filled with busloads of tourists whisked in and out by bored and mechanical guides. The Old World charm that exercised such a profound effect on American authors between the two world wars can now be found only off the beaten paths, still surviving in the nooks and crannies. The best meal I ever ate in Europe, sitting on an oriental rug in the Gritti Palace Hotel in Venice, was a variety of delicatessen meats and cheeses purchased in an obscure grocery and carried up with a fresh loaf of bread in a brown paper bag. Or in the Grande Bri-etagne Hotel in Athens, after a day of sitting in the sun on the Acropolis looking at the Parthenon, some sandwiches and English cake. So one must work at it now, the charm does not just ooze all over, just as one must work hard at lifting one's head above the industrial slime to see where humans are going or not going. The only other alternative is Spenglerian despair.

Perhaps Kierkegaard and Jaspers are correct: Humans must leap if they are to reach either the ethical life or faith, but reason alone cannot justify such a leap. Either one fuses with Being or one does not. Either one chooses to live for others or one does not. The fusion with Being takes place alone in solitude, Heidegger is right about that. It represents a different kind of a leap, from fear to serenity, but contains no implications about how to treat other people. So throughout life we are confronted with two problems unresolvable by reason alone and not related to each other. They have been mixed together in the hope of solving two in one blow but this is not possible. We "know" intuitively that it is bad to hurt someone who loves us and has been devoted and loyal to us. How do we get this "knowledge"?

I am inclined to agree with Schopenhauer on the special place of music in human life. It is mysterious indeed, it seems to have value as a special cipher. At any rate nothing so consistently provides me the feeling of transcendence, especially the music of Bach.

Like Pound, Barry turned to Confucian thought, or at least his interpretation of it, suggesting that obtaining internal satisfaction is the essential way to achieve happiness. He hoped that as long as persons are diligent in making use of their potentiality to obtain knowledge, to develop their talents, to cultivate their personality, to be good to others and to themselves, and to know how to be satisfied with striving while disregarding the outcome of it, then they would gain real happiness in life; he attributed this point of view to Confucius. He agreed with Kierkegaard and Freud that we make the major decisions of our life by irrational leaps, not by rational thought; the latter is used only to justify what we want to think or do in the first place.

He toured the Soviet Union and eastern Europe, incidentally visiting Tolstoy's grave. In Yasna Polanya near Tula, suffering from resistance of the Soviet bureaucracy at every turn, he wrote:

> Tolstoy's estate is a small birch forest now, and he is buried among the trees. One could hear the bird calls in this really inspiring place, far from the reality. Reality is the cluster of wooden houses called villages in which the peasants who are now called collective farmers live in a state of indescribable primitive poverty. These little villages, with the common water well in front, are scattered over a horizon of fields and endless forests of birch that seem to go on forever in all directions. Who is better off, the worker in his little cubicle in innumerable grey high rise apartment buildings that make up the ugly industrial cities of the Soviet Union or the peasant who prefers a wooden to a brick hut because wood holds the heat in better? A great alcohol problem. The people have no freedom whatsoever. Nobody travels anywhere and everybody stays in their grooves and tries not to call attention to themselves. Coming to Budapest was like leaving a dungeon, but Hungary was also the first place where I encountered overt anti-Semitism.

Shortly after his father died, Barry noted his first episode of angina. The notebook entries became fewer and more repetitious and the correspondence dwindled. He seems to have reached a dead end. Returning from eastern Europe, he showed abnormalities in his electrocardiogram during a routine physical examination. The inverted T-waves that developed during his treadmill test demonstrated myocardial ischemia, and he was told to give up smoking and reduce stress. The loneliness and the angina seemed to get worse after his children left for college.

In reading a biography of St. Augustine, Barry argued to himself that the Christian myth was beautiful but obviously a myth. Here was a human dilemma; without revealed knowledge human reason keeps bumping against severe limitations, but revealed knowledge must be taken on faith, and who knows if it is nonsense? None of the usual laws of evidence may be applied, and therefore it is a hopeless situation to look for any overarching scientific understanding of the scheme of things. Without revealed knowledge all ground for tradition is removed as well as ground for conduct and even peace on earth: "In fact I doubt humans can go without some kind of grounding to their existence. Or can they? This is what we are all really searching for."

Many of his notebooks were taken up reporting the difficulties and vicissitudes he endured with his adolescent children, all of whom eventually went through their stormy periods with success. There are also notations of various political crises in the United States, of incidents involving the Vietnam War (that he actively resisted), and of attacks by isolated lunatics on artistic masterpieces such as Rembrandt's *The Night Watch* and Michelangelo's *Pietà*.

He was impressed with how the temple of Karnak at Luxor contrasted with the stagnation, poverty, and filth in Egypt. Cairo, he noted, was certainly what Spengler would have called a megapolis (see Chapter 11). He listened to the otherworldly background call to prayer of the Moslems while watching the color shades of the pyramids change during the day depending on the position of the sun: "The living school children play in its shadow, a spectre of death casting its presence on everything. The grunts and curses of millions of humans cry out from the pyramids over the centuries, a feat of unimaginable human sweat and labor. To what end? To leave a permanent imperial mark, a gigantic monument of jagged stones rising out of a totally inhospitable desert of shifting sand that stretches over a whole continent. A grim picture in a truly desolate part of the world."

Barry's subsequent trip to Jerusalem and the rest of Israel is described in Chapter 16. This was his first trip to a war zone where both soldiers and civilians were walking around with guns, everyone living on a knife edge. Returning home he wrote,

> Listening to Donizetti's *Elixir of Love*. Entranced by the music, crying for the longing that the hero feels. Much reflection on what it is to love and my terrible loneliness. I

want to have a passionate love affair, to feel alive again . . .
but my brain tells me this is crazy. Is love only sexual lust?
What makes a person fall desperately in love? Why throw all
away for such a passion? If you gain your object then what
happens? When the aura shifts what do you have? But what
else besides religion can give life meaning? What makes a
woman look stunningly beautiful to an individual man? Is it
some sort of creative act? The moment of possession of the
loved one is the peak experience of a life. But then the price
is to be paid. To spend a weekend with Ruth in Jerusalem!
Mysticism and ecstasy mixed together at a fevered pitch! But
then what?

Here we experience phenomenologically Kohut's (1991) notion
of a fragmenting self watching helplessly as it is replaced by a
feverishly intensified longing for pleasure experience, by the as-
cent of a pleasure-giving erotogenous zone, and thus of the drive
over the self. So in his fifties Barry began his relationship with the
woman named Ruth. He wrote to her quoting Ezra Pound's
(1949) short poem " 'IMEIPΩ" [I desire]. She replied, "See the
bottom of page 25, the second verse of his poem *The Garrett*."
Barry read,

> Dawn enters with little feet.
>   Like a gilded Pavlova,
> And I am near my desire.
> Nor has life in it aught better
> Than this hour of clear coolness,
>   The hour of waking together.

The devil pours honey into other men's wives. Kernberg
(1975) pointed out that careful observation of the productivity of
narcissistic personalities over a long period of time gives evidence
of superficiality and flightiness. In middle age they develop com-
plicating symptoms that worsen their functioning and lead to
chronic depression and a sense of emptiness at having wasted
their lives. In such films as *Still of the Night* and *Lovesick*, reaching
very large audiences, psychiatrists are shown as unable to hold
their marriages together and as violating a basic taboo of their
profession by becoming romantically involved with their patients.
Barry was a man trying unceasingly to communicate with a world

ever more indifferent to him, he was frustrated, and his voice weakened and the world no longer took any notice of him at all. He disappeared from it, and his circle grew smaller. Barry was, as Tom Lehrer so eloquently put it, sliding down the razor blade of life. His response would have been that of Dickens's Ralph Nickleby: "I know the world. I know people. I look right through the face into the grinning skull underneath." But he did not, like Pound, engage in radio broadcasts in a more and more bizarre exhibitionistic effort to gain recognition. His reality testing was better.

Barry traveled repeatedly to Germany and also visited Vienna and the Salzburg Festival. He spent a little time in the Freud museum which was then mostly empty, since when Freud was chased out of Vienna what he left behind was impounded and stolen. He was impressed with the prosperity and power of Germany, entering it on his first visit through the city of Munich and then later repeatedly by flying into Frankfurt. In Cologne he wrote,

> Walking around the cathedral again and again in the twilight. From the immediate side angle it rises massive and towering into the sky, very heavy, dark, and Gothic. From the straight side with buttresses it looks more like a delicate Renaissance work of art, one of those remarkable wonders that changes with every light and with every direction from which one looks at it.

He traveled down the Rhine and repeatedly visited Heidelberg, Weimar (the home of Goethe), and Jena, where Hegel once taught. He spent time in Berlin before the Wall came down and also afterwards, marveling at this magnificent city, one of the most exciting in Europe today, and saddened by what the Germans brought on themselves in its destruction. He was horrified both by East Berlin with its police state and by souless materialistic West Berlin. But he found German psychiatrists to be the most hospitable and welcoming to American colleagues in all of Europe.

In Vienna he was reminded of Freud's statement that nature gave him a dauntless love of truth, the keen eye of an investigator, the right sense of the values in life, the gift of working hard, and the pleasure of doing so. But Barry compared himself to the provincial poet Lucien Chardon in Balzac's (1837-1843) *Lost Illusions*, who sold out for money.

13 LATER STAGES ON LIFE'S WAY

My conversation with the poet took place in the summer before the war. A year later the war broke out and robbed the world of its beauties. It destroyed not only the beauty of the countrysides through which it passed and the works of art which it met with on its path but it also shattered our pride in the achievements of our civilization, our admiration for many philosophers and artists and our hopes for a final triumph over the differences between nations and races. It tarnished the lofty impartiality of our science, it revealed our instincts in all their nakedness and let loose the evil spirits within us which we thought had been tamed forever by centuries of continuous education by the noblest minds. . . It robbed us of very much that we had loved, and it showed us how ephemeral were many things that we had regarded as changeless.

— *Sigmund Freud,* On Transience

Earlier I mentioned the importance of Proust's (1981) *Remembrance of Things Past,* which in English probably should have been titled *In Search of Lost Time* (see Chapter 10). Proust's writing shows acute sensitivity and perspicuous sensibility to both artistic and natural sensations, weaving the reader into the text so that each reading is in a sense a reliving of one's own life. Proust attempted to capture the past eternally in art and experienced it as a remedy for being-towards-death and the evanescence of everything; for Proust, art on the phenomenologic channel attempts to achieve a triumph over time.

Kohut (1977) argued, using the self psychology channel, that Proust never succeeded in his task of attempting to reunite the fragments of his self with the aid of *Remembrance of Things Past:* "His creative effort, it is true, held him together for many years after the loss of the parental self-objects (especially of his mother) that had sustained the cohesion of his self. Yet, his monumental novel

225

contains much evidence of his persisting fragmentation . . . as it contains evidence of his reconsolidation" (pp. 180-181). Kohut claimed that although it seems Proust's "narrator" has to keep Albertine a prisoner and appears to be desperately preoccupied with regaining possession of her when she leaves him, "he is actually attempting to restore his own self" (p. 181).

Among the books that make up Proust's masterpiece, *Swann's Way* with its "overture" contains the themes and sets the tone of the entire work, concluding with magnificent unforgettable literary passages. Swann fails where the "narrator" succeeds, and Swann dies a dilettante and wasted person. The "narrator" almost reaches that point when he returns at the age of fifty to postwar Paris, but in Volume 7 of the novel he suddenly finds the secret of his existence and his goal in life: to triumph over time and art. He hopes to capture a life by connecting all the shifting and misleading images together. *Cities of the Plain* illustrates the disintegration of Culture into the decadence of Civilization, as described in Chapter 11.

The centerpiece of the novel is the narrator's need to possess Albertine, his yearning for a soothing selfobject, or what Lacan would call *objet petit a* (discussed further in Chapter 14). By this he of course stifles Albertine and drives her away, since she appropriately experiences his behavior as suffocation. In *The Sweet Cheat Gone,* the truth is revealed about Albertine who actually loved little girls, about St. Loup who was gay, and about Gilberte who really loved the narrator. Proust (1934) explained, "A large part of what we believe to be true (and this applies even to our final conclusions) with a persistence equaled only by our sincerity, springs from an original misconception of our premises" (p. 841). In *The Past Recaptured,* Proust offers a famous and shocking description of what time does to the degenerate Baron de Charlus.

The crucial theme of the novel is that only art endures and reality is within us under our sensations, a theme reminiscent of the philosophy of Bergson. It should be kept in mind that the narrator considers himself old at the age of fifty. This chapter of the present book briefly examines some of the later stages on life's way and some of the later stages in the development of our understanding of Spirit or our achievement of the transcendence that Hegel was looking for and claimed to have found, and that Ezra Pound and Barry were unsuccessfully looking for, remaining mired in endless epics that led only to a dead end.

Hegel's Concepts

There are a few concepts from Hegel worth keeping in mind for the rest of the present book. I will review some of them here and discuss them again in Chapter 18 because they are difficult, especially for readers in our current era. The philosopher Dilthey at the end of the nineteenth century announced that the generation that can read Hegel is dead, and that is why Hegel is rarely taken seriously anymore. His terrible writing style and conceptual obscurity have caused him to be much referred to but little studied. I assume the reader is aware of Hegel's dialectical method in philosophy, in which each contention or proposition or orientation is a retrospective comment on what is implied in the previous contention or proposition or orientation, a progression that Hegel believed was necessitated by what went before. For Hegel this was a rigorous process of continuous development, determined by "the cunning of Reason," studied by a systematic science (*Wissenschaft*), and terminating in Absolute Spirit. In this German Idealistic philosophy only Mind is real, not substance, and consciousness is primary and always changing, as illustrated in his most famous work, *Phenomenology of Spirit* (Hegel, 1807).

Hegel believed that Mind, both of Man collectively and of each individual human, evolves, and in a parallel way, through a series of unfolding levels in a process during which each level is incorporated into the next. Thus, the mind is an inner force shaping outer observable forms and not, as Kant believed, a disinterested judge. It follows from this that Truth can only be reached by a historical or genetic approach, showing the evolution of it up to any particular stage as a necessary outcome of a series of conflicts and discrepancies and their corrections. Hegel attempted to prove that an inevitable dialectic of self-consciousness would end with a monism of Absolute Spirit, where thought and its object, originally perceived as separated, are transcended through first art, then religion, and finally philosophy.

Hegel was the first to focus on the problem of alienation, as illustrated, for example, by Dostoevsky's (1864) "underground man." This was an unknown problem for the philosophy of the Enlightenment, which assumed that humans could through rational activity live in a congenial and reasonable world. This state of "otherness" for Hegel was a driving force to advance consciousness to higher levels, but Marx and Dostoevsky interpreted it in socioeconomic and psychological terms. Marx hoped this basic need to overcome alienation would function as a force that eventually would enable individuals to have the freedom to create and make their lives, to carry out their basic project.

Hegel believed that human beings are not just rational animals but are also spiritual; they aspire to freedom and have a sense of values and a destiny. He argued that history has significance and represents the progress of the consciousness of freedom, as even feebly illustrated by the so-called consciousness-raising movements prevalent today. He (Hegel, 1821) maintained that our wants and desires are shaped by our society and that therefore an organic community is needed, one that fosters desires that benefit the community and form one's identity as being part of the community. He stressed our lived experiences, our being-in-the-world, and he claimed that what makes a form of experience appear to be "necessary" is the social context of it at any given time. It follows that ideas are ways of dealing with the times in an effort to grasp the contemporary world of the thinker.

Metaphors and visions as an attempt to make sense of the world are in disrepute in most philosophy today, and although Hegel's metaphysics as a system has few adherents, there are many corollaries of it that are extremely valuable in the understanding of humans, of mental illness, and of creativity. For example, Hegel claimed that the sense of self exists only by being acknowledged, and therefore, contra Descartes, preconditions for the self do exist. This is because self-consciousness emerges out of a struggle with the world—it is not an immediate intuition. Conflict and opposition as well as recognition and approval are required for self-formation. In this, Hegel's phenomenologic viewpoint comes close to Kohut's self psychological viewpoint.

Of special interest to us here is Hegel's concept of the ascending order of adequacy of the form of Absolute Spirit. He maintained that art was a nonrepresentative form of it, religion represented it in images, and philosophy was the end point, articulating Absolute Spirit in rational and logical terminology. But Taylor (1975) presented an argument I agree with, that today art is a higher representation of Absolute Spirit than religion. For Hegel religion meant mainly Christianity, and he tended to ignore or be prejudiced against other religious beliefs.

In art Absolute Spirit *(Geist)* is presented to us in what Hegel called "sensuous reality" or Beauty. As in Schiller's (1965) letters *On the Aesthetic Education of Man,* Hegel believed that modern humans have the crucial enforced preoccupation of trying to attain expressive unity and a radical autonomy. Toward this goal, art has to take on a quasi-religious function, so that even in the Preface to *Phenomenology of Spirit* he (Hegel, 1807) made the famous statement that the True is the "Bacchanalian revel in which no member is not drunk" (p. 27), that is, Spirit *(Geist)* lives by affirmation and denial, by contradiction in transitory, insubstantial, sensuous, finite things. The metaphysical aspect of this, proclaiming that *Geist* or Spirit realizes itself through the action of humans who only see through a glass darkly what they are doing and are guided by the "cunning of Reason," leaves much to be debated. But the central importance of art, religion, and philosophy, to which I would include among the arts the important category of mythology, is very significant in Hegel's thought and shines through in the strivings of both Ezra Pound and Barry. So also Heidegger (1971a), in one of the most important philosophical essays of the twentieth century, maintained that Being and Truth reveal themselves in art.

Each age has its own set of values, and according to Hegel these are determined by the phenomenologic or ontological structure of that age, which provides standards of truth and propriety and is determined by the form of consciousness of the age. Since this is always imperfect, contradictions are recognized and overcome, and in this manner new ontologies form. Beginning with Sophocles' *Antigone,* the earlier lack of separation between a person's identity and a person's social role begins to break down. Early society had no form of recognition for the human person empty of social content, as described in Chapter 11 of the beginning stage of a Culture.

Hegel would say that the work of Ezra Pound and Barry represented "bad infinity," an endless epic that implies some things are not ever explainable, understandable, or resolvable. He would contrast this to "good infinity," a circle like Einstein's finite but unbounded space or, as in Hegel's philosophy, a process that recapitulates the whole series and method by which the circle has been generated and ends with a rational explication of Absolute Idea. In the philosophy of Hegel the characters in the human drama eventually become aware that they are just characters in a drama, and the final scene of the drama is the awareness of the author-director's (or Spirit's) production of the drama (Inwood, 1983).

For Hegel, self-understanding and self-actualization evolve through a dialectic of forms shaped by cultural traditions. Thus, the process of any individual's self-actualization must be understood in its social and historical meaning. He adds that the whole of humanity is a collective subject with its Mind, and there even exists "national spirits" and a "World Spirit," but it is not necessary to adhere to such metaphysics to understand the contemporary value of what Hegel is driving at.

The present book could be called, following Hegel, a *Bildungsroman*, a story of *Bildung* (formation) precipitated out of culture, education, and self-formation, a deliberation through self-discipline out of which emerges the true volitional subject or moral self. The individual freedom required for such self-actualization is what was impaired due to the psychopathology of Ezra Pound and of Barry. It is this psychopathology that interfered with their attainment of "good infinity," reaching the calm and peace that accompanies a sense of transcendence, and condemned them to a "bad infinity," an endless, meaningless epic with no focus and no resolution, as reflected in their literary creations.

Hegel (1833) correctly maintained that human history is a slaughter-bench on which the happiness of peoples, the wisdom of states, and the virtues of individuals have been sacrificed. His work may be read as an attempt to understand this slaughter-bench, just as Ezra Pound attempted to explain it through a paranoid crystallization. I have always been fascinated by the fact that Hegel received his Ph.D. for a closely reasoned logical dissertation that proved there could only be seven planets. This is the problem of rigid metaphysical systems; the world is too complex and cannot fit into any fixed eternal system. Such systems close one's mind and do not, as was once believed, indisputably justify action. As Nietzsche (1886) put it, metaphysical systems are groundless and just express the personality of the systematizer; in fact, they do not even answer the question of why one would prefer truth or have a system to begin with. But, as I have now repeatedly stated, humans always need systems, myths, religions, art, and philosophy, and they will not tolerate the absolute nihilism implied in the destruction of these things; even Turgenev's (1948) Bazarov (in my opinion) committed suicide.

For Hegel (1905), art lets truth radiate forth; unity and harmony shine brightly through and art gives us a breathing space to feel at one with ourselves and with the world. It tempers and refines our activity in the world. Architecture is the least adequate. Sculpture reconciles humanity with nature but it cannot contain complex human experience. Painting offers us illusory space so it can bring us farther toward transcendence. Music is restricted to feeling. Poetry is the best for these purposes, but it forms the limit of art as art, said Hegel, and so due to this limit art inevitably evolves toward religion and then eventually into philosophy. Hegel erroneously stated that art had reached its end because it no longer expressed the deep interests of humanity in our civilization; this conclusion was reached because he incorrectly maintained that art was inevitably dialectically replaced by religion and eventually philosophy (see Biezer, 1993, p. 369). For Hegel, art, religion, and philosophy are outside history and represent for each age the form of self-awareness attained by Spirit through its objective striving for self-actualization.

Although Hegel was not a relativist and he believed that Truth is universal and eternal, he was the pioneer thinker who began historicism as a method of philosophy to be used against the pretenses and illusions of systems of philosophy before his time and their claims to have reached Truth. So thoughts, ideas, and concepts by which we think about the world, the subject matter of philosophy, undergo constant development and transformation; even the object of thought is not given to us but is created by our thinking about it, a view exactly opposed to Plato. Hegel claimed that laws or values once believed to be eternal are culturally relative, and are stages in the unfolding of Spirit, and the same is true for ideas that were once thought to be innate. Institutions that were once thought of as having supernatural origin are now seen to be culture-bound. Entities reified as independent of human consciousness are actually the product of the unconscious; intuitions that were once thought due to intrinsic genius are the products of education and culture, and no one can create a presuppositionless philosophy. In his lectures on aesthetics Hegel (1905) maintained that art offers metaphysical knowledge by revealing Truth through perception, but it is inadequate because there are conceptual modes higher than the sensory perception that is central to the appreciation of art. Artistic beauty needs to be understood in historical terms, said Hegel, because the context in which art is produced is indispensable, and we must always examine the purpose of the production of art by any given artist at any given time.

The Curve of Life

Schopenhauer (1970) presupposed that society is a network of latent hostility and reciprocal ill will (Safranski, 1990). Dostoevsky (1872) maintained that the whole second half of a person's life is most often made up only of habits accumulated during the first half. Maugham (1992) said that the central problem of human life is the step-by-step abandonment of ideals, a process that enables one to attain total realism. In his novel, which borrows its title (Of Human Bondage) from Part IV of Spinoza's (1955) Ethics but presents an entirely different philosophy, the protagonist Philip is the symbol of a man born into a society that indoctrinates him with what Maugham considered to be illusions, such as Christian theology and morals, and the idea that happiness is the greatest good. Because he is crippled and intelligent, society appears to him in an unmasked light, enabling him to cast off these illusions.

Freud also became increasingly pessimistic in his older years. He believed correctly that happiness arises from loving and being loved, but he recognized that such a state also makes one the most vulnerable. Freud said one must continuously re-win serenity in the unceasing struggle of life, but he added, "life at my age is not easy, but spring is beautiful and so is love" (Schur, 1972, p. 480). Feibleman (1982), in a gloomy look at the twilight of

Western civilization, stressed the senselessness of human life that to some individuals seems apparent when one reaches old age, and he emphasized the importance of self-containment. Life is a long process of the decreasing of one's options; the road gets narrower and narrower. He expressed a kind of wry despair about the modern world.

Others have offered a much more upbeat attitude for the second half of life. Churchill insisted, "Never, never, give in" (Manchester, 1983, p. 7). He made no concession to weakness and no complaint of fatigue, even though he suffered all his life from depression, fathomless gloom, and fits of rage as well as probable alcoholism. He knew how to stand alone and clung tenaciously to his ambitions. He needed outer excitement to ward off melancholia, and the only subject that really interested him was himself. He claimed that one should never abandon life because there is a way out of everything except death.

Einstein (Sayen, 1985) said that a teacher must love his subject and bring it to life, and that only a life lived for others is a life worthwhile at any age. The psychoanalyst Greenson (1992) wrote that at the age of sixty-three one's friends and colleagues begin to die, which means that one had better enjoy one's family, one's friends, and the activities one loves, and provide time for quiet work. He felt the latter was very important in aging successfully.

After one has a coronary occlusion as did Greenson, one asks whether one should change, what is important and what is trivial, what gives the greatest pleasure, and what one will not give up even if there is a risk of further disease. Greenson suggested that one must be more selective, do more of what is enjoyable, productive, and worthwhile, treasure one's loved ones more, work effectively, do good for others, and help one's children. I believe the issue Greenson did not address is *how* to achieve this help while protecting the independence and autonomy of one's children, to render the aid with "no strings attached" consciously or unconsciously. From the age of sixty on, death is a steady companion, he said. For Greenson the key to old age is whether one will face the day with zest, vigor, and vitality, and whether one will take up activities one never had the time for and explore new areas of pleasure. One must adaptively meet change and endure pain and defeat. In order to do this one must be honest with one's self about one's abilities, capacities, and limitations. He concluded that it takes courage, honesty, and modesty to grow old with dignity.

Ezra Pound's older years were a good example of disastrous failure to negotiate the curve of life in its second half, and Barry's demise represented a similar tragic failure. When psychiatrists were interviewed about aging (Pollock, 1992), they agreed that reminiscence in old age is an adaptive ego function and helps maintain identity and self-esteem in a civilization that discards old people like Kleenex. Some of Pollock's subjects got tired of doing much professionally when they passed the age of sixty-five because they were unwilling to endure the output of energy and the sacrifice of other activities it required:

> So, it came to pass that after more than forty stimulating, re-warding years with every minute filled I began to feel tired of doing so much professionally. The output of energy and the sacrifice of other activity no longer seemed worth while and I wanted a different pace with more variety in my activity, al-though not "retirement" in the meaning of doing little or nothing. This difference in perspective between sixty-five and seventy is not unusual, I find. It may be identified as transient, or as a sign of a disease for which treatment is sought. Sometimes it is vigorously denied and provokes ob-vious attempts to recapture a lost youthful elan. I think such different perception of self may be an early endopsychic awareness of definite physiological alterations with concur-rent psychological responses. In fact, it may be a relatively dependable sign of the phase specific aging process. (Clower, 1992, p. 81)

Pollock's (1992) respondents seemed to feel that aging was espe-cially difficult for the mental health professional, and this is il-lustrated in the case of Barry. Pollock concluded that one should know what one wants and "if you can and as long as you can, ig-nore the passing years, and surrounding yourself with knowledge of your mortality, travel on as if you have forever" (p. 223).

The sixth decade is when the finitude of life is realized acutely and painfully. One's coping style tends to change. Galatzer-Levy and Cohler (1993) emphasized the tendency in males to become more passive, develop alcoholism and somatic complaints, and become interested in young adoring women. The midlife crisis occurs as one realizes the loss of options and regrets not having used them, a feeling of having missed life, leading to chronic depression and/or subtle despair. For example, parents are forced to doubt their performance as parents and have to receive the condemnation of society when their children turn out badly or are less successful than hoped and expected.

All this is illustrated in a novel by Klíma (1993), who asked, "But what is one to answer when one has never found sufficient freedom or courage, and one has allowed the light that maybe once burned within one to go out?" (p. 361). He emphasized the problem of people whose whole life consisted of doing things because someone else wanted them to do it and in order to oblige other people. He suggested one should live one's life in such a way that one would enjoy meeting one's self. Klíma reminded us that one cannot climb out of one's own life or start over regardless of how many resolutions and assessments one makes, such as those Barry packed into his repetitive jottings. So, as might be expected, Barry had copied into his notebook the comment from Iain Pears' (1998) novel, *An Instance of the Fingerpost*, "It is cruel that we are granted the desire to know, but denied the time to do so properly. We all die frustrated; it is the greatest lesson we have to learn" (p. 554).

Similarly, the novels of Anita Brookner (1994) deal with the late part of the curve of life, with people who wait too long and who fear old age not merely for itself but for its humiliations: "Time gave one an initial endowment which it then progressively canceled, and Time's ally Nature equally progressively imposed humiliations" (p. 159). How true! The great American transcendentalist Emerson emphasized the ecstatic experience as being outside of time and believed as he became older that the universe and human life were essentially tragic. As Freud said at the age of sixty-five in a letter to his son, "A peaceful old age appears to be as much of a fable as a happy youth" (Newton, 1995, p. 246).

One should never forget, however, that the search for transcendence goes on throughout life and, in the words of that tragic genius Oscar Wilde (1988), in his play *Lady Windermere's*

Fan, "We are all in the gutter, but some of us are looking at the stars" (p. 59). In order to understand the phenomena of the next chapter, the later poetry of Ezra Pound and the final writings of Barry and their later life events, it is necessary to keep in mind the important and vital discrepancy between the deterioration of the body and the closing of options in old age on the one hand, and the flickering flame that remains in some individuals, motivating them to continue looking at the stars, on the other. For example, Alfred North Whitehead's retirement from the Department of Mathematics at Cambridge offered him time in London and then, after the age of sixty-three at Harvard, to develop one of the most significant metaphysical systems of the twentieth century (Schilpp, 1941). So it is possible that old age can even offer a certain repose that permits the individual to release his or her creative capacities in an artistic direction; these capacities may have been kept inhibited because of the demands of middle age and youth to meet with the everyday exigencies of living and raising a family.

Another antidote to the pessimism of some of these authors about old age is found in the example of the not so rare individual who even in his or her nineties can continue running a major business and immerse himself or herself in financial activities or community and voluntary organizational work. The only limitation on this kind of old age is one's health; as long as it holds up there is no reason why the individual cannot go forward seeking ciphers of transcendence or losing himself or herself in commitments of all sorts, including religion or business or academic pursuits to the end of one's life.

The secret of success is in the commitment. So, using the self psychology channel, Basch (1980) wrote, "The hallmark of depression is the sense or the attitude that life is meaningless— an indication that the perception of the self is no longer a unifying focus for ambitions and ideals" (p. 136). Basch believed the various symptoms manifested in a depressive or dysthymic disorder are efforts to get around a sense of helplessness and to get assistance in restoring some kind of meaning to one's life or, in Basch's terms, "to recapture a sense of direction for the self" (p. 136) . His comments about "George and Betty" are quite relevant to Barry's predicament:

George had been raised to be a perfectionistic, obedient little boy who worked hard for approval, and in adulthood he was filled with rage and shame when he failed to achieve preferment and recognition. Betty was much more easy-going, able to enjoy the moment, and take pleasure in a situation for itself. Unlike George, she did not take herself so seriously and react to every situation as if it were a mirror that showed her either in a favorable or in an unfavorable light. (p. 158)

Galatzer-Levy and Cohler (1993) explained, "Anne Frank used her diary as an essential other, maintaining her courage and capacity to face each day, just as the residents of the Venice senior center . . . had their stories, rituals, and concerns for each other. Similarly, Mary Hamilton . . . horribly alone in a frontier region, remained sane by keeping a diary" (p. 337). Not only can the diary serve as an essential other, but religious rituals can be extremely important in maintaining the integrity of the sense of self even in very great old age. In this book I try in a phenomenologic approach to focus on the presence or absence of various factors that foster morale and inspire a sense of coherence through cultural and aesthetic participation. This phenomenologic point of view differs sharply from the Freudian perspective in that it emphasizes the inestimable self-cohesive value of myths and religion and art instead of concentrating on and exploring the irrational and infantile factors in religious rituals and artistic production, which of course are also important, and surely appear when one listens on the traditional psychoanalytic channel.

Using the self psychology channel, Galatzer-Levy and Cohler (1993) concluded, "Essential others constitute the central means by which people maintain meaning, personal integrity, and morale" (p. 357). They emphasized the centrality of society in culture and in individual human life, rather than the usual alternatives of religion or the mechanistic rationality of the Enlightenment. Religion, they said,

attributes significance to human experience based on its relationship to an overarching, intrinsically valuable, ultimate reality. But this position has been difficult to maintain because it is so hard to find convincing evidence for meaning and value outside of human activity, and the clarification of the nature of the material world has interfered with the most satisfying anthropomorphic pictures of the deity, leaving would be believers a choice between ever more abstract visions of God and the active suspension of concerns for contradictions between scientific data and religious precepts. (pp. 357-358)

I believe these authors did not recognize the enormous capacity people have, when necessary, for maintaining entirely contradictory beliefs side by side in their psyche without anxiety or conflict when they need to do this. I have already discussed at length in Chapters 5 and 11 the failure of mechanistic rationality as a way for humans to maintain meaning, personal integrity, and morale, that is, the failure of the project of the Enlightenment. Let me turn now to further description and exploration of the failures of Ezra Pound and Barry as a function of their psychopathology, utilizing all five psychoanalytic listening channels whenever possible.

14 THE INTRUSION OF MENTAL ILLNESS

Perhaps you know me well enough by now to realize that I see the major issue of life not in the terms of the outcome of the struggle for dominance, but in the terms of the outcome of the struggle to maintain active creativeness. Creativeness, however, depends in the last analysis on the ability to be in touch with the playful child deep in the personality, and thus on the ability to maintain the freshness of the child's encounter with the world. All mature creativity . . . depends on our capacity to encourage the growth of that inner freedom.

—Heinz Kohut, The Curve of Life

I have always found the tortuous writings of Kohut to be exciting, stimulating, and highly influential in my practice of psychoanalysis and intensive psychotherapy. Even his published lectures (Kohut, 1996) show a certain charisma, while at the same time he preserves a chilly, distancing formality. There is something about the way Kohut communicated that is not usually present in the writing of his followers or of most psychoanalysts, who tend to be more scholastic and focused on less interesting minutiae. Somehow Kohut managed to place in psychoanalytic perspective the grand sweep of our culture of narcissism (Lasch, 1978) and the development of what he called Tragic Man, earning credit for a major creative accomplishment.

A whole variety of clinical phenomena such as various addictions, perversions, eating disorders, personality disorders in general, and even borderline and psychotic states may be discussed from an orientation that rests on Kohut's notion of the self, what I referred to in Chapter 3 as the self psychology channel. In the writings of self psychologists, the precise definitions of concepts such as "nuclear self" and "fragmentation" are never clear, but anyone who investigates his or her own life experiences is well aware that these concepts have immediate application. A number of hitherto unexplained phenomena, such as why the ego in the perversions should be so helpless against those perverse urges whereas it is comparatively more in charge of the genital drive and why delay can be tolerated so much less easily in perversions and addictions than it can be with regard to the same person's genital drive, become explainable and fall neatly into Kohut's conceptual framework (see Goldberg, 1995).

Although there is an ambiguity about what Kohut considered to be the curative factors in psychoanalysis, because sometimes he maintained that empathic understanding and explaining the genetics and the dynamics of the patient's disorder of the self constitute the essence of the treatment and at other times he claimed empathy itself is curative, all of this influences the way one practices psychoanalytic therapy. In contrasting his view with that of Kernberg (1975, 1976, 1980), Kohut complained that Kernberg's approach rests on the Kleinian view of the baby as evil and a powder keg of envy, rage, and destructiveness. Aggression in Kernberg's view is something that must be expressed, tamed, and sublimated, whereas for Kohut it is secondary to lack of empathic responsiveness.

Kohut's (1994) attitude of urging the analyst to consider the greatest possible number of explanatory configurations (pp. 110-111) is compatible with my (Chessick, 1992a) five-channel approach to psychoanalytic listening described in Chapter 3, and is especially important when determining whether one is dealing with a narcissistic personality disorder or an individual who has regressed from crucial oedipal conflicts to a narcissistic defensive organization. Patiently waiting and examining the unfolding of the transference yields the answer in each case, said Kohut, and I believe he is correct.

I find Kohut's concept of the nuclear self parallel to Sartre's notion of the basic project, and to my knowledge there has been little published comparing and contrasting Kohut's concept with the emphasis Sartre placed on the unique basic project developed by every individual and which can only be completely understood retrospectively. It must be kept in mind when examining an individual's apparent basic project that what appears to be a strong narcissistically invested self actually can represent a false self that has been developed out of the grandiose expectations of the mother (or father), while the person's true or nuclear self has remained deeply repressed and enfeebled. This involves a person in great difficulties. For example, Kohut discussed the mother who is unable to respond to the child's increasingly independent self, responding instead to the child's physical needs, gratifying the drives continuously but not permitting a mirroring of the whole child. Such individuals as adults become fixated on drives because their budding selves were overlooked and not responded to, and drive gratification becomes an antidepressive and compulsive necessity. Such use of the drives is compared by Kohut to eating with a gastric fistula, since it never achieves the formation of structure but only temporarily restores narcissistic equilibrium. It is this endless search for the restoration of narcissistic equilibrium that superimposes itself on the sexual pleasure involved in the perversions (Goldberg, 1995), or in the eating disorders, or alcoholism, and gives these activities such an incredible predominance in the life of the individual.

Walter Benjamin

An outstanding example of Kohut's concept of Tragic Man, as well as an extreme illustration of the thesis presented in this book that psychopathology seriously constricts if not entirely destroys creative capacity, is found in the story of Walter Benjamin. He was a brilliant German-Jewish literary critic who showed self-defeating tendencies at a very early age. When Hitler rose to power he fled to France, and his friends attempted to bring him to Jerusalem or New York, but he resisted all such efforts. After the fall of France he struggled through innumerable places of refuge and finally tried to escape to Spain. When the Spanish at first refused him and two other companions permission to enter their country, he injected himself with a fatal dose of morphine. The next day his two companions were allowed into Spain.

He carried with him at the time a heavy briefcase which contained the manuscript of what was to be his major work, *The*

Parisian Arcades, a historical critique that was probably some sort of mixture of Marxism, mysticism, theology, and metaphysics. Throughout his flight he clung to this briefcase with its precious manuscript as his selfobject, like a child with its treasured toy among displaced refugees. Benjamin was truly a man of letters, so rare in our era. His (Benjamin, 1994) correspondence contains scholarly analyses of ideas, books, and articles, multiple suggestions for future projects, and all sorts and kinds of literary criticism and cultural studies. Yet Benjamin, who seems to have been a severely obsessive individual, finished very few of these projects, in some ways flitting from creative idea to creative idea as Pound does in his cantos.

Benjamin's reputation was rescued after his death by a few devoted individuals. His letters (Benjamin, 1994) reveal him as fragmenting more and more in his isolation as he moved furtively from place to place to avoid capture and the inevitable subsequent concentration camp. In addition, he shifted from his focus on theological, metaphysical, and mystical themes to a spurious sort of Marxism that was not accepted by anybody. In 1930 the scholar Gerhard Scholem, who was probably his best friend, wrote to him, "Given how your life is constituted, it is certain that you, more than any other person, will always arrive at some place other than where you intended" (Benjamin, 1994, p. 364).

In many ways Benjamin was the model of Kohut's Tragic Man and yet he was able to produce some remarkable cultural and critical documents in a fragmentary form under the worst possible conditions. Parini (1997) presented a biography of Benjamin in the form of a novel that illustrated quite well the constricting effect of Benjamin's obsessive psychopathology on his capacity to create and bring his creative work to fruition. It is even doubtful if *The Parisian Arcades* ever would have been completed had Benjamin lived, since he was almost never satisfied with any of his own work. Sadly for Western civilization, the briefcase containing his precious manuscript has never been found. Benjamin suffered from an even more extreme form of the destruction of creativity by psychopathology than that demonstrated by the career of Ezra Pound. I will now turn to the autumn of Pound's career, at a time when he found himself alienated and alone in Italy during World War II.

Pound as Traitor

The outbreak of World War II begins a period of Pound's most reprehensible behavior. He volunteered to speak over the Fascist Italian radio, and he began a long series of virulent broadcasts marked primarily by anti-Semitism and innumerable slurs on the United States government and President Roosevelt, whom he regarded as a tool of the Jews. In January 1940 Cantos LII-LXXI were printed, but only in a thousand copies in England and a thousand in the United States. These cantos reflect his confusion between Confucian ethics and Eleusinian and sexual mysteries, which Confucius would surely have disapproved of. They are spattered with anti-Semitism and abuse, and again in this 1940 batch many parts are simply incomprehensible, suffering from a fragmentary approach to material that makes it impossible for the reader to have any sense of historical cause and effect. Carpenter (1988) concluded, "The impression prevails that Ezra did little more than rush through his source-material, picking out randomly such economic or political facts as appealed to him. At times, he even admits to being bored himself" (p. 572).

There followed a weird episode in Italy between Ezra Pound and the conservative philosopher George Santayana. Pound could not accept the fact that Santayana had no wish to collaborate with him or to be one of his disciples. He pushed himself upon Santayana, visiting without invitation and writing many letters in spite of very few responses. Although Santayana shared his anti-Semitic views and was also pro-Fascist, he was very detached, uninvolved, and aloof in contrast to the strident aggressiveness of Pound. In 1937, when Pound was fifty-two and thrust himself on Santayana, the philosopher was already seventy-four years old, and he soon became convinced that Pound was completely mad. Pound, with his poor reality testing, mistook Santayana's distant courtesy for cordiality and approval (for details see McCormick, 1987).

Pound became increasingly strident and repulsive in his remarks, writings, and broadcasts. He remained isolated in Rapallo, where the only predominant source of news was the heavily censored Italian and German media. When he listened to the BBC he could not believe what he heard. He also began publishing articles on economics in the Fascist (and some Japanese) newspapers, where his articles were almost always placed on the front page alongside speeches by major Fascists. But the editor of the Italian paper had the impression that Pound was an amusement, a bizarre poet, and not a serious authority.

Friends began to notice that Pound was somewhat out of control, and there seemed to be almost a manic intensity to his efforts to get on the Italian radio and change the world by his speeches. He sounded very unusual with his many strange speech mannerisms when he began his serious broadcasts in 1941, and numerous listeners began to believe that Pound was insane. The payment he received for these talks helped to make up for the fact that he could no longer receive money from his wife's inheritance in England due to the war. His broadcasts were bizarre, manifesting the numerous idiosyncratic pronunciations and peculiarities that have been described previously, and it is quite obvious that no one listening could have been persuaded to change allegiances by Pound's absurd, slanderous, downright vulgar, and disgusting commentary, which at times was so obscure as to be unintelligible and at other times sounded like the worst type of racial and religious hatred. The theme, however, was clear. He hated the Jews, he hated the American and English governments, and he supported the Axis powers in World War II to the best of his ability on these radio broadcasts. Nothing could hold him back; his reality testing was so impaired that he proposed to print his broadcasts and make them available in England and America where, he assumed, they would have a profound impact.

The broadcasts in many ways mirrored the cantos. They flitted from subject to subject, with all sorts of images from Pound's personal life mixed in with crackpot economic theory and slanderous statements about racial and religious groups. He did not seem to be aware that what he was doing would constitute treason. Also, "anti-Semitism was the chief motif of one of Ezra's 1941 broadcasts . . . As the war and the broadcasts went on, he seemed to feel less need to mince matters about the Jews" (Carpenter, 1988, p. 594). He began to sign letters with "Heil Hitler."

Although it is true that there were American organizations at the time that had the same prejudices as Pound, they were not broadcasting over the enemy radio and advocating the Axis cause. Even the Italians did not understand why he was bothering to interest himself in economics and why he was undertaking the broadcasts. It seems clear that by this time he was suffering from grandiose delusions and living in a world largely of his own construction.

From December 7, 1941, Pound's broadcasts led to his being accused of treason against the United States, since our country was now at war with Germany, Italy, and Japan. He seems never to have entertained the possibility that legal charges might be brought against him and he insisted that he was simply exercising his right of freedom of speech, without any apparent recognition of the reality of what he was doing. Hemingway suggested in a letter to Archibald MacLeish that Pound should shoot himself and that he probably should have done so after publishing the twelfth canto, or maybe earlier.

Although he was aware of what was being done to the Jews in Germany, Pound felt this was for the public good, and he completely accepted the truth of that notorious anti-Semitic, fake *Protocols of the Elders of Zion,* which he urged his listeners to read.

On July 26, 1943, Pound was formally indicted for treason by a federal grand jury in Washington, DC. No one reading his broadcast transcripts can doubt that he was mentally unbalanced, his reality testing was seriously impaired, that he was aiding and abetting the causes of anti- Semitism and Fascism, and what little effect his broadcasts had was certainly against the Allied war effort. He continued these broadcasts even after the downfall of Mussolini. When the Allies landed and the Germans invaded Italy, Pound headed north to stay with his daughter Mary, who was living in Gais up in the Tyrol, a 450-mile journey he made by himself.

After Mussolini was abducted by the Germans and the Salò Republic was set up by the Germans, the deportation of Jews began; over 10,000 Jews were arrested by Christmas 1943. Most of them were deported to Auschwitz and murdered. But Pound contacted the officials of the Salò Republic as soon as it was set up and asked to broadcast again, which he did at first in person and later by scripts that were read by others. He also found a Fascist bi-weekly journal that was willing to print his articles.

As the Allies began their victorious march up the Italian boot, Olga Rudge, Dorothy Shakespear, and Ezra Pound were in an extremely precarious financial and psychological situation. They found it difficult to find food, and they all lived together in Sant'Ambrogio. Olga and Dorothy had a cold hatred for each other, producing a poisonous atmosphere for all three of them. Pound wrote Canto LXXII and LXXIII in 1944 in Italian at that time, but Pound's family preferred to keep these out of sight because, as a take-off on Dante, they cursed the "shit" of multi-Allied forces, the Jews, and so forth.

Pound wrongly assumed that the Italians would bravely fight for the Axis cause, but the reality was that between 1943 and 1945 strong partisan groups were attacking the Germans and aiding the Allies. In spite of all this and the collapse of the Fascist government, he continued to write articles on economics for the newspapers. He was arrested by the Italian partisans as a traitor and taken away, slipping a copy of Confucius in his pocket.

Surprisingly, they did not shoot him but released him. As an aftermath of this episode he decided to surrender to the Americans. Still grandiose, he expected that he would swiftly be taken to Washington to impart to the Americans his alleged detailed knowledge of the Italian situation and explain to them what he decided was the true nature of the international war of Jewish usurers against humanity, hoping preferably to speak directly to the President. He was surprised to discover that the president in January 1946 was Harry Truman, not Roosevelt. Pound was now fifty-nine years old, he was not senile, and he was strongly in favor of Hitler and Mussolini, openly expressing his contempt for Stalin, Churchill, and Roosevelt. He began shifting his story to concentrate on his hatred of usury, because it was obvious that his advocacy of Hitler and Mussolini was going over very badly with the Allied officials.

When he was handcuffed he thought he was going to be put on a plane to the United States, but instead he was placed in a prison camp in the maximum security compound in Pisa. He was kept in a cage with stout wooden frames and strong steel mesh so he could be under continuous observation to prevent suicide or escape. The steel mesh in his cage was reinforced; he considered it to be a gorilla cage and felt proud of the fact that he was being treated like a dangerous criminal. The treatment was unnecessarily cruel, in that he was not protected against the weather and not able to go out for exercise like the other prisoners. It gradually dawned on him that no plane was waiting to take him to Washington. All night long powerful floodlights poured into his cage. He immersed himself in Confucius. The cruelty of being exposed to the elements was assuaged by his conviction that eventually he would be sent to Washington where he could exonerate himself.

Pound was a clever prisoner who made efforts to exercise himself and preserve what sanity he had; his eyes became inflamed and he began losing weight very fast. Two psychiatrists at this time in Pisa reported that he was circumlocuitous but exhibited no paranoia, delusions, or hallucinations. They felt he was simply anxious and tremulous due to the environment in which he was being forced to live. They feared such an environment would precipitate a mental breakdown, so they at least had some idea Pound already showed preliminary symptoms of psychosis. Because of this he was moved into the medical compound and given a tent to live in. He seemed obsessed with economics and under severe pressure of speech whenever anyone attempted to interview him. Using an old broom handle as a walking stick, he went endlessly around the perimeter of the medical compound to the point where he wore a path in the grass; there is again a hint here of hypomanic behavior. He was allowed to use a typewriter and soon ingratiated himself with both prisoners and authorities because of his skill with words.

In this setting he wrote *The Pisan Cantos LXXIV-LXXXIV*, with allusions to the previous cantos and expressing regret for the downfall of Mussolini. Enormous controversy has developed over what Pound was trying to express in these *Pisan Cantos*. It is a mistake to think they express remorse or any attempt at contrition; any sadness in them is more related to Pound's realization that Fascist Italy would not be the place where he could build his political and economic dream: "For this worldly dream, Ezra begins now to substitute his own ideal city or community of the mind, chiefly expressed in mythological terms" (Carpenter, 1988, p. 672).

Phenomenologically we experience here a withdrawal into the poet's own private mental world where he attempts, by exploring his own mind and memory (he has no library or books available in this place except Confucius), to search for a perfect city. This is one reason why there are a plethora of personal memories and references that make up the greater part of *The Pisan Cantos.* Canto LXXXI, containing the famous "Pull down" stanzas, again amazingly reaches the height of poetic achievement. My view is that as Pound gradually realized he had been out of contact with reality in his hopes about Facism producing an ideal state, and as he endured the painful physical experiences of his captivity, there was a temporary cohesion of his self that enabled him to get in touch once more with his genius, perhaps for the last time. Kohut (1978) repeatedly described patients on the verge of fragmentation, who pull themselves together by suffering or inflicting upon themselves pain such as body mutilation, head banging, and so on, that seems to have a temporary consolidating effect on the sense of self. I have also experienced such individuals in my clinical work with borderline patients (Chessick, 1977b, 1997c).

Pound followed up *The Pisan Cantos* with some idiosyncratic Confucian translations that he entitled "The Unwobbling Pivot" (see Chapter 2) and, his sixtieth birthday having come and gone, he now became gradually depressed. In November 1946, Pound was returned to the United States to stand trial on his indictment for treason. No one reading the transcripts of his radio broadcasts (Doob, 1952) can have anything but a sense of revulsion mixed with the feeling that Pound was completely out of touch with reality. Enmeshed in his grandiosity, Pound did not seem to understand what he was doing, and out of the same grandiosity he did not seem to realize how offensive and vicious were his statements. A good legal case was possible to justify his permanent incarceration or even his execution.

A good case can also be made that Ezra Pound defies classification in *DSM-IV;* his pathology can be much better explained as slippage back and forth on the ego axis, as described in Chapter 1. Ackroyd (1987) observed, "The general effect of reading the [broadcast] transcripts is devastating: rambling, Jew-baiting, self-deluded, often sickeningly brutal" (p. 85). Further, Ackroyd maintains that in *The Pisan Cantos* "the obscurity is often portentous and clumsy: madness, at least Pound's madness, is saying what he means without reference to any other context, whether social or linguistic" (p. 90). Heymann (1976) reported that even *Poetry* disclaimed Pound, "denouncing him as a supporter of the enemy, if not an outright traitor. . . . Pound seemed to revel in his role, enjoying immensely the attention and notoriety he was receiving" (p. 103); "his radio speeches elicited the same shock and sensation among the intelligentsia as did his previous cavalier theories on literature and the arts" (p. 103).

Many have noted the relationship between Pound's treatment in Pisa and the sudden temporary reopening of his creative life. This man on whom the sun went down (as Pound described himself) was somehow able, after he collapsed when he realized the peril of his situation, to communicate with a passion and a personal poetic power in a way different from the previous cantos. Tytell (1987) argued that *The Pisan Cantos* release feeling, while the earlier cantos preserved an attitude of Jamesian restraint, in which feelings were qualities that other people had, and one never articulated them or exhibited them: "In the final inferno, Pound's pain and the openness about it made that hell full of dimension and reality" (p. 281). He concluded that *The Pisan Cantos* remind us, "Pound's greatest strength as a poet was his lyricism, an ability to register sharp pictures of nature which evoke feeling" (p. 282).

Mullins (1961) defended Pound's behavior, considering him the only individual who attempted to stop the war and refused to become a barbarian. He wrote,

> The Radio Rome broadcasts contain much interesting biographical and philosophical material of Pound's which is not presently available elsewhere. Perhaps a volume of these broadcasts, which are of as great interest as his published letters, will be issued in the future. When I read some of the texts of these broadcasts, after having known Pound some five years, I was surprised at how much of this material continued to reappear during our daily talks. . . Some of the material appears in the *Cantos*. (pp. 204-205)

So much for the idea that Pound later recanted or regretted what he had to say over the Rome radio. The reader interested in this controversy is advised to read the transcripts of Pound's broadcasts (Doob, 1952). For example, according to Stock (1970),

The Jews were a favorite subject: the Jews who were behind Roosevelt, the Jews who were ruining England, the Jewish religion. . . . "Don't start a pogrom," he said on 30 April, 1942, "that is, not an old style killing of small Jews. . . .Of course, if some man had a stroke of genius and could start a pogrom up at the top. . . there might be something to say for it. . . . The sixty kikes who started this war might be sent to St. Helena, as a measure of world prophylaxis, and some hyper-kikes or non-Jewish kikes along with them." (p. 394)

Stock concluded, "Whatever his intentions were, some of his words must have sounded highly treasonable coming from an enemy station in wartime" (p. 395).

But consider this: If Pound, who described Hitler as a martyr, would have been shot by the partisans, we would not have *The Pisan Cantos:* "Out of a life of bright achievement and miserable failure he rescued the rare pieces and the broken columns, transforming them as with the pale light of a late afternoon in autumn. *The Pisan Cantos* are a man of sixty remembering, against a background of life in the Disciplinary Training Centre at Pisa" (Stock, 1970, p. 412). Although there are boring passages in *The Pisan Cantos,* "Unlike earlier sections, the bad passages are seldom tiresome and if we read on we are sure to be rewarded. For, stripped of all but himself and his one mastery, control of speech, he created a world which astonishes and delights, whether it be by sudden shock. . .or by straggling procession, in which dignity and solemnity are matched with neat disorder" (Stock, 1970, p. 413).

There is no better example I can think of than how Pound's harsh treatment in Pisa resulted in a temporary cohesion of the self and the volcanic production of *The Pisan Cantos,* and then his subsequent depressive and quasi-psychotic collapse, to illustrate the difficulties with *DSM-IV*—the importance of understanding psychopathology in terms of shifting back and forth on the ego axis rather than in terms of specific symptoms of a "disease"—and the intimate interrelationship between psychopathology and genius. When Pound shifted to the right on the ego axis he was capable of intense creative activity producing transcendent beauty; when he shifted to the left on the ego axis he demonstrated hypomanic defenses, depressive collapse, ultimate schizo-affective and paranoid psychotic manifestations with a loss of appropriate reality testing and a quasi-psychotic grandiosity. It is this capacity to shift back and forth that caused so much controversy over settling the subsequent fate of Ezra Pound after he was brought back to the United States to face trial on his indictment as a traitor.

Barry as *Flâneur*

The suicide of Walter Benjamin, who fragmented more and more in his forced isolation so that his late productions often read like an S.O.S. from a sinking ship, is considered symbolic of the losing battle fought by an alienated and isolated rational human against the weight of irrational, tyrannical, brutal, fanatic power, an overwhelming practico-inert. Benjamin may be thought of as the last representative of the man of culture, a literate European philosopher and intellectual involved in the pursuit of truth and meaning for its own sake. Neither his grave nor the precious manuscript he carried with him have survived. Attempting to read Benjamin is not easy because his material is very obscure; for this reason it has an attraction for current academics who enjoy immersing themselves in jargon and obscurity, which they seem to equate with profundity. Like Barry, his letters range over a wide spectrum of thinkers, books, various articles he has read, and concepts that he is working out in unpublished form.

Although Benjamin had an auspicious start, even being invited in 1916 when he was only twenty-four to contribute to Martin Buber's journal, and receiving by 1924 important support and encouragement from the famous poet and playwright Hugo Von Hofmansthal, something quite early in his career obviously went wrong. He began sending out frequent announcements of papers he was going to write on every conceivable subject, dispersing his creative energies in all directions rather than focusing them in one or two larger, more integrated achievements. This seems to have had something to do with his wish to feel continuously independent and his disdain or inability to do the ordinary work that is required to bring a creative idea to fruition, as described by Kohut (1978); see the quotation beginning Chapter 10 of the present book.

In Benjamin's (1968) *Illuminations*, he called attention to Balzac's concept of the *flâneur*, the individual aimlessly strolling through crowds in big cities in contrast to the hurried purposeful activity of the people around him. It is to the *flâneur* that Benjamin believed things reveal themselves in their secret meaning, and certainly the arcades of Paris invite such strolling! Barry, as we shall soon discover, had recourse to a similar process in his travels.

Benjamin saw history as a catastrophe showering wreckage upon wreckage. He had a cardiac problem similar to that of Barry. Both were collectors of books and quotations, and both kept notebooks and correspondence filled with much unpublished material. Benjamin had an illusory idea of independence, arguing that persons of letters live in the world of books, do not write for a living, and maintain a detachment from social and political affairs. Barry would not have agreed with this. He often pondered the question raised by Benjamin (1968), whether the artwork withers in our current era as the art object is detached from the domain of tradition, placed in museums alongside of many other works of art from scattered traditions, and reproduced and distributed everywhere through modern methods of communication, now even on the Internet.

When Pound was fifty-four years old he began his broadcasts for the Italian Fascist radio, but he had ahead of him a great creative spurt that appeared in *The Pisan Cantos*. By the time Barry was fifty-four years old his material had become increasingly repetitious, and he was turning more and more to international travel as a *flâneur* to try to find a sense of Spirit that would manifest itself through the common brotherhood of mankind and the community of cultures as it had been envisioned by the founders of the United Nations; an important ideal when it was established during Barry's adolescence. He maintained this ideal throughout the Cold War (which he regarded as an aberration of history), and he was not surprised when the Soviet Union collapsed. It was shortly after the reunification of Germany that he died at the age of sixty-two.

He died convinced that humans cannot live without myths, art, religion, and philosophy, and that Spirit unfolds itself irresistibly through human history, although not through a kind of steady progress but rather through a process of clashing contradictions and over regressive as well as progressive eras. In his last decade of life, his humanistic writing became increasingly repetitious except for the sudden outpouring that produced the play presented in Chapter 16, a composition that in a way summarizes the entire last decade of his thinking.

Whitehead wrote,

> Beauty, moral and aesthetic, is the aim of existence; and . . . kindness and love, and artistic satisfaction are among its modes of attainment. Logic and Science are the disclosure of relevant patterns, and also procure the avoidance of irrelevancies. . .This outlook. . .directs attention to the periods of great art and literature, as expressing the essential values of life. (quoted in Schilpp, 1941, p. 8).

Barry hoped to teach the great works of authors like Whitehead or Freud over and over again. He wanted these texts to be made to come alive, and to develop a living or imaginary ongoing relationship with their authors. The secret of Heidegger's great success as a teacher of philosophy was in his ability to do these things. Barry did not have such ability. He asked,

> What is mind, if anything? What makes it up? What is truth? What is metaphysics and of what use is it? What are values and where do they come from? Why is it that the old "parental shoulds" lose their former reasonableness but not their tyrannical power? Why do people throughout their life always make the same ungratifying choices, culminating in an existence which does not allow pleasure and predisposes them to chronic depression with definite paranoid and obsessive features?

He was convinced that eventually Spirit would somehow unfold itself and there would be a reflowering of humans at some future date beyond his lifetime:

> Humans would have to radically transform into being personally hurt by the condition of others. Actually, humans are now going the other way, as the death of God has removed the last barrier to total self-centeredness. I cling to Platonic values: mathematics, philosophy, music, and truth to be pursued for their own sake, although my lack of talent brings me

no success at these and other practical burdens constantly interfere. Humans have boundless possibilities and it is not necessary to be as pessimistic as Freud. There is too much scatter in my work, no clear plan, no vision of where I want to go. The philosopher who contemplates the κόσμος (cosmos), actually an untranslatable term involving order, becomes κόσμιος, well ordered, moderate, regular, divine and orderly, in his own soul. Thus κόσμος represents perfect arrangement, beauty, the world, and the universe. Philosophy should be studied above all, because through the greatness of the universe philosophy contemplates, the mind is also rendered great and becomes capable of that union with the universe which constitutes its highest goal. So the mind of man can be focused on either κόσμος or on trivia. This is somewhat similar to Heidegger's (1962) concept of an authentic or an inauthentic existence, but with a metaphysical twist. The crucial question remains whether there really is anything besides trivia; of course, Plato said that the existence of mathematics proves there is. The task of education is to pull the mind from preoccupation with fleeting shadows and trivia to κόσμος. Corruption is being pulled the other way.

Barry's unsuccessful struggle with coronary artery disease risk factors went on to the end of his life. He suffered from insomnia, travel anxiety, and a chronic depression, for which he never sought treatment. The last decade of his life was marked by the death of many of his close relatives, almost always from coronary artery disease, as well as the death of a number of his good friends and the retirement and moving away of others. Like Pound, he became increasingly isolated. He was aware of his poor social skills and had a number of experiences with scientific presentations that resulted only in a lack of mirroring and appreciation. He suffered from mild angina but, even though he was a physician, he did nothing about it. Barry was attempting to stem an impending fragmentation and possibly even suicide, which was never very far from his conscious mind: "If I am going to be ignored I might as well contemplate and arrange for κόσμος in my soul. These would be the consolations of Greek ideals of virtue and balance, and I would patiently wait for the end. I should live like an exile, constructing a routine as did the old Prince Bolkónski in Tolstoy's (1868) *War and Peace*."

Barry's psychopathology, which is worth studying from the self psychology channel, is explainable as well on the object relations channel. Kernberg (1980) discussed normal and pathological narcissism in middle age, beginning with Melanie Klein's contention that the successful resolution of excessive envy and rivalry (such as Barry experienced even as a child with his unfortunate girl cousin, described in Chapter 4) are a precondition for normal adjustment to adulthood and old age. An increased narcissistic cathexis of the superego and ego ideal can lead to rigidity, compulsiveness, intolerance, and depression, while a narcissistic cathexis of the ego produces an increased expectation of admiration and self-affirmation. If limits cannot be accepted, one may develop denial, resignation, cynicism, and masochistic self-blame. The acceptance of limits requires the painful realization of where one's creativity will lead next and where it will not.

In middle age the abiding ideals of adolescence are now put to a definite test. If things go well, pleasure in creativity and achievement now fuses with pleasure in giving and dedicating one's self to those one loves and to the ideals for which one stands. One attempts to become "the generous parent" and accept the inevitable loss of power and control that goes with aging and death. In pathological narcissism there is no protective libidinal reserve available, and the individual longs for narcissistic refueling, but lasting satisfaction is never found. Greed becomes relentless and success is quickly spoiled. The defense of denial by hypomanic undertaking of activities that would ordinarily diminish or be restricted by the aging process appears, or a desperate clinging to wealth and possessions ending in a cynicism, bitterness, and distrust that I have previously described as the outcome of corruption in the individual.

Barry also asked, "Why do the abstract disciplines such as mathematics describe the working of nature with such accuracy? Why should long chains of reasoning produce remarkably applicable conclusions?" Like Benjamin, he was spinning his wheels over many questions. He was much more inclined to the Platonism of the mathematical physicist Penrose (1997) than to the reductive materialism of that remarkable mathematical physicist Hawking. As Barry began formulating his play, he remembered Melanie Klein's (1958) statement that "terrifying figures in the deep layers of the unconscious make themselves felt when internal or external pressure is extreme" (p. 243), and Franz Kafka's explanation of neuroses as desperate attempts to find anchorage in no matter what maternal soil.

He listed in his notebooks some of the various "high points" of his travels, for example, leisurely viewing a room full of El Grecos at the Metropolitan Museum of Art (now in Gallery 29) in New York. He added, "When you go over the pieces in the museum's Greek collection only a whisper reaches you from 400 B.C.E. What is impressive is that art and culture were every bit as beautiful and sophisticated as they can be now. Man has not changed in his capacities and potential—and his tragedy." He spent some time in a hotel room with a clear view of the great pyramids of Egypt and also visited Luxor. He found dehumanized tradition and stagnation everywhere in Egypt, symbolized by a shocking, one-legged, no-handed beggar jumping on the street among the cars, asking for money. Barry wrote,

> The great pyramid changes its shades of color all day like Monet's haystacks. School children play in its shadow. Cairo traffic at a deadlock with these silent monuments of death always in the background. The remarkable clarity and cleverness and beauty in the wall paintings and the Sakarra Step Pyramid coming from the first four dynasties. No real improvement since then in Egyptian art. When sitting in front of the Great Pyramid, watching the constantly changing shades of brown, one can hear the grunts and curses of millions of humans crying out from it over the centuries. A feat of unimaginable human sweat and labor. To what end? To leave a permanent human mark on brutish evanescent human life in the boiling sun. A gigantic monument now of jagged stones, rising out of a totally inhospitable desert of shifting sand that stretches over a whole continent.

Beginning with a trip to Mexico, the notebooks are filled with experimental starts and pieces and drafts. For example,

> A beautiful red sunset into the deep blue sea in Puerto Vallarta . . .a dirty sandy primitive road into the jungle dotted by shacks, no electricity, unbelievable squalor,

people just sitting in the shade, especially women and girls. Lush jungle, scrawny banana plants, magnificent parrots, all kinds of colored flowers, but mainly greenery, bushes, and palm trees. The dry season now, a sense of desolation and uninhabitable areas for eighty million people. Soil poor quality, hard to grow crops; an occasional scrawny corn plant. Real poverty and in spite of magnificent scenery and climate of tropics, a problem for humans to thrive.

Barry identified with Krapp of Samuel Beckett's (1960) *Krapp's Last Tape*. Krapp was an unwashed old failure, an unread writer who every year made a tape of the events of the previous 12 months and now reads aloud with sighs and groans and acerbic comments the tape he recorded thirty years ago at the age of thirty-nine. He has bursts of rage and impatience at his young self and at times stops the tape or winds it ahead with laughter. At the age of thirty-nine Krapp says farewell to love in a beautiful passage about himself in a punt with a young woman, and he plays this tape again and again. But Barry did not remember the famous Italian Marxist Gramsci's saying that to beat one's head against the wall is to break one's head and not the wall.

His experiences in Africa as well as those from the Middle East and Greece (see Chapter 16) are incorporated in his play. In Japan, he felt that the Great Buddha of Kamikura, a very impressive thirteenth-century bronze cast, was one of the first objects with spiritual meaning he observed. The Hiroshima Peace Park, a monument to man's inhumanity to man and the unspeakable evil of war, overshadowed everything in Japan. He visited the Ryoanji Zen temple and its famous rock garden with a twelfth-century pond, and then the Koryo-Ji temple, a museum in which he watched a light play on the Miroku Bsatsu, a most delicate seventh-century statue:

> If there was any sense of religion at the altar before this statue, there it should have been. To me the sensation was primarily aesthetic, a truly beautiful and delicate object, the best of a number of superb wood carvings in this museum. But not of any Western-style transcendence; pri-

marily these are a pantheon of gods and idols. Of course Easterners would not agree.

He concluded something was wrong in current Japanese civilization:

> Incredible overcrowding in a beautiful place mixed up with the grafting on of Western materialism which somehow does not integrate with Buddhist and Shinto practices. A continual ambiguity, a blurring of reality, a confusion of practices, keeping true messages and thoughts concealed, all constitute a different form of thought. The cutting edge of Japan is changing, becoming more international and slowly developing a more realistic approach and away from insularity and fooling themselves.

When the sun came out over Mount Fuji he saw a high-towering peak, not so flat on top as Mount Kilimanjaro but equally as snow-covered: "The apparition rose like a god just as my daughter and I were discussing her need to be among artists, even though they are notoriously unstable and can hurt her. She said Paris is out of date, and the future belongs to Japan and the Pacific Rim countries."

Barry believed that humans have the potential either to be species-focused with communal conscience, as Marx thought, or to be totally self-centered, materialistic, and infested with the money spirit (Weber, 1930). Both developments have evolutionary adaptational value. Society shapes humans by bringing out, encouraging, and rewarding one or the other of these potentials but not both, since they basically contradict each other. Harrington (1989), one of the most perceptive and socially conscious writers of our time, pointed out how Aquinas believed in an economic life regulated by justice and not merely a play of the market, but from the time of Luther and afterwards God became more distant, and the Protestant ethic led to the money spirit (p. 267). Society then became an unsocial aggregate of egotistical individuals and forgot the Greek tradition that society has a goal beyond just providing the rules for individual striving.

Hegel said that as Spirit unfolded itself, greater and greater freedom became available, and then society was enabled to help people toward a good quality of life and to unite for the common good. Barry believed, and I agree, that fellowship and global solidarity are needed, along with planned cities and participatory democracy. Unification must occur on the basis of ethical value, not class, and this is consistent with both the French and American revolutions, in contrast to the rampant capitalism that prevails today. In midlife Barry became increasingly concerned about the growing inequality between the rich and poor, the permeation of our culture by military values, the absence of effective international peacekeeping mechanisms, the domination of foreign and domestic policy-making decisions by corporate interests and elites uninterested in democratic processes, the rise of transnational media conglomerates controlling international information and unaccountable to the public, the failure of the conservation of the environment, and the lack of decent health care for all Americans through a system of universal insurance. Even today, in the richest country the world has ever seen, over forty million Americans have no health insurance coverage at all.

But as his last decade moved toward an end, Barry became increasingly preoccupied with death rather than social improvement. He visited the cemeteries where his grandparents and parents were buried and noted, "Here I felt the most eerie, the most eternal, like time has stopped . . .this was *transcendent,* eternity, I am the only person left in the world who fondly remembers the two people that were my parents. When I die they will pass on to utter nothingness in their small graves. I can't get over it. I can't get over the incredible mystery." He remembered the lines from Tennyson's (1886) poem"Locksley Hall 60 Years After":

> In my life there was a picture, she that clasped my neck had
> flown.
> I was left within the shadow, sitting on the wreck alone.
>   (p. 148)

He repeated over and over again to himself the poem "Riders Song," written in 1924 by Frederico García Lorca (1991, p. 447). These continual thoughts of death are woven into Barry's preoccupation with the unknown beloved whom he can never fuse with, as in the beautiful seventeenth-century poems *Exequy* by Henry King (1657, pp. 358-359):

> Stay for me there; I will not faile
> To meet thee in that hollow Vale.

And think not much of my delay;
I am already on the way. . .

The thought of this bids me go on,
And wait my dissolution
With hope and comfort. *Dear* (forgive
The crime) I am content to live
Divided, with but half a heart,
Till we shall meet and never part.

and *Definition of Love* by Andrew Marvell (1681, p. 37):

i

My Love is of a birth as rare
As 'tis for object strange and high:
It was begotten by despair
Upon Impossibility . . .

viii

Therefore the Love which us doth bind,
But Fate so enviously debarrs,
Is the Conjunction of the Mind,
And Opposition of the Stars.

Barry's preoccupation with ecstatic love is best expressed by Ann Sexton's (1981) poem "When Man Enters Woman" (p. 428).

In the final year of Barry's life his first grandchild was born, and the Soviet Union collapsed. Germany voted to make Berlin its capital again, and he visited Germany for the last time. The contemporary German philosopher Gadamer emphasized the importance of Plato's *Seventh Letter,* and Barry agreed that the True and the Good and the Beautiful (aspects of Hegel's Spirit) can only be glimpsed after proper preparation, as Plato (Hamilton and Cairns, 1973) said: "Acquaintance with it must come rather after a long period of attendance on instruction in the subject itself and of close companionship, when, suddenly, like a blaze kindled by a leaping spark, it is generated in the soul and it once becomes self-sustaining" (p. 1589).

Gadamer blamed Heidegger's Nazism on a lack of courage and quoted Schelling on how anxiety decenters a person from himself or herself. He objected to Hegel's dialectical method as too rigid and compartmentalized and, like Heidegger, Gadamer hoped that eventually we would be able to supersede the age of technology. On the road in Germany, Barry wrote,

> The weather cleared, and I could see the Black Forest. (The forest nearer to Heidelberg is the Odenwald, where Hagen killed Siegfried and the Niebelungs dwell). First I saw it immersed in fog and mist, and then the villages appeared among the pine trees which grow even at the top of the hills. So again, with Heidegger, the Black Forest both revealed to me and concealed from me because I never did get to Freiburg. I never got into the Black Forest, I never saw Heidegger's hut, but I can imagine Heidegger in his hut in the forest becoming a mystic, far from the world of technology. Germany is a whole new mystical world, totally different from France, where the sun shines. Heidelberg is wonderful and really grows upon a person. Würzburg of course has the greater art, including the *Residenz* with its marvelous Tiepolo, his gigantic ceiling fresco of *The Four Continents* (all that were known at the time), the final outpouring of Baroque art.

He visited Prague, a gloomy shabby city at the time under the Communist heel. Like Budapest in the same situation, everything was very run down, including the majestic old buildings, some of which were quite beautiful but in a pitiful state. Barry stopped at Frankfurt to change planes and took advantage of the time interval to visit Goethe's house. That was the last time he was able to stroll comfortably through a major European city.

Clearly, Barry was keeping what are ὑπομνήματα (*Hypomnēmata*). This is a type of copybook that was in vogue in Plato's time, carrying quotations, fragments of works, examples and reports of witnessed actions, reflections, and reasonings for a training of one's self by itself. I found there his clumsy translation of lines 357-362 from Sophocles' *Antigone:* "All-resourceful to flee the inhospitable piercing frost under the clear wintry sky, he has contrived to run away from dreadful diseases. He meets with nothing that will be very difficult for him, but death alone he will not devise how to flee." Some other entries were:

- From the Oxford Bible: Proverbs 15:13. "A glad heart makes a cheerful countenance, but by sorrow of heart the spirit is broken." 17:6. "Grandchildren are the crown of the aged." 17:22. "A cheerful heart is good medicine but a downcast spirit dries up the bones."

- From the novelist Davies (1990) : "During your illness I suppose you did a lot of thinking about your situation. That is what these illnesses are for you know—these mysterious ailments that take us out of life but do not kill us. They are signals that our life is going the wrong way, and intervals for reflection . . . To *write:* that is to sit in judgement over one's self" (pp. 433, 448).

- From the *Ajax* of Sophocles, lines 644-648:

Strangely the long and countless drift of time
brings all things forth from darkness into light,
Then covers them once more. Nothing so marvelous
That man can say it surely will not be—
Strong oath and iron intent come crashing down.
        (Grene and Lattimore, 1959, pp. 237-238)

- From *The Iliad,* Book 16, lines 852-853:

ἀλλά τοι ἤδη
ἄγχι παρέστηκεν θάνατος καὶ μοῖρα κραταιή
(Benner, 1931, p. 145)

- From his last trip, to Germany:

At Eisenach one sees the house where probably Bach was born, and the Wartburg Castle shrouded in mist (from *Tannhäuser*), and the rundown houses with their Schreber gardens. On a chilly bright day with the autumn sun beating down and the last brown leaves falling, we struggle through the huge traffic jam on the Autobahn and take the cutoff to Buchenwald. Here are mostly stones, cold, grey, horrible in every respect, showing man's inhumanity to man beyond comprehension. The wife of our German host started to cry and we left. There were groups of teenagers there from German schools and I hope they were listening to their teachers, but I doubt it. Nearby in Jena was the old university where Hegel, Schelling, and Schiller taught. The students at the adjacent new university, when I spoke with them, were not even aware of it. The Goethe house in Weimar is much more interesting than the one in Frankfurt. Goethe had what today would be called a modest collection of art and antiques in various rooms, and a small garden. From this he built a renaissance life. East Berlin now just open and fused with West Berlin to soon produce a city that will be the most magnificent in Europe, perhaps in the world. The *Unter der Linden* is already beautiful with the autumnal ambience and the yellow leaves. Here I met my colleague, Dr. H, who in my fantasy looked like a tank commander in Rommel's desert army, smoked cigarettes incessantly, and was deeply interested in the work of Hegel. The magnificent museum in East Berlin contains artifacts and pieces of a temple stolen from Pergamum in Turkey, a Hellenic temple, and a Babylonian temple of astonishing beauty. There was a remarkable contrast because the Greek work is much more somber and the Babylonian joyful and pleasant, a juxtaposition in this museum of Hegelian opposites. Here our conversation led to the novel *Jennie Gerhardt*, a book where Dreiser (1989) poses the central question, "What was this element in life that could seize and overwhelm one as does a great wind? Why this sudden intrusion of death to shatter all that had seemed most promising in life?" (p. 95)

Proust believed that the writer has two selves. A body of writing is the product of a different self from the one we manifest in our habits, our social life, and our vices. He thought that the act of writing should be a matter of making contact with the deep self, rediscovering it only by abstracting one's self from other people and the self that knows other people. It is the self that has been waiting while one has been with other people, the self one feels is the only real self. Artists end up by living for this alone, like a god whom they cease to ignore and for whom they have sacrificed a life that serves only to honor him. Writing emerges from an underground stream of deep reflectiveness. Meanwhile, the everyday transactions of the creative person are as superficial as those of everybody else. Ibsen said living means fighting within you the ghosts of dark powers; writing is putting on trial your innermost self.

Finally, in Berlin Barry wrote, "At Hegel's grave, an icy abstractness, and yet I feel I have reached the end of my quest, like the Spirit unfolded. It is odd."

15 UNDERSTANDING CREATIVITY

I say unto you: one must still have chaos in oneself to be able to give birth to a dancing star. I say unto you: you still have chaos in yourselves.

It is by invisible hands that we are bent and tortured worst.

You aspire to the free heights, your soul thirsts for the stars. But your wicked instincts, too, thirst for freedom. Your wild dogs want freedom; they bark with joy in their cellar when your spirit plans to open all prisons. To me you are still a prisoner who is plotting his freedom.

But the worst enemy you can encounter will always be you, yourself; you lie and wait for yourself in caves and woods.
— *Friedrich Nietzsche,* Thus Spoke Zarathustra

Nietzsche correctly characterized himself as an enigma that is hard to solve. He compared his life as a lonely ignored outsider to that of the scholar who has adjusted to society, and he presented many masks and experiments with various belief systems. These masks demonstrate his denial of the absolute unity of the personality (Morgan, 1965) . For Nietzsche, nobody is ultimately any one thing, there is no essential self. He would argue that our "sense of self" so emphasized by Kohut is a myth, an illusion, a prejudice.

The curious back and forth movement in Nietzsche between intimately personal comments and significant philosophical thought makes him impossible to classify (Stern, 1979). A man of tremendous intellectual energy who kept starting over, he experienced the world as fragmented and conveyed it to us as such; this experience of fragmentation suggests that Nietzsche belongs in the realm of self psychology. Kohut (1978) wrote that the modern artist heralds the coming fragmentation of his or her civilization, and Nietzsche in his superlative literary prose and poetry clearly heralded the breakup of European civilization in World War I, just as *Les présages*, choreographed in 1932 for *Ballet Russe de Monte Carlo* by Leonid Massine to Tchaikovksy's Fifth Symphony, was an eerie forecast of imminent World War II.

Nietzsche and Freud

Elsewhere I (Chessick, 1981) discussed the relevance of understanding Nietzsche to the study of Freud and Kohut, and I (Chessick, 1983) reviewed Nietzsche's life and work in detail. Nietzsche used letter writing as a substitute for personal contact, and he became increasingly isolated and alienated. It is interesting that, like Heidegger, he was very involved with the poetry of Hölderlin and even called Hölderlin his favorite poet. There is a curious parallel between Nietzsche's course to madness and that of Hölderlin, as well as a parallel situation in which the thoughts and insights of these writers were clearly wrestling with the invading darkness of insanity. Whether the last writings of Nietzsche represent the grandiosity of a psychotic or have philosophical value is disputed. I believe that, like Pound's cantos, they are a mixture of both.

Although there are many statements in Nietzsche's work that seem to have intuitive psychological truth to them, there are other statements that seem incredibly obtuse. Nietzsche stopped barely short of postulating an unconscious area of the mind; he recognized that consciousness is only the tip of the iceberg and that we find reasons for what our instincts want us to do. Nietzsche and Freud agreed that civilization is founded on the suppression of instincts. As Hayman (1980) explained, "It is a point that Robert Musil makes when his man without qualities, Ulrich, observes that if humanity could dream collectively, it would dream Moosbrugger, the rapist-murderer" (p. 301). (See Chessick, 1996c, for a discussion of Musil's work.)

Nietzsche said that in dreams we resemble savages and gratify impulses. Our cognition is unreliable and colored by wishes, as is our memory. Remarkably he (1878) wrote, "The unresolved dissonances between the personalities and dispositions of the parents go on echoing in the child's character, forming the history of his or her inner sufferings" [my translation], and,

"Everyone bears within him a picture of a woman derived from his mother; it is this which determines whether, in his dealings with women, he respects them or despises them or is in general indifferent to them" (p. 150).

Both Golomb (1989) and Ginsberg (1973) depicted the similarities in Nietzsche and Freud involving the unconscious, repression, sublimation, projection, the ego, overdetermination, psychic energy, and the view of dreams as manifestations of the person. But it is misleading to primarily approach Nietzsche as a proto-Freudian, although he was at times a great intuitive psychologist. Nietzsche's focus was quite different from that of Freud. Freud was attempting to develop what he thought of as a scientific medical system, whereas Nietzsche condemned all scientific systems as simplistic "prejudices." It might be better to think of Nietzsche's epistemology as taking a postmodern jump over that of Freud's nineteenth-century epistemology (see Chessick, 1980, for an investigation of Freud's epistemology.)

Nietzsche's prescription for what is necessary for sick humanity—dancing near an abyss and developing a creative life using life-enhancing perspectives—is quite different from Freud's notion of how psychoanalysis cures. Nietzsche's predominant topics were those of perspectivism (see Chapter 17), the disintegration of human life, and the nature of the self; he was immersed in general concerns about the plight of contemporary humanity after the death of God rather than any concern for curing individual psychopathology.

Nietzsche should be compared not with Freud but with Rousseau, who longed for something beyond himself, calling on nature and trying to diagnose and overcome the current mediocrity of his civilization. Freud was not that sort of a visionary, believing much more in the power of reason and science to achieve slow progress. Freud never envisioned a superior form of man, and embraced the pessimistic Schopenhauerian view of human life that Nietzsche dramatically turned away from and tried to counter.

Nietzsche on Creating the Self

Nietzsche offered each of us a horizon of infinite perspectives from which to survey one's life and mold it accordingly (Golomb,

1995). For Nietzsche (1874), the individual is "a thing dark and veiled" (p. 129), using masks over a hollow core. Nietzsche claimed unmasking takes place through looking back on life and asking what one has truly loved and revered. In helping a young person to do this, he said, educators can be liberators. For Nietzsche we are merely drives, memories, and mental states determined by society, and our beliefs are never free from our place in the world (see Tanner, 1996).

In Nietzsche's (1884) *Thus Spoke Zarathustra*, the instinctive self has hegemony over the self-conscious ego, which is never autonomous; Smith (1996) noticed the parallel with Freud's view on this point, but, "*Zarathustra* further asserts that the fervent unconscious wish of the self is to create beyond itself" (p. 102). Freud does not go in that direction in his theories at all, and Kohut would argue that the fervent unconscious wish of the self is to remain as cohesive as possible under stress. But Nietzsche believed that "at the deepest level man is a nothing that must be constituted and reconstituted as a work of art" (Smith, 1996, p. 102). So Nietzsche insisted self-unity has to be created as a work of art; innate nature does not determine the self. For Schutte (1984) this implied that Nietzsche was trying to overcome his own fragmented self; the recovery of the self is Nietzsche's crucial task: "The importance of healing one's fragmentation and self-division is the main life-affirming message imparted by Nietzsche's critique of metaphysics. Without the recovery of the self it is impossible for a person to turn into a genuine free spirit and authentically to affirm life" (pp. 74-75).

Schutte (1984) also criticized Nietzsche's moral and political theory because of his statements involving power and violence, and claimed that his "unsystematic method and enigmatic teachings. . . are bound to generate controversy regarding how he ought to be read" (p. x). Allison (1985) presented a collection of critical essays that similarly stressed the ambiguity of Nietzsche's proclamations. There is no common ground for the interpretation of the work of Nietzsche. As I (Chessick, 1983) pointed out, there are "hard" and "soft" interpretations of Nietzsche's writings. The hard interpreters call him a kind of proto-Nazi emphasizing suffering and cruelty, but the soft interpreters claim his focus is on the artistic creation of the individual, who must by self

overcoming give a meaning to his or her life out of inner
strength. Nietzsche's "Overman" is the rare individual who can
do this; it has nothing to do with that ridiculous Nazi brute, their
fictitious Aryan superman, or Wagner's hero Siegfried, a perpetually adolescent monster.

Many authors insist that it is a great mistake to rely on Nietzsche's unpublished notes later gathered by his demonic proto-
Nazi and dishonest sister and published as *The Will to Power*,
(Nietzsche, 1883-1888), and that doing so will be inevitably misleading. It should be kept in mind that the selection, arrangement, and chapter headings in *The Will to Power* are not the work
of Nietzsche and "contrary to Heidegger . . . the entire thrust of
Nietzsche's work is opposed to the understanding of philosophy
as systematic and system building" (Smith, 1996, p. 39). The notions of "the will to power" and "the eternal return" are not crucial in Nietzsche, claimed Solomon (1988), because they appear
much more in his unpublished notes than they do in his published work. The Overman is mentioned only at some length in
Zarathustra. This view is in direct contrast to that of Heidegger
(1979, 1982, 1984, 1987), who leaned heavily on these well-
known concepts of Nietzsche in labeling Nietzsche the last metaphysician (see Chessick, 1991, for discussion of Heidegger's
arbitrarily shifting views of Nietzsche.)

Nietzsche's commentators may be divided into "lumpers"
and "splitters" (Magnus, Stewart, and Mileur, 1993). The lumpers
include *The Will to Power* and treat such unpublished material as
final versions in an attempt to make an ontology out of Nietzsche's thought. The splitters are more postmodern; they emphasize only his published work and believe he spoke out with
"many voices in his many published texts, not with a single voice
governing every concern" (p. 46). The splitters argue that the
use of all Nietzsche's fragmented and unpublished notes to interpret him is a mistake (e.g., see Tanner, 1996; also Chapter 17
of the present book).

The Creative Process: Traditional Views

Albert Schweitzer stated that his philosophy of humanity, as he
called it, or "reverence for life" came to him in a daydream on a

river in Africa during a three day voyage. He never responded to any attack on his philosophical position because he felt rather mystically that silence was invincible. Relaxing by immersion in philosophy and playing the organ, he gave Nietzsche credit for maintaining his interest in the ethical precept about kindness and mercy toward all living things (Schweitzer, 1992). How he got this from Nietzsche is never explained. Throughout the present book I have emphasized the basic principle of reverence for human life from birth to death, an emendation of Schweitzer's unrealistically idealistic notion. I believe that if this precept could be a worldwide and fundamental premise of all human relationships, we could enter an era where Being manifests itself in a new way, beside the worn-out extreme materialism and untrammeled capitalism of our present age.

Aristotle denoted ὄρεξις (desire) as a general name for the mode of force to which animals are subject. He believed that in animals either anger or the pleasure principle prevails, whereas in rational beings there is also a desire for the good. All desires involve both judgment and impulse, and the differentiation between humans and animals is not that animals are creatures of pure impulse but that they are guided only by sporadic imagination of things pleasant or painful, whereas humans can also have a rational concept of the good. Aristotle viewed humans at the top of a scale of life, capable of reasoning, creating, and expressing forms of Truth, Goodness, and Beauty (Allan, 1952), although of course, contrary to Plato, he did not believe such forms have any separate existence.

Let us turn now to a deeper understanding of the creative process and briefly review some of the well-known attitudes of famous creators. Of course I have selected for the purposes of the present book from a vast and conflicting literature on this subject (for example, see Young-Bruehl, 1991, and Rose, 1996; the former appends an outstanding bibliographic list on the topic and the latter offers a controversial sample of a recent psychoanalytic approach). Bergson (1950b) maintained we are free only at those moments of crisis when our true self comes out; only then we get back to ourselves. Roland (1988) explained that in Japan one cultivates the inner self through a variety of aesthetic and other activities; the private self is communicated only indirectly, and others are expected to sense it. For Ortega y Gasset (Marias,

1967), life is a poetic task. One must invent what one is going to be in view of one's circumstances. Each person must do this for himself or herself, a contention similar to Nietzsche's.

At the heart of nineteenth-century philosophy was an antagonism between the creative imagination and the critical intellect. For example, Arnold saw modern humans as crippled and incomplete (Trilling, 1939). Convinced that both rationalism and romanticism had failed, Arnold tried to weave them together. He viewed culture as an attitude of spirit, a perfection of an inward condition to receive the truth. He correctly claimed that science could not take the place of humanistic study because science loses sight of the issue of how to live. Although Arnold condemned the middle class as Philistines who were stiff necked and resistive to aesthetic light, viewed the aristocracy as barbarians who pursued power and pleasure, and described the working class as masses bawling to do what they like, marching, meeting, and smashing, he maintained that humans with a bent for culture emerge in all three classes. These latter humans are the "aliens," led not by a class spirit but by a general humane spirit (Trilling, 1949). Freud's colleague Ernest Jones once said that neurotics are the torchbearers of civilization, but I think Jones meant that because neurotics are alienated they have to create their own projects and as such they open new options, develop new ways of understanding, and offer different solutions from existing ones, thus advancing and liberating humans.

Two other colleagues of Freud, Rank and Sachs (1916), maintained that affects which in life are painful are made pleasurable by art. A great work of art arouses strong unconscious mental affects and permits discharge and gratification in fantasy and in a censored form. Thus, artists belong to the leaders of humanity in the struggle for taming and ennobling the instincts that are hostile to culture. Rank and Sachs also believed that an artist must have a strong need for an audience.

Rank (1932) went on to argue that art springs from the personal consciousness of the individual and that the impulse of the creative genius arises from the human tendency to immortalize the self. He thought art represented a constructive victory over oedipal experiences, in the form of individual new creation. Rank claimed that the neurotic (like Barry) is a failed artist who cannot overcome irrational fear. He believed there is a kind of primeval conflict in the artist between the lower and higher self that is intense because he or she cannot merely fall back on the collective or social forms at hand, but has to build up a personal creation of collective values. Sachs (1942) added that the successful artist brings up emotion from the id with little loss of freshness and with directness and impact, but at the same time must conform to the demands of the ego by avoiding the unfettered and irresistible emotions swamping the ego through repetition and sometimes by too much structure (as one sees, for example, in Egyptian art). He maintained that a bond forms between the audience and the artist, bringing the artist out of isolation through self-elimination of the artist in the artwork. Similarly, Rank (1932) said the aesthetic pleasure of the person who enjoys art is enabled by a oneness with it when that person participates in the artwork. Both the artist and the audience, by simultaneous dissolution of their individuality in the greater whole, enjoy the personal enrichment of that individuality through the feeling of oneness. Notice the parallel to ecstatic love, as discussed in Chapters 7 and 9.

In Kris's (1952) traditional psychoanalytic view there are two processes in artistic creation: inspiration, the feeling of being driven by an outside agent, and elaboration, the purposeful organization and intent to solve a problem. This is superficially similar to Kohut's (1978, pp. 815-816) more recent self psychological view of the creative process. Kris maintained that art serves the purpose of communication; the id communicates to the ego in inspiration and is then submitted to others in an elaborated form. Using Freudian metapsychology, Kris postulated that these stages are characterized by shifts in psychic levels, in degrees of ego control, and in the cathexis of the self and the audience. In addition, such shifts also occur in the observer or audience and are pleasurable. The artist tries to endow with secondary public meaning what was meaningful originally only to himself or herself, an important task that Pound's psychopathology impeded. Kris, in a much-quoted phrase, spoke of the temporary ego regression or regression in the service of the ego that occurs, for example, during inspirational creation. Plato in the dialog "Ion" called this a kind of productive insanity (see Hamilton and Cairns, 1973, p. 220).

In Kris' s view, the normal artist depicts the world for others, and the task of artistic production has a realistic meaning, whereas the psychotic artist creates in order to literally transform the real world, seeks no real live audience, and utilizes an unchanging, unelaborated mode of expression. He believed that art as a social and aesthetic phenomenon depends on the intactness of the ego. I hope I have already demonstrated that the production of art requires this intactness, a functioning of the ego on the relatively healthy side of the ego axis; when the individual slides into the relatively unhealthy side of the ego axis, artistic production deteriorates and is interfered with by the intrusion of autistic thinking, obsessions, or even delusions.

All authors seem to believe that artistic creation flows from the great psychic reservoir of the unconscious (Ghiselin, 1952). Tapping and transforming the unconscious by a combination of intuition and cognition allows for a creative thrust from the unconscious and creative mastery by the conscious. The artist is driven by imagining the possibility of a newer and greater interpretation; the power of this visionary insight can even be blinding (Schneider, 1954)

The great Thomistic philosopher Maritain (1955) divided the mind into the preconscious life of the intellect where poetic intuition is born, which he called the imaginative region, and the region of conceptual and logical reason. He did not believe any mechanistic concept of the psyche, such as Freud's structural theory, does justice to aesthetic activity (but neither did Freud, as I will quote him later). For Maritain, poetic knowledge is the grasping of the objective reality of the outer and inner world, that knowledge arising through affective union embodied in ourselves, and the looking at what we are in our inner bents and in the properties of our own inner being. Beauty is both aesthetic beauty perceived by the senses and transcendental beauty perceived by the mind, so, for Maritain, poetry is the divination of the spiritual in things of sense. This resembles Hegel's (1807) view. Rilke (1962) had a similar intuitive orientation, advising a young poet to forget aesthetic criticism and allow himself an unhurried inner growth in the unconscious, making art actually a way of living. This latter is a very important Nietzschean concept.

In many ways artists seem to have a deeper understanding of the creative process than psychoanalysts, a wider and more phenomenologic vision of it. For example, Kundera (1986) viewed the novel as a meditation on the enigma of existence in which novelists draw up a map of existence; in a novel no one possesses the truth. He correctly maintained that the mass media crush individual thought, smothering the very essence of European culture, and he expressed the highest respect for the individual and his or her right to original thought and an inviolable private life. Again, a creator advocates reverence for human life from birth to death. The novelist Davies (1988) viewed music as the language of the dream world. He hoped to open the door to the underworld of feeling and suggested the term *sprezzatura,* representing a contempt for the obvious and for beaten paths, and a sudden leap in art toward a farther shore, an extremely important idea if one is to understand the shining forth of Truth in art and the creative process.

For Bertrand Russell also, creative striving is toward the point of light, just as the plant reaches to light (Ryan, 1988). He placed loneliness at the heart of the human condition and maintained that passionate love (see Chapters 7 and 9) is the only escape from an indifferent universe and is the most important thing in the world. Steiner (1989) insisted that the aesthetic act of bringing art into being is an imitation of the "Big Bang" with which our universe began: "Deep inside of every art act lies the dream of an absolute leap out of nothingness" (p. 202). For Steiner the arts relate us most directly to what in Being is not ours, a concept grasped phenomenologically, for example, in experiencing the slow movement of Schubert's C Major Quintet. He insisted that the arts are the evidence Russell was looking for in his quest for transcendence and his search for evidence that there was something beyond the material world, something absolutely certain.

The Creative Process: Current Psychoanalytic Views

Psychoanalysts more recently have advanced their study of the creative process, especially focusing on ego functioning in creativity. The usual metapsychological description of creativity declares that it is facilitated by regression in the service of the ego;

at least, the inspiration part of creativity involves this process. But Weissman (1967) argued that repressed id content can reenter the ego for inspirational creative purposes without ego regression. He maintained that alteration from personal enactment to creative enactment can be ascribed to the dissociative function of the ego, making the capacity for dissociation a predominant feature of ego functioning in the creative process. The artist would then have a creative self and a more conventional self:

> Applied to the creative person, the dissociative function reemerges whenever he is in search of a creative state. The dissociative function liberates him from his customary mode of operation and permits emerging drive-derived cathexis to new treatment by the ego and the superego. It is probable that the dissociative function (rather than ego regression) is receptive to the new id-derived cathexis available for the ego. This constitutes the optimal state of the ego for creative inspirational activity." (p. 43)

He did not consider the dissociative function a regressive phenomenon. As we have seen in the case of Ezra Pound imprisoned in Pisa, there is evidence for Weissman's implication that psychotics may achieve respite from a psychotic regression due to the effects of the dissociative function during their creative activity.

I agree with Giovacchini (1968) that although there is a phenomenologic similarity between the psychic structure and behavior of creative persons and those of disturbed noncreative patients, these similarities are not so deep and there are important fundamental differences. For example, Kafka (1973) wrote that his talent for portraying his dreamlike inner life thrust all other matters into the background. He described himself as having strange, deep, inaccessible powers and compared the process of creative writing to the sleep of death. Neurotics do not experience this; they are preoccupied with their gratification and/or the prevention of fragmentation and alienation and/or their ontological insecurity (Laing, 1969).

Bush (1969) carefully criticized the lack of clarity and specificity of the entire concept of regression in the service of the ego. He claimed that it fails (1) to differentiate sufficiently between the various aspects of adaptive ego regression, (2) to differentiate regressive phenomena that lead to creativity from those that accompany the creative process, (3) to differentiate shifts of energy among ego functions that are regressive in nature from those that constitute normal ego functioning, (4) to take into account the individual characteristic mode of ego functioning as a baseline from which to estimate regressive or progressive alteration in the level of ego functioning, and (5) to explain the relationship between the structural and topographic aspects of regression in the service of the ego (see Bush, pp. 159-160). He concluded,

> There has been an overemphasis on the role of regression in psychoanalytic discourse on creative thinking. This has occurred for several reasons: an overschematization of the polarities between primary-process and secondary-process functioning; a failure to appreciate the range of individual differences in characteristic modes of cognition; and the lack of an adequate conceptualization of the distinction between a reversion to primitive cognition as it once existed and the elaboration of primitive forms of mentation into highly advanced, adaptive resources. (p. 180)

Creativity and Psychopathology

Freud (1928) referred to the unanalyzable artistic endowment of the writer and later to "the riddle of the miraculous gift that makes an artist" (Freud, 1930b, p. 211). He asked in the former essay, "How is one to find one's way in this bewildering complexity?" (Freud, 1928, p. 177). There appears to be a number of themes that keep coming up in the psychoanalytic literature on creativity:

> Some try to demonstrate that genius and gross mental disturbance go hand in hand; others separate the psychopathology so frequently encountered in the lives of highly creative individuals from their productive propensities and achievements; and between these opposing approaches, variegated blends and opinions are set forth in an effort to understand the conditions and trends that allow for an emergence of the powerful impulses—be they libidinal,

aggressive, or both—and their actualization by way of the creative act. (Niederland, 1976, p. 186)

A controversy still exists as to whether psychopathology is essential to true creativity (see Maher, 1993, for a fine summary of the psychoanalytic literature on this topic). I am firmly in agreement with Kubie (1958) that psychopathology "corrupts, mars, distorts, and blocks creativeness in every field" (p. 142), and that resolution of psychopathology will certainly not cause atrophy of the creative drive. Although I disagree with his explanation of the creative process itself, I think his notion that the creative process in science or art is metapsychologically similar to any other form of conflict resolution, pathological or not, is correct. In contrast to the production of crippling neurotic symptoms as a way of solving unconscious conflicts by compromise formations, the creative process transmutes "unconscious conflicts into some socially and artistically acceptable symbolic form" (p. 143). But Kubie's view is still a metapsychologically reductionistic conception of the creative process. It ignores phenomena such as Kafka's experience of his strange, deep, and inaccessible powers, representing the complementary process in which the artist and the artwork partake in the shining forth of Beauty and Truth, and it also ignores the role of the audience in completing the artwork by its participation (see Chapter 20).

The artist is able to perceive relations and images that most of us do not or cannot perceive. Creativity is an innate capacity, a rare characteristic of certain endowed individuals, involving both the tendency and the ability to perhaps playfully take apart and put together again, to break established patterns of relationships and replace them with new ones. Niederland (1976) claimed that frequently there is a history of significant traumatic experience in the early lives of creative individuals, and he agreed with Kris (1952) that this traumatization plays an unusually great part in creativity. But these are undocumented anecdotal reports based on their clinical experience and not necessarily from a representative sample of creative people, some of whom do not want or need psychotherapy. Gedo (1996a) proposed that creativity is not a reaction to childhood depression or narcissistic injury, but rather due to the injury of nonrecognition of special talents and of the problems involved in adaptation to unusual endowments.

Niederland (1976) wrote, "Creativity is a solitary activity. It is usually accompanied by a withdrawal from complex emotional involvements with the external world and the latter's replacement—in the mind—by ideas, projects, fantasies, and personal, artistic, cultural, or religious strivings" (pp. 193-194). This is similar to Bush's (1969) depiction of a self-insulating sanctuary that the artist lives in at least for periods of time. Niederland (1976) called this "a walled-off garden away not only from the turbulence and strife of the outer world but also from irksome emotional problems and involvement with people. It is under such circumstances that, in the gifted person, the world of repressed visual, auditory, and kinesthetic memories emerges, which the artist transmutes into the creative act" (pp. 193-195). I believe this to be very accurate, but it is equally applicable to the story of both Ezra Pound and of Barry. For successful creativity there also has to be the spark of genius, and that endowment, as Freud complained, is what we have not yet adequately explained.

Gedo (1983) said creative work is not regression in the service of the ego, but rather a dialogue in which the idealized representation of one's own mind restores self-esteem. He maintained that geniuses underestimated as children develop a demonic creative effort and a fragile self-worth. Great art can even be produced by wicked individuals such as Wagner, because they can isolate off their pathology. So Gedo also maintains that psychopathology interferes with creativity if it cannot be walled off or somehow transcended. Gedo (1996b) shifted the study of creativity from the Freudian libidinal to the self psychology channel. He viewed the pleasure of the creative artist not as due the satisfaction of sublimated drives but to the "enormous boost in self-esteem provided by any sense of unusual competence" (p. 82). This by itself may offer such intense pleasure that it can provide the necessary emotional sustenance to continue creating even in isolation.

In a view also influenced by self psychology, Pollock (1982) claimed that creativity in later life has to do with mourning for one's own losses and the transformation of these through creative processes as one ages. Similarly Hanly (1986) maintained that the integrity of art cannot be understood adequately in terms of either ego functions alone or primary process alone:

"When viewed from a multifaceted perspective, the function of art can be recognized to include not only catharsis, but also, as in the play of children, the quest for maturation, reparation, restoration, and psychic integration" (p. 21).

In the last decade psychoanalysts have returned again to examining the process of creativity in its relation to psychopathology. Trosman (1990) discussed Eliot's *The Wasteland* as a series of images depicting the state of a depleted psyche in an empty bereft world. Eliot was attempting to reverse a temporary self-fragmentation experience by creative activity, and Trosman claimed that the creative act "not only gives expression to the deepest unconscious wishes; it also offers the creator opportunities for the reparation of loss, conquest and competition, and cryptomnesic incorporation through the experience of being influenced and influencing" (p. 57). The audience for a work of art has a chance in the response to meet the artist halfway and resonate with the artwork, combining the latent fantasy of the artist with resonating fantasies of their own.

Oremland (1997) claimed art is related to universal experiences and primal concerns. The viewer of art is brought into contact with aspects of himself or herself that are fleeting, distant, or disorganized and often fear laden: "It is art's economic dialectic with the universals, birth, separation, dependency, autonomy, involution, death, fear, anxiety, and rage, to name several, that gives art its overarching evocative power and accounts for its enduring place in history" (p. 39). Oremland continued, "The interpersonal world of the artist is but a part of the larger world of configurations, colors, tones, forms, and the like and not as singular and central as it is for most individuals" (p. 86). I think this is a very important point. In my clinical psychoanalytic experience working with artists, I have been impressed by their unusual visual capacities, enabling them to see things in the world that are ordinarily overlooked or to see things from a remarkably original standpoint. It is this extraordinary way of seeing or hearing that is the mark of real artistic talent, but it also carries the disadvantage, as Oremland points out, that creative individuals of this sort do not find people as central to them as the ordinary individual does: "The lessened centrality of persons as *objects* with its concomitant lessened centrality of interpersonal relatedness often earns the artist pejorative labels such as self-centered, infantile, or within a psychopathological lexicon, narcissistic" (p. 87).

Oremland, like numerous other authors, objects to the assumption that psychopathology must be present for creative generativity and artistic production. On the contrary, it is clear that analytic treatment can help solve inhibitions, blocks, and paralysis which prevent the free use of creativity. He views sublimation as much more than a defense and follows Winnicott's location of the creative process somewhere in the transitional space where subjectively each person interacts with the process of the social reality in which he or she is immersed. He offers an ontogenetic metapsychology of creativity in which "creativity recapitulates the major developmental levels of ontogenesis" (p. 103). He views the creative process as a dialectic between the past and present, and between intrapsychic and social processes, "a kind of inner dialogue. . .part of the quest for immortality" (p. xii).

Oremland emphasizes the importance of engagement with an imagined audience or imagined effect of his or her ongoing artistic work as activating various stages of the artist's development. He writes, "the primary anxiety of creativity is the anxiety of aloneness" (p. 55). He refers to the "primal other" (p. 102), the mother whose representation he believes is at the basis of all subsequent self and object representations, functioning as a mediating presence or what self psychologists would call an archaic selfobject, allowing the artist to have sufficient support during the isolating experience of rearranging perceptions of the surround in a unique and sometimes idiosyncratic manner. He concludes that creativity seeks a representation of the primal object and this leads to the creation of a new object that is a derivative version of this primal object. This seems to be a speculative overgeneralization hard to apply to the enormous variety of artistic productions over the centuries.

There is no need here to review innumerable biographical examples of this problem among artists, as summarized in the conductor George Szell's famous comment about Glen Gould: "This nut is a genius." (For an example of bizarre eccentricities in the field of musical genius that can even border on psychoses, see Ostwald's [1997] account of his experiences with Glen Gould.) The highly neurotic Proust insisted there is no art without neurosis, implying that inner conflicts increase the pressure to focus within, to enhance the power to symbolize, and to achieve liberation of expression. But no one is ever free from inner conflicts. I believe the pressure to create also comes from the necessity of all primates to communicate, deeply built into our species along with the need for mirroring.

Noy (1979) maintained that the problem of the creative artist is to cross three censor stations in order to transmit the meaning inherent in his or her work of art from the deep unconscious to the audience. These censors are the artist's own defenses or controls, the barrier that the audience has, and the external defenses and controls of the audience. He explained, in an exceptionally important statement,

> Not only do the defenses that keep the message of the artist from reaching the public change from time to time, but also the psychological needs of the public that the artist has to satisfy, which change from one historical period to the other and from one culture to the other. In addition to the basic universal needs that are satisfied by art, every period and culture is characterized by specific needs and patterns of defenses. This requires that the creative artists continually renew their tactics and keep searching for new means to fulfill their main function, that of addressing themselves to the depth mind of the public and satisfying their psychological needs . . . .Thus the search for creative forms becomes a never-ending endeavor which will continue as long as human beings continue to create art. (p. 243)

Understanding Noy's position helps us to understand the great impact Ezra Pound's new methods in poetry had on his contemporary poetic colleagues, and why Hegel was wrong when he claimed that the creation of art was over and inevitably superseded by religion.

Noy maintained that neurotics and creative artists differ not in their basic psychopathology but in the way they succeed in coping with it. As Freud (1924) said, "The artist, like the neurotic, had withdrawn from an unsatisfactory reality into this world of imagination; but, unlike the neurotic, he knew how to find a way back from it and once more to get a firm foothold in reality" (p. 64). According to

Noy (1979), "The solution found by creative artists is the exact dynamic opposite of the neurotic solution" (p. 253). There is redundancy and repetition and freezing in a neurosis with a tendency to resist change, whereas creativity is characterized by never-ending attempts to originate new and daring patterns of adaptation. Yet creativity and neurosis may both represent attempts to solve the same problems, and there might even be a dynamic fluctuation between neurotic and creative states, so a problem solved in the creative way at one time may be resolved by neurotic psychodynamics at another time. Like many psychoanalytic authors, Noy viewed the creative act as an attempt to resolve fragmentation or a step toward the reattainment or attainment of mental health. Later Noy (1984-1985) mentioned Kohut's (1971) concept that creativity is one of the transformations of narcissism and argued that the motive for creativity is always a self-centered one.

To my knowledge no psychoanalytic author has utilized Popper's (1994) posthumous book, in which he labeled objective knowledge and all autonomous products of the human mind as "world 3." For him "world 2" is constituted by our mental states and "world 1" is the physical world. Through world 2, world 3 also acts on world 1. World 3 is constituted by the aggregation of products of the human mind, including architecture, visual arts, music, scholarship, theories, problems, and so on. The way in which world 3 acts on world 2 is as follows: As the artist produces art it feeds back with unintended consequences that suggest new ideas to the artist, a give-and-take interaction between a person and his or her creative work. This is phenomenologically correct. The question examined in Chapters 18–20 of the present book is whether there is also a "world 4," a world perhaps consisting of Truth, Beauty, Moral Norms, and Reality. This is in various forms the central question of all the great philosophers.

Is world 4 merely a human construction or does it have an independent existence? Have we ciphers on the way to discover it? For example, Bloom (1994) argued that a literary work breaks into the Western canon by its "aesthetic strength." This strength is measured by its mastery of figurative language, originality, cognitive power, knowledge, exuberance of diction, and being the kind of work that demands rereading. Is the presence of "aesthetic strength" a cipher?

Some Examples of Psychopathology in Creators

We know that art and, especially, music were crucial for the misanthrope Schopenhauer (Safranski, 1990) as a form of temporary transcendence offering an escape from Will, although he felt that in the end everyone was alone. His schedule was to spend three hours early in the morning in intellectual work, play the flute, have an enormous lunch, and then read the newspapers. In the afternoons he took a long walk and in the evenings during his early adulthood he went to the theater and parties; later in life he stayed home from parties but continued the theater, opera, and concerts. Embittered and alone, he slept with a loaded pistol under his pillow. He believed that art was nearer to Truth than intellectual concepts and he produced a number of memorable essays written with admirable artistic skill. The contemporary philosopher Magee (1997) cites his discovery of Schopenhauer's philosophy in mid-life as a therapeutic turning point in Magee's depression and obsessive lifelong quest to understand the relationship between our empirical experience and underlying Reality, what in the present book I have called Truth, Beauty, and Being.

For Schopenhauer, as well as Einstein (Bryan, 1996) and many other thinkers, the motive that drives humans to art and science is to escape the monotony and rawness of everyday life, an attempt to take refuge in a world with images of a human's own creation. For example, Dickens (Kaplan, 1988; Ackroyd, 1990) sought images from his study of infancy to express the primal fear of the frightened child. He was always alert to the dark side under farce and to the absurdity of human behavior. Dickens argued that human identity cannot change and that travel only confirms the prison of the self in which each one of us is perpetually trapped. Proust at the age of twenty-five, in 1897, slept during the day from 8 a.m. to 3 p.m. and stayed up all night. He lived with his parents but actually escaped from them in this way, spending more and more time in bed. Finally in 1910 he took a second step of withdrawal by removing himself from society into a cloistered, ascetic life (Hayman, 1990). Thomas Wolfe in 1926 said that he wrote a novel in an effort to find "a breech in the wall somewhere," a theme or pattern in a life that was characterized by a terrible childhood (Donald, 1987). Anaïs Nin (1966) remarked in her diaries that the world of the artist contains joy, creation, freedom, and altruism, and she contrasted that to the world of reality containing greed, power, self-interest, war, corruption, dullness, and hypocrisy. Franz Kafka cherished those hours when his dream life could come forth (Krarl, 1991) and he was always trying to communicate an incommunicable fear. Writing became his life; he was the first child of a money-oriented businessman and a mother utterly devoted to meeting the ceaseless needs and demands of her husband. As a result he was an abandoned firstborn infant whose younger brother died when he was four years old and who lost another younger brother when he was five years old (Pawel, 1984), leaving his parents devastated and Kafka with a heavy burden of unconscious guilt.

Artists who have committed suicide are a special problem. Mark Rothko, who ended his life this way, maintained that the artist must steal a place on the rich man's wall (Breslin, 1993). His paintings pull us to a preverbal inward and difficult conflicted state. He was an alien figure who stepped outside a repressive social environment in an attempt to uncover a core human presence, a presence that survives massive fragmentation, violence, bureaucracies, and trivialities of life—all that constitutes the practico-inert in the twentieth century. An incredible number of artists have killed themselves in the twentieth century (Alvarez, 1971). The sense of chaos in our time is a pervasive artistic theme, an era of unlimited technological violence, absurd death, and the potential for annihilation of our species. This ambience of disaster is the phenomenologic context in which our contemporary arts are created: A destruction of the old traditional structures of social relations and beliefs, and a spinoff of technology that makes death random and absurd, all perhaps best symbolized today by the so-called "mindless" drive-by shooting. Perhaps the most dramatic demonstration of all this comes from the life and work of Jackson Pollock, whose capacity to disengage his mental illness (depression and alcoholism) from his artistic creativity suddenly snapped on the eve of the greatest exhibition of his work in his life, after a season of spectacular success and achievement, sending him "off the edge of a spiritual sinkhole from which he will, in essence, never emerge" (Varnedoe, 1998, p. 61). The violence of Jackson's most successful paintings was desublimated and manifested itself subsequently in his premature self-destruction.

For Beckett, all life is a disease (Bair, 1978). Creativity, a seizure of the conscious by the unconscious, is the only way we can preserve ourselves from death. Otherwise the loneliness, the futility, the disillusionment we experience when we think about Being-towards-death robs us of all enthusiasm. Beckett believed that art helps us emerge from the darknesses of time and habit and passion and intelligence (Cronin, 1997). The whole of human life, that of the supposedly fortunate as well as of the unlucky, involves inevitable disappointment, he said, modified and alleviated only by illusions of various sorts, the recurrence of false hopes, and briefly welcome deceits. Knowlson (1996) pointed out that Beckett experienced a surge of creative energy and anxiety attacks *simultaneously* after his mother died, resulting in the writing of *Endgame*, which is probably his best play and is loaded with images of death and ambivalence toward the dying. By a combination of artistic creativity and neurotic mechanisms operating simultaneously, Beckett tried to work out his endless struggle with his strong-willed mother. With these considerations in mind the reader is now prepared to examine the only completed but unpublished humanistic work written by Barry, exhibiting a variety of his neurotic efforts to reverse the fragmentation process and operating *pari passu* with his creative strivings both to communicate and to reverse this lethal fragmentation.

16 BARRY'S "FRAGMENTATION"

Christmas Inscape

She stands there
black eyes, black hair
slim in red dress, picturesque.
A beautiful vision she
takes my breath away
heaven sent.
The yearning, the longing
so powerful it transcends
all passion; it is poetry.
A whole holiday season
compressed in an hour
with her.
Must life be
so painful?

—Barry (notebook)

Introduction

This chapter offers the only completed artistic work found in Barry's notebooks. It is an attempt on his part to present a phenomenologic study of the fragmentation of a psychotherapist, including an affair with an ex-patient. The play juxtaposes the disintegration of the protagonist psychiatrist Barry with the disintegration of Ezra Pound. Gabbard (1989) collected essays on every conceivable aspect of sexual relations between therapist and patient, and I (Chessick, 1997a) have described the "love/lust obsessed therapist." A middle-aged therapist, typically (but not always) male, gets involved sexually with a female patient an average of 16.5 years younger than he is. Intrusive thoughts of the loved one force their way into the therapist's dream and waking life. They have a great need for each other's presence. Gutheil (1989) pointed out that patients with borderline personality disorder are particularly likely to evoke boundary violations (Gabbard and Lester, 1996) from the therapist, including sexual acting out, but of course the responsibility is solely on the therapist.

As illustrated in the play, the therapist is sometimes in a "drugged" or dreamlike state when he is with the "beloved" patient, and so he takes extraordinary risks with her that may irrevocably damage his career, incur legal penalties, and ruin his personal life. He may claim that he is trying to heal the tormented patient's psyche, perhaps in the experimental manner tried by Ferenczi (1988)—although Ferenczi soon admitted this did not work—or on the basis of numerous other rationalizations. The psychodynamics involve regression along the ego axis to blurred ego boundaries with a consequent blurring of the therapeutic boundaries, and often only with this one patient. The therapist is usually a well-functioning narcissist like Barry who may work satisfactorily with other patients, but in his personal life he has typically entered into some sort of midlife crisis. His susceptibility to using the patient to resolve this crisis often shows itself first by maneuvers such as inappropriate self-disclosure to the patient, which can sometimes result in an actual reversal of roles.

The patient wants to be "special" in the most desperate way, out of an intense archaic need for mirroring that is often generated by regression in the transference, or that is present to some extent even in all her relationships. The therapist, on the other hand, because of the narcissistic disequilibrium from which he suffers, wants sadistically enforced control of an archaic selfobject in order to restore that equilibrium. For example, the situation may represent a reversal of roles in which the therapist as a helpless child was sadistically controlled in every aspect of his mental and bodily functions by a narcissistic mother who used him as a selfobject for the purpose of maintaining her own narcissistic equilibrium, or, even worse, to prevent a total fragmentation of herself.

This play is an imagined drama of fragmentation and failed attempts at restitution, created by the therapist (Barry) at a time when his own self was threatened. The autobiographical aspects are evident, but creating the play clearly performed a selfobject function for Barry, allowing him to discharge in his imagination what fragmentation symptoms he might have otherwise acted out to his own self-destruction, place them on paper, and separate himself from them. This chapter presents the play for your direct phenomenologic experience. In the first section of the next chapter I will discuss the psychoanalytic aspects of the play in greater detail.

The Play

ACT I

(As the curtain rises we see a bourgeois dinner party in progress. There are four people at the table: Alice, a feather-headed gossip; Eva, a sad and uncertain mature woman; Bob, a somewhat pompous fundamentalist minister who is convinced that religion has the right answers to all questions; and Ken, a rather arrogant surgeon and a "take-charge guy" who looks to science for answers. They are all middle-aged and dressed in a middle-class fashion, their suits and dresses of modest price. It is the home of Bob and Eva, as a prominent Bible on a side table and a crucifix on the wall indicates. The Arkansas State flag hangs on the wall, with the sign "Arkansas: Home Sweet Home" next to it.)

Ken: The stupid psychiatrists saved him—the Russians would have hung him, I am sure.

Alice: They stuck him in a madhouse where crazy poets belong—what do poets know, they are nothing but a public nuisance.

Bob: Paranoid! Obsessed with money and money-lenders.

Eva: Really?

Ken: Anti-Semite!

Alice: Fascist!

Bob: Ugh! This wine is sour; I could spit it out.

Eva: Mind your manners, dear.

Bob: Eight years in this little parish and they can't come up with a decent bottle of wine for me for Christmas. Bah! They think God lowered the Bible to us from heaven on a golden thread and that psychiatrists do the devil's work. Maybe they are waiting for a good bottle of Chablis to come down on a golden thread for me.

Ken: Psychiatrists! They are an odd bunch. It's lucky a surgeon like me doesn't have to bother with them—they are not even doctors, I say. The psychiatrists who work in our hospital are all creeps. They don't fit in.

Alice: I heard of one once who was crazier than his patients. They are obsessed with sex.

Bob (uneasy about the discussion moving to sex, changes the subject.): So we are going to Africa.

Eva: Yes, it's agreed. A toast! *(She raises a glass and the others follow.)*

Ken: I have our reservations all set. We are staying in deluxe accommodations and the food is going to be magnificent.

Bob: Two weeks among the heathens—ugh!—but it is also the rainy season so maybe the rains will clean up the place. A dirty place. Disease and pestilence, the Bible says. I wonder how it will compare with Arkansas.

Alice: Rainy season or not, it was a bargain rate for us; our first vacation together. I can't wait to buy a safari suit!

Bob: Eva has a pen pal named Barry who is a psychiatrist. He went to medical school with John, her first husband. Barry used to read Ezra Pound's poetry in the medical student's lounge while all those around him were boning up on their anatomy textbooks. When John died—what a tragedy—twenty-five years ago—from cancer—it suddenly destroyed him within a few months—he asked this guy to look after Eva, but *he's* the one who needs looking after, if you ask me.

Alice: What do you mean? Why does he need looking after?

Bob: He writes these crazy letters to her. I tell her not to answer but she feels sorry for the guy.

Ken: That's nice of you, Eva. What's his problem?

Bob: Come on, Eva, read his last letter to them.

Eva: It's too long-winded.

Alice and Ken (together): Oh, come on, be a good hostess, entertain us.

Eva: It's not entertaining.

Ken: Well then, shock us.

Alice: Come on, Eva, let's have a little gossip.

Bob: Don't be a stick-in-the-mud, Eva; it's all in fun.

Eva (pensively): We will be meeting him at last, although in what a strange place—the International Hotel in Nairobi! *(She gets up rather reluctantly and hesitatingly to find the letter. Taking the letter from a far corner, she slowly comes back to the table and begins to read.)*

My dear Eva: It has been so long—I was delighted to hear that our paths will finally cross, even though it will be far from home. What good news that you and Bob could find such clever friends as Ken and Alice, who seem to have produced a bargain tour to fit a minister's salary. I look forward to meeting all of you. My journey is not for a vacation; at this point I couldn't stand it anymore—I had to go far away to escape the curse on my house that torments me with one disappointing blow after another.

Bob (unbelieving and superciliously): A mysterious fellow.

Alice: I don't understand. He sounds like a medieval man.

Eva (reads on): What I really want to tell you about now is an extraordinary event that has taken place in my family. As you know, my daughter Anna for several years now has been studying for a doctorate in Eastern religions. All she needs now is to write her dissertation and she will graduate.

Ken: What could be more useless? She would make more money as a waitress.

Eva (reads on): Even before Mary and I separated, we noted to our discomfort that each summer Anna left her husband and went off to study Japanese. For two summers she attended a special college in Vermont; last summer she spent in Tokyo. I could never understand how someone who was studying medieval Chinese and Japanese Buddhism would need to know anything special about modern Japanese—but she insisted it was true. We did not have a very high suspicion index. It turns out she was having trouble with her husband; going away for the summers apparently represented some sort of trial separation.

Alice: Well *I* certainly would have caught on a lot faster. What is the matter with these people? They seem to be living in a world of their own, outside of the good old American scene.

Eva (reads on): Last summer she apparently met some Korean students in Japan and between their broken English and her broken Japanese they were able to communicate. A friendship developed with one of the Koreans that apparently led to a love affair during the summer which continued into a correspondence. My wife and I did not know . . .

Alice: Well *I* would have known about it. My daughters and I are on the phone every day and we talk about *everything,* and I mean everything; clothes, food, quarrels with our husbands—everything important to us. How could a psychiatrist and his wife know so little about their own daughter's marriage?

Ken: Alice, will you stop interrupting?

Eva (reads on): Last Christmas Anna announced her plan to go to Japan for about nine months and applied for another grant—which she will probably get because she is a brilliant scholar . . . followed by another announcement that she decided to go perhaps even for two years. At this point our suspicion index became extremely high, and she finally declared that the correspondence with this Korean was blossoming by mail into a continuing love affair.

Ken: She must be crazy. I would belt her one. Only a psychiatrist's kid . . .

Eva (interrupts and reads on): I am trying hard to decide what to do. Some strategy needs to be devised . . . perhaps she and her husband can receive some counseling. This is the new ambience in our society; if people don't get along right away, they think more about divorce and separation than about trying to work out their problems.

Bob (angrily): He means the godlessness of our society! You have to start when they are young. If he would have brought that child to my church every Sunday. . . . How absolutely disgusting! The little . . .

Eva (interrupts and reads on): Eva, my old friend, I am not used to matters working out this way. When our children were young Mary and I had our ups and downs, but on the whole we operated in a fairly standard middle-class way. We lived an ordinary life in an unpretentious suburb. In addition, my parents and grandparents were inner directed; even through hard times and persecution in the old country they held on to a very strong sense of honor. We simply did not do things that were flagrantly dishonorable . . .

Bob (angrily): What sort of morality is that? People laugh and sneer at our looking to the Bible for answers, but there *are* answers clearly given to us, there *are* statements from God about what is right and what is wrong, about what is good and what is bad. Look at the results of the relativistic morality that this psychiatrist—this so-called expert on human affairs—has offered to his children.

Eva (reads on): Anna shattered this tradition . . . just flagrant adultery baldly announced to her husband . . . something has happened. In my family this is probably the first incident of profoundly dishonorable behavior—and our record goes back several generations, at least on my father's side. Women didn't count in the old country. I am the first son of a first son, and Anna is my firstborn child, the apple of my eye.

Alice: Poor foolish man . . . and rather stupid, also. A medieval man! I wonder what his parents were like? It's hard to feel sympathy for him.

Eva (reads on): What do I do? For example, I might eventually go to Japan and find them—but can I take action that would hurt my own daughter? Should I do nothing at all and just continue to let events take their own course—which is what Mary would be inclined to do? Now that she has moved out we don't talk much, even about our grown children. I am uneasy and restless. It is not in my character to sit still, say nothing, and make no efforts to influence Anna's activity. I find myself torn and conflicted among alternatives.

Bob: And with no minister and no God to turn to. That is no medieval man, it is a man who has lost his way, who is confused.

Eva (reads on): Awakened by a midnight nightmare, I tried my hand at *haiku:*

When the leaf falls
can it return to the tree?
What would it take?

The tree is older.
The leaf does not yet feel it
dancing in the wind.

I sometimes believe the worst part of all of this is the heavy moral burden Anna's behavior places on my already overloaded shoulders. I find myself sagging—unable to sleep at night, and living in a greater and greater sense of despair. Something will have to be done to achieve a restitution of the profound disequilibrium and internal disorder that her situation has produced in me . . .

Ken: What fancy language! He should knock their heads together . . .

Bob (shocked): That is brutal. He must find a way to bring religion into their life. It is not too late . . .

Alice: The little tramp! He should disown her . . . never speak to her again until she behaves ... the very idea!

(All are thoroughly aroused by now and repeat their views as expressed above, interrupting each other.)

Eva (out of patience): You asked me to read the letter. Will you be quiet and let me read it? *(They fall silent.)*

Eva (reads on): I realize that the person suffering the most here is my daughter, who must have been extremely desperate and unhappy to have made such a rash move that can only bring down on her all kinds of difficulties and problems. But I cannot rest ... strange music keeps running through my head . . . something has broken loose inside of me . . . I don't know why . . . I don't know how . . .

Eva (stops reading and looks at Alice): You know Alice, in a way you are right. Why can't he leave it alone? What is all this other stuff? Why does he pile all this "curse on my house" nonsense onto himself? Life is hard enough. Why not take it as it comes and do the best you can? Enjoy what you can, suffer when you have to, cry when your children are sick or unhappy—but why look for abstractions and spooks?

Bob: And why not the consolations Jesus has to offer? Did He not suffer for us all? This man is arrogant—almost blasphemous—to take such a burden on himself. *(Grouchily)* I like him less and less; he is a troublesome ghost from Eva's past.

(Eva picks up the letter and moves toward center stage, ignores the others, and reads more slowly and dramatically now. The spotlight is on her.)

At night in the dark a haunting vista keeps unfolding in front of me. I face my relatives in Elysium, and the formative individuals in my young life—now all dead—my teachers, my best friends, including your John, and of course the generations of male relatives—my grandfather, my father, and a couple of my favorite uncles—all standing there, old, decayed, some with beards and yarmulkes and some without, and pointing their bony fingers at me and saying, "What happened?"

How will I ever answer them? What will I tell them that I did to make restitution? Can I just say I was passive and did nothing?

What will I say to them? How will I justify myself? They will ask me, "What took place in your life that suddenly one of your children exploded in this fashion?" And they will not point to her, they will point to *me*, because by the ancient code from which we come it is the fathers who must shoulder the disgrace of their children and this is passed down from generation to generation. Have I placed this curse upon my house?

Ken (standing up and talking to Eva): You know, the trouble with this guy is that he takes himself too seriously. I bet nobody else does. He thinks he's so profound. He's gonna get himself crucified—he thinks too much. One has to take action and deal with the problems of life the best one can. You assess the situation coolly, realistically, do what advance tests you can do, make a decision, and act on it. This fellow introduces all sorts of complications that nobody else would come up with. He should learn to fit in *(sits down disgustedly)*.

Alice: Does he ever laugh? Does he ever tell a joke? I can't imagine him relaxing and having fun or watching TV. What on earth is he so guilty about? I don't get it.

Bob: I think he is trouble. I don't look forward to meeting him. He sounds like an arrogant unbeliever and he certainly is not a Christian. *(Slowly and ominously)* He is not one of us.

Eva: (reads on): All this has rent the entire fabric of my self. And Eva, it has set me questioning, endlessly questioning, in a very fundamental way. What went wrong? *(She reads slowly.)* You know, Eva, I am tired, I cannot sleep, and I am so tired . . . so tired. *(Lights fade out and the curtain falls; there is darkness. Spotlight goes on as Barry appears at the far right side in front of the curtain.)*

Barry (somberly):
His soul approached the region where dwell vast hosts of the dead. He was conscious of, but could not apprehend their wayward and flickering existence. His own identity was fading out into a grey impalpable world. The solid world itself, which these dead had at one time been reared and lived in, was dissolving and dwindling.*

---

*Joyce, 1947, pp. 241–242.

(A low-pitched voice is heard chanting from the off-stage area, a kind of booming chant.)

Tho' my errors and wrecks lie about me
And I am not a demigod,
I cannot make it cohere.
If love be not in the house there is nothing.*

(Spotlight out; stage dark: Curtain)

ACT II

(As the curtain rises we see a rather typical looking psychiatrist's office. At the right end of the office there is a couch and a chair as well as a small desk. A very large picture of Freud with his penetrating look hangs on the back wall, looking out over the scene at the audience. A substantial area of rug-covered floor lies before the door that leads out of the office, which is situated on the left side wall. When the curtain rises the light is extremely harsh, cold, and white. Two people are lying on the rug in the relatively open area. Barry, a middle-aged doctor, is naked to the waist and is lying on his side with his back toward the audience. He has his arms clasped around Ruth, an attractive woman with black hair and black eyes, about fifteen years younger who is dressed only in panties and bra and who in turn has her arms and legs around him. Their bodies are belly to belly and Barry is clearly very sexually aroused and passionate. Ruth is relatively indifferent and simply servicing the man, who is rubbing himself up and down on her abdomen as part of the embrace.)

Barry: Oh . . . Oh . . . Oh! *(Moves as if he has ejaculated.)* Oh, this is glorious, Oh!

Ruth (soothingly): There, there, my dear.

Barry: Oh, what a glorious experience. But it's not enough. I want it all.

Ruth: I would feel guilty. I have made marriage vows, you know, and what we are doing is almost like incest.

---

*E. Pound, 1950, p. 796.

Barry: I know. I can't help it. I want it all. I can't stand it anymore. It's so humiliating to be limited like this. I can't trust you if I don't possess you.

Ruth: I thought you did.

Barry: I have to possess all of you, body and soul, property, everything, always.

Ruth (soothingly): You do, dear, you do.

Barry: Prove it by letting me have it all.

Ruth: I can do it, but I will feel guilty.

Barry: I have to have more . . . more.

Ruth (somewhat exasperated): What has gotten into you anyhow?

Barry: Ever since the paranoid husband of that battered woman patient I helped to get a divorce threatened to kill me, the tension has been unbearable. He said he would wipe me off the face of the earth and I never know when he will appear. There is nothing anybody can do, and so far he has only made a lot of empty noise. I have never seen him; I don't even know what he looks like.

Ruth (soothingly): There, there. Don't suffer alone. Let me help you. You don't have to suffer alone. Remember Rilke's* "Love Song"? Does it not speak directly for us?

> How shall I keep my soul
> from touching yours? How shall
> I lift it over you toward other things?
> Ah, I would like to lodge it
> in the dark with some lost thing
> on some foreign silent place
> that doesn't tremble, when your depths stir.
> Yet everything that touches *you* and *me*
> takes us together like a bow's stroke
> that from two strings draws *one* voice.

---

*R. M. Rilke, 1984a, pp. 8–9.

Across what instrument are we stretched taut?
And what player holds us in his hand?
O sweet song.

Barry: You have already helped me. I feel much better. I couldn't even talk about it before. It has been a terrible week.

(As they talk further they begin slowly to get dressed without particular excitement or embarrassment, like a couple that has been together for quite a while. Ruth wears a red dress. Barry wears a suit.)

Barry: Ever since Mary left me, it is harder and harder to sleep and think. I don't blame her, though; it must have been terrible to live with me.

Ruth: Thank God we found each other. We are two lonely people and these times together seem to be the only happiness that each of us ever has. What led up to all this, Barry? You have never done anything like this before, I am sure. What brought you to such an extreme state of agitation?

Barry: There is a story in the *Wall Street Journal*, of all places, from December 1986. One day last winter an old bum appeared at a busy street corner in an affluent Chicago neighborhood. He sat down on a bench, folded his hands, bowed his head, and remained there in the worst rains and bitterest cold.

He would never say what brought him to that particular bench and talked to no one. He refused spare change or offers of help and just sat filthy and disheveled day after day, stirring unease and resentment in the neighbors.

A priest approached him and he said his name was Jim, but, says the article, "in his tattered poncho and grey beard, he looked more like an unwashed Moses." There were piles of junk and a lot of old books next to him which he guarded carefully and stacked beside him in rusted shopping carts. Sometimes he muttered to himself:

For two gross of broken statues
For a few thousand battered books. . .*

---

*E. Pound, 1949, p. 64.

The residents in this fashionable neighborhood regarded him as an eyesore and frequently complained to the police.

Even on subzero days there were very few invitations to Jim to sit inside the warmth of nearby stores, because shopkeepers claimed that his odor drove customers away. He even infuriated many bridal parties because he would show up uninvited at a nearby church to huddle for some warmth while weddings were taking place.

The newspaper reports that one night last summer Jim and his belongings were mysteriously set on fire. He survived and moved to an alley in another neighborhood a few miles away, but the bench remains as a monument to him, bearing on it an angry charcoal-black burn.

Ruth (pensively): Our cultural metaphor in a quick glance— there was a famous conversation between Simone de Beauvoir and Simone Weil. When de Beauvoir said that the problem of the modern human condition is the problem of self-identity, Weil replied, "It is obvious that you have never been hungry." Is this what the old bum was trying to say? *(pauses)* Barry, you have never been the same since you came back from that professional meeting. What happened there?

Barry (pensively): I arrived twenty minutes early. The empty chairs were lined up in neat rows. I walked down the middle aisle, climbed the three steps up to the podium, and looked over the deserted room. A faint haze of tobacco smoke from the morning meeting hung in the air, producing a dismal smell and lending a dingy cast to the whole scene. At the back of the room on a small table covered with an ugly green cloth were several pitchers of ice water and a scattering of glasses prepared for those during the afternoon who needed an excuse to stretch themselves.

Ruth: What were you supposed to do there?

Barry: I was at a meeting of our psychiatric society and would be permitted twenty minutes to read a brief talk. There were four or five other speakers for the afternoon "panel" in addition to numerous assigned discussants, so that in order to read this twenty-minute paper I had to sit on the podium for three hours.

Ruth: That sounds deadly.

Barry: The panel chairman was a fat administrative psychiatrist, a successful veteran of many political encounters, who occupied an established high-salaried chair at a university department, serving on innumerable committees all over the United States. Since he had never heard of me, he simply called me to the podium as the first speaker, even while the audience was still coming in.

I rose to my feet, glanced over the half-filled room, and dodged the cigar smoke of the chairman—this was not easy to do, since the ventilation in the hotel was dreadful. As I read my paper—more to myself than to the audience—it was not possible for anyone to detect the lonely intense intellectual and psychological investment I had made in trying to answer certain questions for years, over and over again.

I am sure that something is missing in the standard descriptions of therapeutic process that have dominated the reports in psychiatric journals for the last fifteen years. I asked myself over and over again, "How does one help the mind to heal?" Binswanger* quotes Freud as unexpectedly answering, "Yes, spirit *(Geist)* is everything." What did Freud mean? Was he thinking of Hegel?

Ruth: You tackled that in a twenty-minute talk? Vanity!

Barry: I dimly realized that even in this brief period I lost the audience. Some were drowsy after a big lunch perhaps punctuated with alcohol; some wanted it simple, looking for a "how-to-do-it" manual; some were tired after three days of meetings—away from home and sleeping in an unfamiliar hotel room, in no mood to think intensely about anything; some clearly were there to hear another speaker on the program.

My moment to exhibit myself came and went, marked by a ripple of polite applause. The discussant of my paper used his assigned five minutes to make a little speech of his own. There was no further discussion. I had failed. I was unappreciated and unknown. I would now have to sit on the podium out of courtesy while the rest of the papers droned on. I yearned to go home.

As the participants went through their motions I defended myself against the pain of the disappointment by withdrawing in-

*Binswanger, 1963, p. 1.

creasingly into my own thoughts. I was of an age past the time when, as Schopenhauer remarked, a man begins to spend his capital. What were my aims? Using the pencil provided by the hotel, a souvenir advertising the name of the hotel in big letters, I scribbled on the pad in front of me: To be fully human. To think one's own thoughts. To reach a point at which, whether one's ideas are different from or similar to other men's ideas, they are truly one's own. To discover one's nature and one's place in nature. To make good intentions effective in the world. To be in touch with Spirit.

There was a scratching of chairs and a ripple of applause as another speaker finished, and I could not hold to this idealistic plane of thought. Despair began to set in and I concluded, "My mind is filled with fantasies that cannot be actualized; only tedium is my reality."

Ruth: You are working too hard, Barry. You need a vacation. You are under too much stress and strain.

Barry: The long hours, the demanding patients, home late for supper, the ready access to narcotics are much less of a problem to a doctor whose childhood has been happy and who has appeared psychologically sound by the time he reaches college. Football, not poets! But a doctor from an unhappy childhood may gain great comfort and strength from his patients' grateful recognition. He, not the literally overworked doctor, resorts to all sorts of measures to alleviate what he calls "fatigue," his own chronic depression. I don't know which comes first.

Ruth: Barry, the meeting was terrible! Come, let me hold you. *(She holds out her arms.)*

Barry (continues slowly as if she were not there): That night I dreamed I was at the cemetery with my children. Unburied bodies were laid out in a row resembling a big city morgue, and they were twitching and twisting and groaning and quite shriveled. One nearby corpse reached out for me, an old woman. I tried to explain to my children that this was the normal process of decay after death, but finally I decided it was too scary for them and led them away with their eyes covered.

I could not get the picture of the old lady out of my head.

As I went through the labors of the day there was a sense of dread and I tried over and over again to analyze the dream, but I failed. The following afternoon I still felt depressed by the dream. I kept seeing that corpse from the dream in front of me. I could not tell if it was beckoning to me or not—the hand is reaching out, but does it want to pull itself up on me or pull me to it, or is it only contracture and death? I cannot tell. It is unusual for a dream to persist into my waking life. Am I going crazy? Is my dead mother the corpse? Or is it something within myself?

Ruth: Barry, why don't you take a vacation trip? Travel, see new sights, hear new sounds, meet new people . . .

Barry (dreamily): One morning bright and early I took a bus south from Athens to view the castles of the Mycenaean kings. While the others had lunch at the base of the hill, I climbed up all the way to the impressive castle itself, which probably at one time was the home of Agamemnon, the castle with the famous lions on the gate, a castle with the cyclopean walls. At the very top, surrounded by natural beauty, I thought for just a moment in the eerie hush that I could somehow hear the voices of men long ago.

The next day I split off from the group to visit the completely ruined temple of Aesculapius, the compassionate and kind demigod of healing, the son of Apollo and a mortal mother. The ruins of his temple are ignored by everybody, and yet this was the starting point of psychological healing. The air was scented from the pine trees. The blue sky contained an occasional wisp of a cloud and a radiant sun, but it was not a hot day. . . . Generations of men with their dramatic history all crammed together on top of one another from 3000 B.C.E. to the very present in Greece. Ugly black smoke and fire-belching monoliths of oil refineries and shipyards line the Corinth-to-Athens highway. *These* represent the Acropolis of the twentieth century.

That night I watched the sunset from my hotel in the harbor of Nauplia. Shimmering pure green colors of all shades came and went in the mirrorlike water. The colors kept changing as the sun went down and I thought, "This is not the age of Aquarius, it is the age of the death of Apollo! Dionysius rages unchecked."

Ruth: Barry, you are not making sense! Was all this stirred up by the failure of your little talk at the meeting? Surely this is vanity. Is this why you called me?

Barry: No! When I returned from the meeting—the last straw! I told you about that, Anna's crazy affair with the Korean, the breakup of her marriage, gone to Japan. She was the apple of my eye, the pride of my older years. My firstborn child. I couldn't stand the tension. I had to have you. So I called you.

I wanted you to become my mistress—"no, my lover, for 'mistress' is too circumscribed, too curtailed. My lover, my confidante, my soul-mate. Yes, my soul-mate."* My soul, alone too long, needed you, my beloved fellow wanderer, like the lonely Henry VIII or like Odysseus, marooned on Circe's isle.

How can I explain it? There was something in you which drew me to you, as if lying on your breast I would know everything in life I desired to know, and unopened doors would open for me. . . . At base it is inexplicable. Something deep within you called to something deep within me. And the calling was powerful; it was undeniable. When we pressed together this afternoon, even as it happened, in some far off corner of myself I heard an inner voice saying, "You will never be the same. It is all gone." Yet at that moment I felt as though all had just arrived. For a moment I burst upward into a new fresh life—freedom, euphoria, . . . and light.†

Ruth (sings to the accompaniment of offstage recorder or flute):

The greatest cosmic hopelessness of all
Is the illusion of erotic love.
Promising redemption, self-transcendence
It dissolves at orgasm into the clouds above.

I received from you the greatest love
A woman could ever desire.
And yet standing in the stark light of day
We are each alone before a dying fire.

---

*M. George, 1986, p. 258.
†Paraphrased from M. George, 1986, pp. 259, 332.

The night you called I was lying by myself,
My crabby husband sulking in another room.
I hoped the ring of the telephone
Could save me from a lonely doom.

No infidelity or sexual fusion
Intense, ecstatic; then blissful sleep
Can save us each from our own confusion
The gap between us is impenetrable . . . and deep.

Barry: No! No!

(They embrace and kiss passionately. Barry abruptly stops, having glanced at the picture of Freud.)

Barry: Strange, his expression has changed.

Ruth: What?

Barry: For years his look was questioning, penetrating; my ideal. But now it is accusatory, as if he is saying, "Examine yourself. What have you done?" *(pauses)* A curse is on my house!

Ruth: Barry, what is all this! What is happening to you?

Barry (in a dreamlike state): What a vivid dream I had the night I called you! I was back in Jerusalem; a full moon lit up the evening. Near it the planet Venus hung like a blazing white torch in the sky. The scene was hushed, spiritual, eerie . . . I was standing by the Western Wall, leaning over a parapet that blocks access to the square before the wall. There was a long drop down to a concrete pavement on the other side of the parapet—not the way it really is in Jerusalem. *Chasidim* are praying at the wall, swaying, and so forth, some in their fur hats, their male children imitating them like miniature adults. I have my regular work hat on. Some bearded Jews in black hats and black coats come up to me and tip my work hat forward to reveal that I am not wearing a yarmulke. I tell them brusquely to go away, I don't want to buy a yarmulke. I start to write something, perhaps a prayer, following the ancient custom, to be inserted in a crack in the Wailing Wall. Shouting angrily in Hebrew, they beat me fiercely, lift me over their heads, and throw me over the parapet. I land on the concrete and lay there face down in a crucified position. *(pause)* I woke up with terrible anxiety *(pause)* . . . *(continues brightly)*: Afterwards I could think only of the telephone call to you and wonder if you had taped what I said—it was real paranoia. As I thought about the dream I had a visual association of all my Jewish ancestors pointing at me, accusing me of not raising my daughter, the adulteress, in the faith. But I am doing something similar and in some ways worse, for you were once a patient! It is all too horrible to think about, but the guilt over what my daughter has done, far more extreme than anything I ever . . . but like everybody I did have fantasies about doing such things . . . what she has done is really deep, a tribal betrayal, a disgrace, and there has to be punishment. *(pause)* This stuff is just tearing me to pieces!

Ruth: What about your wife? Why did she move out? Couldn't you turn to her? You were married a long time. Does she mean nothing to you? What happened?

Barry: Over and over again my wife said to me, "I tried to understand you but I couldn't. Why all this tension? What is it doing to our marriage?" My wife is no longer content to be a homebody; after twenty-five years of marriage and raising children she wants a self of her own and she is determined to find it now that the children are grown up. So she left me. And who could blame her? *(pause)*

> I have heard the wings beating
> of the grim black angel of death.
>
> Terrified I fall back groping
> for something within or without
> to hold me up.
>
> Mother, I shout, where are you?
> I need you now, don't be away,
> I must have some place
>   where I can stay.
>
> I can't hold out against
>   that grim beat,

that relentless beat,
much longer . . .

(*pause*)

More and more I turn inward, thinking in concentric circles, trying to find what was missing in all those years, and always arriving at a basic visual image. It is my mother's face distorted with rage, gnashing her teeth, out of control, beside herself with frustration at one of my temporary childhood refusals to do what she wanted me to do.

The tension was reflected on my wife; with my children; in ever-expanding circles of tension in my lifeworld, every aspect of my living has become an occurrence of tension and become invested with worry and insecurity. I try again and again to regulate this tension and to fall back on some kind of a compassionate inner core! But at the center of my inner core are those teeth, jumping out of my mother's raging face, that image of those bright glistening teeth, metallic in their luster, gleaming in the white light, stark, merciless, investing the tension with still more tension.

I am moving farther and farther away from the dreams of my youth. Like Sartre's* Roquentin, "I have a broken spring. . . I walk at random, calm and empty, under this wasted sky. . . *I must not be afraid."* I must look elsewhere . . . I must travel. . . I must see new cultures . . . I must pull myself together . . . I will go to Africa; that certainly is far enough away from here and after all, it is probably where the human species began. Albert Schweitzer said, "The clue to the nature of man is at its purest in rural Africa because there is no need to peel off layers that cover more sophisticated societies."† (*pensively*) Was he correct?

Ruth: Barry, I don't know what to make of this. When I was your patient you brought me happiness, relief of suffering, joy at last . . . even with my crazy husband. Now you call me, you are passionate, you are wild for my body, for my very soul, and yet

---

*J. P. Sartre, 1964, p. 67.
†E. Berman, 1986, p. 66.

somehow I feel you are not here, you are distracted, you are holding yourself back. I am grateful to you, I love you, but it is not me, Ruth, that you want. I don't know what you really want except relief for some kind of inner torment. When you hold me I don't feel you are really holding me . . . I don't know what is going on. (*pause*) I must leave; my child is due home from school soon. (*She gets up to leave.*)

Barry: No! No! Wait! (*Hands her a small scissors.*) I need a lock of your hair. Please! (*Ruth cuts a small lock off and hands it to him.*)

Barry: The other hair also, please! (*Ruth turns her back to the audience, raises her skirt, and cuts off a small lock of pubic hair; she hands it to him.*)

Barry (*puts all the hair in a small envelope and pockets it*): Don't leave yet. I need you . . . I can't live without you. Why can't you understand that?

(*Ruth casts him a sad long look over her shoulder and leaves. Barry sits down on the sofa and sinks his head in his hands. Slowly he rocks back and forth.*)

Barry (*wailing*): I am withering!

(*Curtain*)

ACT III

(*As the lights dim a spotlight reveals an old bench with a charcoal-black burn angrily slashed across it, standing at the extreme right front of the stage—well out of the way of the action. It remains there for the rest of the play, illuminated by the spotlight, except when the spotlight is directed on a character as specified in stage instructions. The curtain suddenly rises and the stage is bathed in a harsh bright light. At the right hand side of the stage is a cafe table, round, with four chairs, pepper and salt shakers and an ash tray in the middle. A bottle of wine stands on it surrounded by glasses, as well as plates and silverware, all set up for customers. The door to the room is on the lefthand side wall. Across the back at the top there is a large sign that reads "International Hotel, Nairobi." On a shelf at the back of the room toward the right, stands a radio. At the center of the back wall there is a door-sized opening covered by a hanging drape. A reclining easychair is at the back on the left. Nobody is on the stage. The radio begins to present an announcement.)*

Radio: The government has instituted a massive clampdown in recent months to curb the underground opposition network, *Mwakenya.* As this shadowy movement is as much the spread of a basic idea about the need for further liberation of the people from corrupt and self-serving politicians, from an avidly accumulating ruling class, and from increasing direct subservience to the U.S. military presence, it is not surprising that the government cannot catch this invisible but pervasive spirit of freedom.

What the government is doing is to arrest, detain, and often torture anyone suspected of disseminating such thoughts, especially, teachers, scholars, and students . . .

(At this point Barry comes crashing through the door on the left. He is dressed in a sportshirt, part of which hangs out over his belt, with one sleeve rolled up and the other rolled down. He seems to be in a kind of drunken state and he lurches over to the radio and shuts it off; he then lurches back across the stage and throws himself into the reclining chair. A tall African magician enters through the door calmly with a regal bearing. He is dressed in classical African robes and he carries a small bag attached by a string around his waist.)

Barry: I must have her; don't you understand, I must have her. You are my last hope.

Magician: After all, *Bwana,* I can hardly sprinkle powder from the roots and bark of my magic tree along the entrance of a woman's home back in the United States. We will have to use a more extreme magic! Do you have anything which very personally belongs to this woman? It must be her hair, her fingernails, or a piece of ornament.

Barry (reaching into his pocket): In this envelope are locks of her personal hair. *(Hands it to the Magician.)*

Magician: Good. *(Places the envelope in the bag and now hangs the bag by the string around his neck. Begins walking up and down on the left mumbling to himself.)*

(Just at that point Ken, Alice, and Bob enter. They are dressed in very sharp and snappy safari suits, well pressed and clean, and wearing pith helmets. They walk over to the table on the right. At first they are conversing animatedly and do not notice Barry and the Magician. As they seat themselves Bob bangs on the table shouting.)

Bob: Boy! Boy!

Ken: The old fool, when they let him out of the nuthouse finally, he was mute—never said a word to anybody.

Alice: Even when famous people came to visit him?

Ken: Just sat in Venice and refused to speak. Died and was buried there.

Bob: Disgraceful unchristian behavior to the end. How rude. How ungrateful...the old bum! He will burn!

Alice: He should have begged pardon of everybody and stayed out of the way.

Ken: Nope, he just sat there silently, still and mute as a stone, no matter what.

Bob (pounding on the table again): Boy!

(From behind the curtain emerges a diminutive man dressed in a short-sleeved white shirt and white pants and wearing a smiling brown mask. He comes over to the table with menus, which Bob snatches from him. Waiter stands silently in the background.)

Bob: This place is terrible. It is a dirty place.

Ken: Where is Eva?

Alice: She went to the ladies' room. She will be along in a moment.

(They alternatively study the menu and begin to look to the left, watching the mumbling Magician with wonder and then they notice Barry sprawled in the chair in a somewhat stuporous condition.)

Bob (addressing these words to the waiter): Who is that drunk over there? *(The waiter is silent.)* Cat got your tongue, Boy?

Ken: He seems to be watching that native; I wonder what is going on.

Alice: Perhaps it's part of the local entertainment. Maybe it will be our turn.

Bob (pouring and tasting the wine): Ugh! This wine is terrible! I could spit it out. *(To the waiter)* Don't you have anything better?

(The waiter goes back through the curtain and shortly emerges with another decanter of wine. Bob pours it and tastes it.)

Bob: Ugh! This is just as bad. What an awful place.

Ken: Do you have steak here?

Alice (giving the waiter no time to answer): This is no place to eat steak, Ken. Let's have something native.

Bob (to the waiter): Boy, go back there and bring us some kind of native dish for four people. Everything tastes equally as bad in this dirty place. *(The waiter silently leaves.)*

(The attention of the three now becomes focused on the Magician who is beginning to speak.*)

Magician:

Love magic, your magnetic and hypnotizing power is great.

You are now in my service and you will act as I shall direct you.

My faithful servant, go and enter in the heart of Ruth; make her think of nothing else but me who loves her so tenderly.

Magical power, cause her to dream of my love, join her thoughts with mine, let her hear my whisper so that she may come nearer to my bosom.

O, magical power, I got you through lawful means;

---

*All the incantations in this act are paraphrased from J. Kenyatta, 1938.

in agreement with the ancestral magical spirits.

O, magical power, I recite the spells in magical language;
   you will not therefore fail to serve me faithfully.

*(As he makes this incantation the lights begin to dim; the drape over
the doorway moves aside and Ruth is seen standing silently, bathed in an
eerie yellow light. She is dressed in her panties and bra again and stands
holding her arms out toward Barry.)*

Bob: Dear Jesus, what is this!

Alice: I can't believe it.

Ken: It's some kind of a stage show—you see, it is part of the
entertainment.

Alice: Be quiet. Let's see what happens.

*(Barry rises out of his chair and begins to move toward Ruth but the
Magician stops him. He comes between them and both listen intently.)*

Magician: My beloved, open your heart and get ready to receive my words of love.

Barry and Magician: (chanting together)

I want you to know that I love you. To me you are like the
   rays of the sun, the moon, and the morning star.

When you hear my words of love you will, I am sure, give
   me a positive answer, for there is no room in my heart
   for a negative reply.

I have sent you my love magic wrapped in the rays of the
   sun. This will show my real love to you.

Through the warmth of the morning sun, the magnetic
   power will penetrate into your heart. Do not fail to
   receive my words of love with an open and tender heart.

*(As these words are spoken the light changes from an eerie yellow hue
to a more passionate red until the color seems so intense it will almost
burst.)*

Bob (very uneasily): This is heathen, too erotic.

Alice: I'm getting anxious . . . I'm afraid.

Ken: Be quiet, will you!

(Ruth steps forward, bathed in a passionate reddish light. Magician steps back. Barry moves toward her, and they stand with arms outstretched, hands clasped, the high point of adoration.)

Barry:

While our fates twine together, sate we our eyes
    with love;
For long night comes upon you
    and a day when no day returns.
Let the gods lay chains upon us
    so that no day shall unbind them.
Fool who would set a term to love's madness,
For the sun shall drive with black horses,
    earth shall bring wheat from barley,
The flood shall move toward the fountain
    Ere love know moderations,
    The fish shall swim in dry streams.
No, now while it may be, let not the fruit of
    life cease.*

(An ecstatic pause)

Magician (suddenly stepping between them): Bwana, Memsahib, stop!

(Ruth quickly retreats and disappears.)

Barry (screaming and leaping around the room): Why did you stop it?

Magician: Do you really want this? She was your patient! Do you realize she is a married woman? Evil is in this; reconsider.

Barry (wildly): I must have her. I cannot wait. Do it again. Bring her back. *(He careens around the room out of control.)*

---

*E. Pound, 1949, p. 88.

(Bob, Ken, and Alice shrink back into their seats with some fear as Barry lurches around the room, but the Magician holds his arm outstretched and Barry is pushed away as if by some mysterious force. He collapses sobbing into the chair. The Magician quietly leaves. Just then Eva enters through the door on the left, also dressed in a safari suit and pith helmet. She sees Barry in the chair and, hiding her surprise and revulsion at his appearance, walks primly up to him.)

Eva: Barry, we meet again at last. *Jambo,* how do you do? *(She extends a hand formally.)*

Barry (recovering himself and embarrassed): Hello, Eva, it's so good to see you once more.

Bob: Well I never . . .

Alice: What is going on?

Ken: Who is this?

Eva (turning toward her friends): Alice, Bob, Ken, I would like you to meet my old friend, the psychiatrist Barry, the person whose letter you are familiar with.

(There is a moment of stunned silence during which the waiter reappears carrying several dishes of food which he places on the table and silently leaves.)

Ken (rising politely): Glad to meet you, Barry *(extending a hand).*

Barry: How do you do? *(Shakes his hand.)*

Bob: How do you do, Barry? *(Does not extend a hand.)*

Barry: Hello.

Alice: Glad to meet you, Barry. Won't you join us.

Barry: There is no extra chair.

Bob (banging on the table and shouting): Boy! Boy!

(The waiter reappears.)

Bob: Another chair.

(The waiter disappears and reappears with a chair that fits the others at the table. Barry joins them at an angle so that he is also facing the audience. He has recovered his manners to some extent by this time but is clearly terribly shaken by the magical experience. Eva seems somewhat embarrassed and ill at ease by the whole situation.)

Eva (to engage Barry in polite bourgeois conversation): Well, Barry, it is so nice to see you again. We are having a wonderful tour. So educational! So spiritually uplifting! My mind is filled with the beauty of nature.

Bob: It makes us thank God that we are decent Christian folk living in a decent Christian country. What the early missionaries must have experienced here, God bless them! Open eroticism, women walking around undressed, without shame or embarrassment.

Alice: How long have you been here, Barry? We arrived about a week ago, bought the proper attire, took some tours already, and saw lots of animals. I can't even remember the names of all the beasts.

Ken: I could do without the mosquitoes and the flies. But Nairobi seems relatively free of malaria. It must have been beautiful in colonial days. Barry, don't you agree the incidence of kwashiorkor is much higher now? And the Masai—living with their cattle—what a risk for anthrax! Have you visited the "Flying Doctors" organization on your tour?

Barry: I arrived a week ago also. But I was so shocked by the slums of Nairobi that I went to the university to discuss the matter. I found only despair and a protest movement. Most of the students and teachers were uneasy and afraid to say much about it. I found no answers, only torment and longing; finally I could stand it no longer and sought out the ancient customs and magic. I did not tour or see the animals; I spoke to the people as much as I could and tried to understand their plight.

Eva: Barry, you are missing the whole point of such a trip. Go on safari! Nature is awesome here and one gets such a sense of belonging to a cosmic order, an inextricable order of gods, mortals, earth, and sky...

Bob: You mean earth, mortals, heaven, and one God, and His Only Begotten Son, my dear.

Eva: It was so beautiful out. The sun was shining and the flowers were all so brightly colored! We even got a chance to go into the luxurious swimming pool at the hotel.

Barry: I went down to the huge Mathare State Mental Hospital just outside of Nairobi. In the hospital the roads were only red mud and there were pools of stagnant water everywhere. The patients were kept in cages like animals in the zoo and the smell was oppressive. There were twelve-hundred patients officially, but I guess there were about two thousand and only about ten poorly trained professionals to care for them. I do not think there was a psychiatrist in the place at all. Probably the nurses were doing most of the work. I offered to help them, but my offer was rejected because they had not even organized themselves to accept outside help. This is all part of the beginning of nationalization in Kenya; they are not used to getting themselves together and operating the kinds of organizations that raise funds and get the cooperation of other countries, as they do, for example, in Israel. I left there very dejected and frustrated. They obviously do not want any more Albert Schweitzers in Kenya. But I can't figure out what they do want.

Eva: I tell you, Barry, you ought to go on safari. That's where the beauty is.

Ken: We ran all over the Masai Mara game reserve and I brought three cameras with me. One of them was a new movie camera which even took pictures that you could play directly on your television. We got many, many pictures of magnificent animals, although they seem to be disappearing from Africa.

Alice: The scenery was very unusual but I can't say that it was beautiful.

Eva: As Hemingway wrote so accurately, we were in the green hills of Africa, especially on our safari to Tsavo. The humans and animals were close to the land. Everything was built low down and hidden by the tall grass except for massive animals like the stately statuesque giraffes who stood out on the horizon like tall trees against the clear blue sky. There were herds of huge black buffalo and lions lurking everywhere in the bush; the earth, the sky, the mortals, the gods, all together, mirroring each other. I finally began to understand what Heidegger was talking about.

Bob (peevishly): Well, *I* don't understand what Heidegger was talking about and I have already tried to correct you, Eva. I wish you would pay attention.

Ken: And what about the filth and the disease?

Eva: For the first time I got some understanding of the life force, and what Heidegger meant when he spoke of Being both revealing and concealing itself at the same time; what could be a better example than a group of lions hidden in the bush? You have to get very close. You can spot them and sometimes not spot them even while staring at the same place. It's incredible! And this is true of the other species also. It's only in Africa that you can understand the interrelationship of the earth, the sky, the gods, and the mortals. As Heidegger said, we have become estranged from the planet on which we dwell.

Bob: I still don't understand what you're talking about, Eva. Your mind seems to be turned by your African experience. All I can see here are a lot of primitive people very much in need of more Christian missionaries and hospitals like the one we visited in Kijabe run by the African Inland Church. The chaplain visited every African patient in his or her bed and he boasted of three hundred people who chose for Christ over the past year. How lucky the Africans are to have this kind of attention in addition to the medical attention our decent Christian missionaries give to them.

Eva: And Barry, what about Mount Kilimanjaro that you have always written about going to see? When we approached it on the way to Amboseli we first saw the snow-capped peak and had the greatest difficulty distinguishing it from the clouds. As we got closer, its majestic dominance over the entire Amboseli plain became apparent, and we were transfixed by the majesty of Kilimanjaro, the reaching up of the earth to kiss the cloudy heavens.

In this scene where the earth mirrored the heavens and the heavens mirrored the earth, what was the role of the mortals and the gods? Surely, part of our role is to marvel in awe at such a manifestation of Being; one of the greatest scenes on the surface of the planet on which we dwell. And the spirit of the gods pervades it all . . . ask the Africans.

Barry: All I could see were those tin-roofed shacks that littered the highway with the ragged children crawling around between them, and the women bent over nearly double with huge burdens on their backs. The population of Kenya just grows and grows; the fastest increase in the world.

Ken: On our safari to Amboseli I had the driver stop near the observation tower, as close as vehicles could come. Then I climbed up on the ragged rocks through the red mud to the observation tower and mounted it. What stretched before me, while insects of every kind were buzzing around my head, was a vast wasteland of swamps and desolation, crowned at one end by the harsh, rugged, pitiless Kilimanjaro. What went through my mind was the awesome cruelty of nature and how only the application of reason and scientific medicine has any possibility to help these people; yet somehow they seem too proud to be helped.

Eva: You don't understand. They are not too proud. They have a different way of life and they are not convinced that our way of life is better. But the price they pay for their own way of life is the problem of disease and a short life span. I do not know how we are going to reach them. The gap between the West and Africa is greater than I thought it would be, but I am not sure that we have the spiritual edge over them.

Bob: How can you say that, my dear? Christianity has yet to conquer Africa, as you can see from persisting horrible heathen practices like clitoridectomy that still continues in spite of efforts by missionaries and sometimes even the government to stop it.

Eva: I admit all these things, but sometimes as I watch these people who live so close to the earth I still wonder if we in the West have not taken a wrong turn from which there is no escape. Barry sees only the gloomy side, but there is a message in this safari for all of us, I think, although of course I'm no philosopher.

Alice: Well, I know what *I* came to Africa for. I love to see all the animals and take pictures . . . and every place we stop there is some other trinket for me to buy. Ken will have to get another suitcase to hold all the spears, masks, and souvenirs that I have accumulated in a few short weeks. And won't my friends at the bridge club be jealous! I don't see what all this deep discussion is going to accomplish since each person sees in Africa what he or she wishes to see. The lady sitting next to me on the bus saw giraffes in every piece of wood that was sticking up and elephants in every boulder; as far as she was concerned there were herds of animals everywhere, whereas actually there are hardly any left in Amboseli and you have to drive around for hours in the hot sun to see them. So what is all the fuss about? Isn't it about time that we spend an hour in the bar having some drinks before eating dinner? Don't you remember, we have first-class luxury accommodations and meals on this tour . . . so let's enjoy them. The natives are very polite, it seems to me, and I know they appreciate our presence here and even call the tourist industry "Kenya's oil." Come on Barry, lighten up!

Barry (as if in a trance)

There are some feelings
    that have no words,
There are some thoughts
    that can not be expressed,
There are some moments
    that have such an intensity,
There are some longings
    that are so painful,
There are some situations
    that are so conflicted,
Not even the gods
high on Mount Olympus
all-powerful, all-knowing
rulers of our destiny
are equal to them;
the mighty Zeus himself
ruler of the earth and skies

sheds a tear or two
and the heroes in Valhalla
　　groan in their perplexity
　　　　on and on through
　　　　　never-ending time
　　　　　　until all
　　　　　　　is silence.

(pause)

(There is a banging at the door. Waiter appears from behind the curtain and opens it. Police Inspector enters, wearing frowning brown mask and military uniform.)

Inspector (politely going over to table): Jambo, dear tourists, may I see your passports? *(They hand them over. He thumbs through them and looks up when he reaches Barry's.)* . . . Doctor Barry . . . *(Looks at Barry, who is the only one not in safari suit, and returns the other passports)* you must be the one. *(His tone changes.)* Stand up and come over here, white man. *(Barry rises and comes over as the police inspector places his left hand on his revolver. The others look on in stunned disbelief.)* Are you the one who distributed these protest pamphlets? *(Pulls one out of his pocket with right hand and reads):* "We protest the detention of university staff and students for uttering statements unfavorable to the government. We demand freedom for those held without trial since 1982."

Barry: Yes.

Inspector: You don't even know these people. Why do you protest? Why do you care?

Barry: Citizens of your country are not permitted to protest. Was this Kenyatta's vision of freedom? You Africans have a word for it, *Mantu:* All humankind is one. Reason is Greek, law is Hebrew, feeling is African, but all humankind, *Dasein* is one; the Spirit through which Being unconceals itself in the sudden blink of an eye. Spirit is everything!

Inspector (menacingly): White man, you are crazy and you are lucky. If our military officers did not have such a good relationship with the military in your country, you would disappear. As it is you will only disappear from here. *(Advances threateningly and grabs him by the shirt.)* Foul-smelling white son of a bitch, if you know what's good for you, don't let the sun set on you in Nairobi *(shoves Barry over backwards so he falls with a crash on the table and then stamps out, tossing Barry's passport on the floor. Waiter, who has been silently watching, comes forward, helps Barry into a chair, picks up and returns his passport, and begins cleaning up.)*

Barry (to waiter in Swahili): Asante sana (waiter nods silently).

Bob: Clean up over here, boy. The nerve of these heathen. I will see our ambassador. The State Department will hear about this! The marines . . . *(Waiter cleans up and leaves.)*

Barry (moaning): I can't stand it any more. Something has to happen. What am I to do? *(cries out in despair)*: Magician! Magician!

Bob: Boy! Boy!

(The waiter reappears from behind the curtain.)

Bob: Boy, get the Medicine Man again. It's urgent.

Ken: This is all nonsense.

Eva: It seems as if only a magician can help him anymore.

Alice: I am beginning to be afraid.

(Waiter goes out the door, and soon the Magician reappears, dressed as before. From his bag this time he takes out a small bell which he holds in his left hand and in the right hand he holds a small narrow gourd from about six to twelve inches in length, containing the magical particles with healing power.)

Magician (to Barry): Oh sick one, come over here and lick the healing magic. *(He holds out the gourd.)*

(Barry lurches over and licks the gourd, sinking to his knees in front of the Magician. The stage darkens except for light focused on them. The

Magician begins to chant a healing ritual phrase with a strong voice and a sharp rhythm, accompanied by the tinkling of the bell):

> *Mondo morwaru, ni okeete koingata morima ooyo waku,*
> *ohamwe na ngoma iria ioreheete.*
> *Umbora migiro irea ooe, ona eeria ootoe.*
> *Wethagathage, amu ni okometahika yoothe.*

(At the same time he swings the magical horn over the head of the patient. He repeats this phrase and ritual slowly twice. Suddenly, having achieved a mystical state of mind, he stops chanting and looks Barry straight in the face.)

Magician: Sick man, I have come to chase away your illness. I will also chase away the evil spirits which brought it.

Confess the evils which you know, and also those you do not know. Prepare yourself, for you are about to vomit all these evils.

(He pours the powder from the gourd into a little pool in front of Barry, who kneels over facing the pool as though he was in a state of vomiting. The Magician squats on the other side of the pool, facing Barry. A singsong chant by both of them begins.)

Magician: This is the magic powder *(points to the pool)*. It comes from a root with which I root up the evils that are in your body.

Barry (leans over and licks the powder and pretends he is vomiting, saying): I vomit the illness and the evil spirits that are in my body.

Magician: This is clearing away. I clear away the evils that are in your body.

Barry: This is clearing away. I clear away the evils that are in my body.

Magician: This is a weakening. I weaken the evil spirits that are in your body.

Barry: This is a weakening. I weaken the evil spirits that are in my body.

Magician: Vomit, and vomit the unknown evils that are concealed in your body.

Barry: Vomit, and vomit the unknown evils that are concealed in my body.

Magician: This is a calming. I calm the illness that is in your body.

(Barry begins to rise and attains a trance-like state.)

Barry: Now I am calm. Now I know what I must do. Goodbye, my friends.

(He leaves through the door. The light returns and the Magician also leaves, so that Bob, Eva, Ken, and Alice are left alone together.)

Bob (banging on the table): Boy! Boy!

(The waiter reappears.)

Bob: Bring more wine.

(The waiter disappears behind the curtain.)

Eva: Couldn't you be a little more polite, dear?

Bob: These people understand one language and that is strength and force. If we don't use it on them, they use it on each other. Even that weird infidel poet Blake* knew about Africans:

Night spoke to the Cloud:
"Lo these Human form'd spirits, in smiling hypocrisy
    War
Against one another; so let them War on, slaves to the
    eternal Elements"

(The waiter reappears with another decanter of wine.)

Bob (tasting the wine): Ugh! This wine is terrible. I could spit it out. Let's go; this place is polluted, unclean, heathen. Boy! Our bill!

(Waiter hands him the bill.)

(Bob pays the bill and all leave except the waiter, who silently begins cleaning up.)

(Curtain)

---

*W. Blake, 1974c, p. 364.

ACT IV

Scene 1

(As lights dim again, the spotlight is on the bench and we hear the sound of ocean waves until the curtain rises. When the curtain rises we find ourselves in a very simple Japanese bed chamber. There is a futon on the floor to the audience's left, and a small dresser on the right hand side about the size of the desk in the office in Act II. The door to the room is on the left side wall and there is a very large window at the back. An enormous Japanese flag is displayed on the wall. Two people are lying on the futon at the left of the stage. The entire scene much resembles the opening of Act II. A diminutive Korean wearing a smiling yellow mask is naked to the waist and lying with his back to us. Anna, who resembles Ruth and is dressed in a nightgown, has her arms and legs wrapped around him and they are belly to belly, a pose identical to the opening of Act II. They are clearly in the process of beginning to make love and for a few moments they begin to go through such motions, but suddenly there is a loud banging on the door. They ignore it at first, but the banging continues and the Korean becomes somewhat frightened and leaves through a curtained opening on the right. Anna, with the banging continuing, takes a bathrobe from a hook and wraps it around her. She walks over to the door and opens it. Barry lurches through the door.)

Anna: Dad! You? Here?

Barry: Yes, I have to talk with you. I must right these ancient wrongs.

Anna: Why this distress? *What* is wrong? I have asked nothing from you for a long time . . . since I came to Japan. Why are you here?

Barry(vociferously, barely controlled):

And the running form, naked, Blake,
Shouting, whirling his arms, the swift limbs,
Howling against the evil,
  his eyes rolling,
Whirling like flaming cartwheels,
, and his head held backward to gaze on the evil

As he ran from it,
  to be hid by the steel mountain. . .*

Anna (calmly): Dad, why is it that neither you nor that crazy poet you are always quoting ever paid attention to the very words the poet put into the mouth of Confucius:

And Kung said, and wrote on the bo leaves:
  If a man have not order within him
He can not spread order about him;
And if a man have not order within him
His family will not act with due order . . .
And said nothing of the "life after death."
And he said
  "Anyone can run to excesses,
It is easy to shoot past the mark,
It is hard to stand firm in the middle."†

Barry (trying to recover his professional self): You have a sexual problem.

Anna: You have a sexual problem, but there are some things daughters do not discuss with their fathers.

Barry: It is not heterosexual to stain the family and commit adultery, it is pathological.

Anna: You sound like your mother and you are acting like her.

Barry: I am trying to be helpful, trying to be just like my father.

Anna: You are not helpful; you gnash your teeth like your mother.

Barry: I wanted to replace my father and love my mother.

Anna: You want to replace your mother and love your father . . . and you have done it.

---

*E. Pound, 1950, p. 68.
†E. Pound, 1950, p. 59.

Barry: How dare you talk to me like this? You, the apple of my eye! *(sinks to his knees)* You were the joy of my life, the blessing among my children, my firstborn, my adored child!

Anna: You asked for it . . . you just rant and rave like your patients. Why can't you sit still and be silent? Why do you come bursting in here . . . all the way to Japan! Are you weird?

Barry: To right the wrong you have done. To release the curse on my house. To put an end to this endless pain and suffering and tension. A curse is on my house and I must take action to vomit out the evil.

Anna: Dad, you *are* weird.

(The Korean in the smiling yellow mask now enters the room: dressed neatly in shirt, tie, and jacket.)

Anna (speaking slowly and clearly and pointing politely to Barry): This . . . is . . . my . . . father.

Korean (in halting Japanese): Ko-nichi-wa *(extends his hand and attempts to be very friendly).*

Barry: Don't you *ko-nichi-wa* me, you homewrecker!

Korean (not comprehending the English): Ko-nichi-wa.

Barry: Damn you, I'll wipe you off the face of the earth!

Korean (uncomprehending but recognizing Barry's anger, and more timidly now): Ko-nichi-wa.

Anna: Dad, what is the matter?

Barry (shouting): A curse is on my house! The Nigerian said it best:

> Your houses will leak from the floods
> and your soil will crack from the drought;
> your sons will refuse to pick up the hoe
> and prefer to wander in the wilds;
> you shall learn ways of cheating
> and you will poison the cola nuts
> you serve your own friends.

Yes, things will fall apart.*

Anna: Dad, stop it . . . control yourself!

(Barry shouting incomprehensibly something about wiping the Korean off the face of the earth and vomiting out evil, steps forward and draws a revolver from his coat pocket. He fires all the bullets point blank into the body of the Korean. Korean staggers over to the right hand corner of the room and repeats weakly):

Korean: Ko-nichi-wa. *(collapses on the floor, dead).*

(Anna shrieks, runs over, and throws herself sobbing on top of him. Anna remains in this position throughout the rest of the scene.)

Barry (leaps on the dresser in triumph): Revenge, revenge, revenge at last. Now I can face my ancestors. Now I have righted the ancient wrongs. Now I have done what had to be done. Peace at last!

(There is again a banging on the door.)

Barry (ignoring the banging, deliriously): See what has happened. See how I have redeemed the curse on my house. See my triumph. At last I have found a way to relieve this tension.

(The door bursts open. Four Japanese police enter, two males and two females. Although their uniforms suspiciously resemble safari suits, they now have on police helmets and wear police badges and they carry nightsticks. Barry continues to stand on the dresser with manic shouts of triumph, and the police attempt to get him down and subdue him. A fierce battle ensues. Barry at first lands a few blows, but the men, using Japanese judo-holds, finally manage to subdue him, getting angrier and angrier at his resistance. He is thrown down on the futon. The women begin to scream "Banzai" and the men begin to beat Barry as he lies on the futon. With the women screaming, "Banzai," and egging them on, the men beat him with their fists and sticks again and again. Finally, with a massive scream of "Banzai," the four police raise his body over their heads and hurl him crashing through the window in the back.)

(Curtain)

---

*C. Achebe, 1961, *Things Fall Apart,* quoted in Mazrui, 1986, p. 11.

ACT IV

Scene 2

(When the curtain rises we find Barry with his head facing the audience, lying face down in the position of Christ crucified on the cross. He is lying on a stone floor in a prison cell, dirty and bloody. On the left side wall, as before, there is a door and on the right side wall there are prison bars over a window. A low stool stands on the right hand side which would enable a person to reach the prison bars. There is also a futon on the right hand side. The back of the cell is blank and serves as a large screen, on which an unseen projector projects a huge picture of Emperor Hirohito, bemedaled and in uniform as he appeared during the Second World War, looking out at the audience as did Freud in Act II. His look, however, is inscrutable. Barry is now in an organically damaged and delirious state. He slowly rolls over on his side and, seeing the picture, raises his hand to it.)

Barry: Oh my God, why hast thou forsaken me? Have I not followed the Magician's spell? Have I not achieved the revenge? Let me now speak with my ancestors and receive their blessing, for:

I am almost Extinct & soon shall be a shadow in Oblivion,
Unless some way can be found that I may look upon
    thee & live.
Hide me some shadowy semblance, secret whisp'ring in
    my Ear,
In secret of soft wings, in mazes of delusive beauty.
I have look'd into the secret soul of him I lov'd,
And in the Dark recesses found Sin cannot return.*

Oh, immortal Blake!

(He slowly raises himself to a sitting position. Then he crawls over to the stool and drags it toward the front of the stage. Seated on the stool he stares intently at the picture of Hirohito.)

Barry: Now I understand. This is what Freud meant when he said Spirit is everything . . . The Kenyan† wrote, "The spiritual

---

*W. Blake, 1974b, p. 370.
†B. Ogt, 1961, quoted in A. Mazrui, 1986, p. 50.

part of man . . . is *Jok*, the power which is responsible for conception as well as for fortunes and misfortunes. . . . *Jok* is not an impartial universal power; it is the essence of every being, the force which makes everything what it is, and God himself, the greatest *Jok,* is life-force in itself." . . . I have lost the life-force! There is no clearing for me, only darkness. . . . Oh my God *(reaches out to the picture, which then changes via the slide projector to that of a male lion).*

Barry (addressing the lion): Father, Father, at last you have come. Let us have peace. Forgive me! I have tried to remove the curse upon my house. When you were sick I tried not to neglect you. I did not want to destroy you. I could not help you as you sank into an arteriosclerotic death. I was trying to achieve a self of my own. I wanted desperately to be myself, to help others find themselves. I did not want the responsibility for your death. I tried to escape it. When they told me you had cancer and should have extensive surgery, I objected! I stopped it! Your cardiovascular condition could never have withstood the surgery! I am sure that you did not die of metastases from the cancer! John died of metastases of cancer, but he was young and strong and it was unexpected. What could I do? Forgive me! Let us have peace—let us come together forever *(holds his arms out to the picture and tries to embrace it, at which point it abruptly changes into the picture of a snarling female lion carnivorously guarding its prey).*

Barry (shrinks back, horrified): Mother! You? Here? What have I done? I knew you were lonely. I knew you were old, but I was trying to have a self of my own. Now I am lost in the forest . . . I didn't want to neglect you. *(Shouts)* Don't show me those teeth. *(Screams in a panic)* Don't show me those teeth!

(Barry, now delirious, springs over to the right side of the cell and pounds on the wall.)

Barry (shouting): Mother, my own Anticlea, I have failed you. I have failed you. I have failed you. *(He shouts this over and over again.)* I could not be what you wanted me to be . . . what I wanted to be . . . Oh! Lacan was so right! To be what the mother most desires . . . Anticlea! Mother of Odysseus! Oh!

Offstage booming voice:

And Anticles came, whom I beat off, and then
        Tiresias, Theban,
Holding his golden wand, knew me, and spoke first:
"A second time? Why? man of ill star,
"Facing the sunless dead and this joyless region?
"Stand from the fosse, leave me my bloody bever
"For Soothsay."
        And I stepped back,
And he strong with the blood, said then: "Odysseus
Shalt return through spiteful Neptune, over dark seas,
Lose all companions."* . . . And then Anticlea came.

(Barry covers his head with his arms and the picture on the wall abruptly changes to that of Ruth. As Barry calms down he looks up.)

Barry: Peace, peace at last. Can I possess you at last? Being, unconcealed for a moment?

— Old Ez said,

"What thou lov'st well shall not be reft from
   Thee
What thou lov'st well is thy true heritage"†.

Ruth, you are my last chance. I cannot live without you. Without you I have nothing. I am empty, depleted, collapsed, utterly lost, fragmented. . . . *(He stares enraptured at the picture.)* . . . Ruth I love you. I adore you, you *must* understand. . . . I love you beyond human comprehension. . . . Without you I cannot survive . . . without you Being, the life force, escapes from me . . . forever. . . .

(He rushes over to the picture, but as he does it changes again to an animal family, perhaps of zebras.)

Barry (recoiling): I am an intruder. I am an outsider. I am not wanted. If I possess her I will destroy her family. There is nothing for me; nothing . . . nothing!

(The picture now changes again to a large herd of animals, stampeding away, perhaps wildebeests.)

---

*E. Pound, 1950, pp. 4-5.
†E. Pound, 1950, p. 521.

Barry: They are all moving away and I am left here alone. I cannot belong anywhere. Have I not righted the curse on my house? Why can I not now return to the family of humankind from which I have come? Even Odysseus returned. Why can modern humans never return? Why are we so cut off from Being? Why?

(He rushes to the picture again, which abruptly changes to a menacing herd of elephants, with the bull elephants facing him at the center, their tusks lowered and pointing at him.)

Barry (recoils): What am I to do? What am I to do? . . . I have lost the life force. . . . I am lost forever in the dark woods. . . . No Virgil comes. . . . There is no way out, no light at all. . . . What am I to do?

(As he recoils he stumbles on the stool; this gives him an idea and he carries the stool near the cell bars on the right. As he does this the picture changes to that of Mount Kilimanjaro, no animals. He undoes his belt and his shoelaces and fashions a rope. Standing on the stool, he ties one end to the cell bars and the other around his neck.)

Barry:

I lie on the verge of the deep;
I see thy dark clouds ascend;
I see thy black forests and floods,
A horrible waste to my eyes!*

(As he kicks over the stool and lets out a last dying gasp, the cell becomes completely dark and now only the picture, changed to the inscrutable Hirohito, remains, illuminating the stage. The spotlight is on the bench. As the curtain falls a chant is heard in a booming voice.)

Offstage Booming Voice: Antonin Artaud said, "I am suffering from a terrible sickness of the spirit." And the surrealists said of Artaud, "Let us leave him to his disgusting mixture of dreams, vague assertions, pointless insolence, and manias."

(FINIS)

---

*W. Blake, 1974a, p. 354.

17 PSYCHOANALYSIS AS CREATIVITY

Video meleora proboque: deteriora sequor—like all other human beings, I know what I ought to do, but I continue to do what I know I ought not to do.

—*Aldous Huxley*, Eyeless in Gaza

In this chapter I will first discuss a malignant form of creativity in psychoanalytic therapy, one that occurs when a therapist "falls in love" with a patient, as illustrated in Barry's play. This is a pathological distortion of the creativity involved in "falling in love" (see Chapter 9). Then I will outline the "constructivist" aspect of psychoanalytic treatment, a modern version of Nietzsche's "perspectivism" (Chessick, 1997b), in which the patient and therapist are viewed as inevitably creating together on a moment-to-moment basis the material that constitutes the dialogue of the analytic process. I will compare and contrast that view with "empathy" from the self psychology channel, requiring the therapist to creatively put himself or herself "in the shoes" of the patient, for example, to imagine what it would be like to be almost seven feet tall, or a dwarf, or whatever, and to resonate empathically with the sense of self of the patient at any given time. Finally, I will discuss creative aspects of traditional psychoanalytic treatment that in the practice of the more talented and well-analyzed psychoanalysts have a resemblance to artistic activity.

There has been an increasing realization that all scientific procedures involve a creative process, and that even so-called raw experimental data already carries with it creative choices that have been made as to what constitutes data and how to collect it. The nineteenth-century dichotomy between socially reputable "science" and disreputable "humanities," or between reputable positivistic philosophy and disreputable metaphysical

333

speculation, the latter also a form of artistic creation (see Chapter 19), is gradually breaking down among sophisticated thinkers as we slowly and painstakingly learn that materialism and "unbridled capitalism" (Schlesinger, 1997) are bringing the world to the brink of environmental collapse and nuclear or bacterial terrorism.

Discussion of the Play

Barry's play opens in Arkansas, but it was written before the Clinton presidency, so there are no domestic political allusions. The four opening characters portray four rather typical attitudes toward what our civilization regards as the "Other": poets, psychiatrists, artists, schizophrenics, and assorted individuals who do not seem to fit into the mainstream. Barry is introduced at the time of his disappointment in his daughter. The pathology of his superego is apparent, and he has presumptive symptoms of a narcissistic personality disorder. There is a wide discrepancy between his ideals, which are represented in the play by his allegedly traditional religious deceased male relatives and ancestors, and his actual accomplishments and performance. The disintegration of his daughter's marriage comes across as a narcissistic wound but is probably only symbolic of a series of narcissistic disappointments that have piled up in his life, perhaps culminating with the desertion by his wife. She seems wisely to have outgrown him and found outside interests of her own, once her children left the nest. This is a common story; actually, a woman who does not find a life of her own when her children no longer need her, and who attempts to devote herself to being the nurturing maternal woman her husband would like her to be, his selfobject, often ends up with a depression that is then blamed on menopause.

Barry is also confused, and there is an allusion to the opening of Dante's (1980) *Inferno*:

> When I had journeyed half of our life's way,
> I found myself within a shadowed forest,
> for I had lost the path that does not stray.
> Ah, it is hard to speak of what it was,

that savage forest, dense and difficult,
which even in recall renews my fear:
    so bitter—death is hardly more severe! (Canto I:3)

But, as Barry says near the end of the play, no Virgil appears to guide him.

Throughout the play, the character of Barry is approached in a phenomenologic fashion. Phenomenology comes to understand the truth of something not simply by reference to scientific study and terminology but by moving around it, experiencing it from different perspectives, and letting the manifestations of each perspective communicate the truth of the subject directly, as explained in Chapter 1. In writing this play, Barry was attempting to weave standard psychodynamics and poetry together because he felt, and I agree, that often straightforward psychodynamic presentations lose an ineffable something or exclude the "Other" sometimes found in poetry.

At the beginning of the play Barry is relatively psychologically intact, but he is confused and suffering; his gradual fragmentation is portrayed in stages throughout the play, resulting in his final homicide and suicide. He also has a strange conscience, but one not so unusual in physicians. Parts of it seem hypertrophied and very concerned with the sufferings of this world, while other parts seem blind to the implications, devastation, and self-destructiveness of some of his behavior. He displays a certain narcissistic self-importance.

The poetry ending the first act sets the stage for Barry's subsequent death and presents the lack of love in his house as the precipitating factor in his decline and fall. The enactment of this decline and fall immediately begins to appear in the second act, where the classical, "lovesick" (Twemlow and Gabbard, 1989; Chessick, 1997a) therapist attempts to somehow regain his shattered narcissistic equilibrium by a pathetic kind of masturbation with a patient.

Portrayal of the ex-patient Ruth is in a low key so as not to throw the onus on her provoking of the therapist, because it is the mental set that the therapist brings to the patient that constitutes the central issue in boundary violations. The focus must be on the analytic frame, which it is the sole responsibility of the analyst to produce and maintain. In a safe and secure frame, "empathy and projective identification oscillate back and forth across the semi-permeable membrane constructed by the analytic dyad," allowing what has been called a play space where "more primitive states of fusion and exchange are possible" (Gabbard and Lester, 1996, p. 43). The purpose of analytic boundaries is to emphasize that it is not the function of the analyst to gratify the patient's wishes and needs, but rather to respond to the patient's *"growth needs* (such as the need for empathic understanding, caring, and concern) and, on an ongoing basis, to make sense of the patient's past experience" (p. 45), and so to provide Winnicott's holding environment. But when the analyst attempts deliberate corrective experiences or tries to directly gratify the patient, a serious potential for boundary violations occurs. The safety of the analytic setting along with the analyst's survival of the patient's attacks is obviously very important. The analyst's role is defined by Gabbard and Lester (1996) as:

> relative restraint; an avoidance of excessive self-disclosure; a regularity and predictability of sessions: a devotion to understanding the patient; a generally nonjudgmental attitude; an acknowledgment of complexity in motives, wishes, and needs; a sense of courtesy and respect for the patient; and a willingness to put one's own desires aside in the service of a greater understanding of the patient. (p. 54)

An excellent distinction is made by Gabbard and Lester (1996) between boundary violations and boundary crossings. Although both emerge from countertransference enactments, the former are characterized by having the potential to harm the patient. In current constructivist theory, discussed later in this chapter, boundary crossings take place all the time, and if these are noted and discussed they are saved from becoming violations, but "if an enactment is not discussable for one reason or another, it may bode poorly for the process" (p. 127), and if the enactment is repetitive and unresponsive to the analyst's own self-analytic efforts, we are in the presence of what might well be a boundary violation. It has been my clinical experience that it is much easier to get into boundary violations than to get out of them; it is when the analyst attempts to remove himself or herself from the violation enactment that the patient's rage surfaces and malpractice litigation as well as reports to ethics and licensure committees may result.

Gabbard and Lester's (1996) excellent discussion of post-termination boundaries makes it clear that "once an analyst always an analyst" for any given patient. Research has demonstrated a great readiness for revival of the transference even in patients who have not been seen for a long time, and therefore any involvement of a social nature with a previous patient, as in the instance of Barry with his ex-patient Ruth, is contaminated. It is a disservice to the patient to change roles even after the patient has ceased to be a patient, because the analyst should always be available in the same analytic role for the patient to return to as needed. As Gabbard and Lester pointed out, many patients, "particularly those in the mental health professions, approach analysis with a secret agenda of paving the way for a post-analytic relationship sometimes sexual, sometimes not —that will allow the analyst to be a 'real person'" (p. 153). Termination time is often fraught with loss for both parties and increases the temptation for boundary violation but, as the authors declared, "analysts may not be able to control whom they fall in love with, but they can certainly control whom they fall in bed with" (p. 157).

Barry recognized in writing this play that the entire responsibility rests on the therapist, who in the play is clearly suffering and identifies with the old bum described in the *Wall Street Journal.* The old bum quotes Ezra Pound, fusing together the character Barry, the bum, and Ezra Pound. The narcissistic injuries inflicted on him in his attempt to present something significant at a psychiatric meeting cause Barry to fragment to the point where he begins identifying with a homeless bum and a psychotic poet. The discrepancy between his narcissistic aspirations, which are rationalized in the play as a scientific longing to understand hitherto unknown factors in psychoanalytic treatment, and the casual and indifferent response of the chairman and the audience, presents a severe narcissistic blow to this aging psychiatrist.

In the typical manner of a posttraumatic stress disorder, recalling the psychiatric meeting as he describes it to Ruth stirs up disintegration again. Ruth attempts to hold him in order to soothe him, but it does not work and he continues slowly as if she were not there, in a kind of drugged or dreamlike state. Here he tells us his first dream, a very depressed preoedipal dream that represents his longing for his dead mother, who finally appears in a hallucinatory fashion at the end of the play, as Anticlea, the mother of Odysseus. This represents more narcissism on the part of Barry, a rather grandiose identification with the great and wise Homeric hero.

In the second act comes the usual advice, "Why don't you take a vacation?" Barry responds to this by portraying his alienation, which he regards as having been made complete by the disappointment in his beloved firstborn child. Ruth in a way is the heroine of this act, because she attempts to treat and cure the impending narcissistic disintegration of her ex-therapist. Langs (1982) wrote about the attempt of the patient to cure the therapist so that the therapist may subsequently function as the therapist the patient needs.

The first hint of paranoia appears when Barry imagines a change in Freud's picture. This is condensed together with the Jerusalem dream that portends Barry's demise in the final act of the play. Dreams often portray pathological trends which later, when ego functioning collapses, become a part of conscious life; in this case they appear in Barry's eventual paranoia and hallucinations. The rest of the act demonstrates the increasingly conflictual state of Barry's psyche, moving in a downward spiral toward more and more archaic metaphors and allusions in the style of Pound's progressively published cantos. Projected "all-bad" object representations appear in the form of his raging mother's face. Ruth has failed in her attempt to heal him.

The next phase of Barry's disintegration involves his recourse to magic in the third act. Attempting to get away from his internal conflict he travels to Africa, but he is increasingly depressed by what he experiences there. He externalizes his inner state of conflict, depression, and psychic imprisonment, and attempts to alleviate and rescue the victims of oppression and poverty in whatever way he can, constituting an effort to vicariously rescue himself. This theme is weaved in with his appeal to the Magician to heal him as Ruth, his patient, could not do.

The actual meeting of Barry with the four protagonists from

the opening scene of the first act draws more clearly the distinction between the alienated fragmenting Barry and the ordinary relatively well-adjusted quartet, or at least people who are acceptable in American civilization and are not part of the "Other." The act gains intensity as Barry and the Magician work toward the attempted cure, which fails. After a juxtaposition of the experiences and thoughts of this quartet with the experiences and thoughts of Barry, the act reaches its climax when the inspector threatens Barry with physical harm. From that time on Barry slips into a primitive state and leaves; we are convinced by this point that nothing good is going to happen.

The poetry of Blake is first put in the mouth of Bob, the hostile fundamentalist minister, to demonstrate how an individual can solve his or her intrapsychic problems by the use of fundamentalism, prejudice, and arrogance that relieves the person, at least temporarily, from experiencing the severe and agonizing internal psychic disarray of Barry. Certainly Bob has just as much of a narcissistic disorder as Barry, but he has solved his problems for better or for worse, whereas Barry has not. As the Enlightenment faith in science and reason like that of Ken dissipates in our era, the myth of salvation of humanity solely through science as advocated, for example by Freud, is increasingly replaced by Bob's dangerous regressive solution, intransigently utilizing various religious myths.

The final act opens with an oedipal-like scene, but has an odd twist to it. By this time Barry is psychotic and has no order within him, as Pound paraphrased the recommendation from Confucius' *Analects* in his *Canto XIII*. Barry's psychosis is related to an archaic identification with his mother and the inevitable conflicts produced by that sort of gender identification when it occurs in a male. Anna correctly labels the regressive identification or fusion with his mother as the final step in his disintegration. The price of this archaic identification is a loss of reality testing and a blurring of bodily boundaries. At this point the fragmentation becomes unbearable and Barry attempts to project his internal rage and psychosis onto the Korean as an enemy and to kill it by killing the Korean, a very common dynamic in psychotics who commit murder.

By the second scene of the fourth act Barry is identifying with Jesus in a quasi-psychotic fashion. He begins to experience animals as metaphoric representations of people, and as the fragmentation has become irreversible, he realizes that he has lost all hope of communication and contact with the human race. In another behavior characteristic of psychotic patients who are in that state, he commits suicide, choosing death over total isolation in his psychic inferno.

In the play we see how a sexual relationship with a patient may be a last-ditch defense against the danger of melancholia (Bak, 1973) or even against an impending breakdown of the self of the therapist; similarly, falling in love with the patient, a pathological distortion of the creativity described in Chapters 7 and 9, may also be a last-ditch defense against the same psychic disasters. This breakdown may have begun well before the therapist started treatment with the patient and can occur regardless of whatever provocations the patient does or does not offer. Even very slight clues from the patient, for example, resemblance to an individual from the therapist's childhood, may become a precipitating factor in the formation of disintegration symptoms in the therapist, such as "falling in love at first sight." The roots of all this are firmly planted in infantile psychopathology and should not be confused with a mature love relationship.

Kohut's self psychology has been criticized (Schwartz, 1978) because it lacks a clear definition of the term "fragmentation." The fragmenting self occurs when the patient reacts to narcissistic disappointments, such as the patient's perception of the therapist's lack of empathy, by the loss of the sense of a cohesive self. Signs of this impending fragmentation are disheveled dress, posture and gait disturbances, vague anxiety, time and space disorientation, and hypochondriacal concerns. Barry demonstrates some of this in the play. The concept of the fragmentation of the self seems to be equated with psychotic-like phenomena, at which time reality testing is in danger of being lost. It is characterized as a regressive phenomenon, predominantly autoerotic, a state of fragmented self-nuclei, in contrast to the state of the cohesive self (Kohut, 1971).

Aspects of complete fragmentation are illustrated phenomenologically in the final part of the play. In his early work Kohut (1971) called fragmentation of the self "dissolution of the narcissistic unity of the self" (pp. 120-121), and explained how it is often accompanied by frantic activities of various kinds in the work and sexual areas of the person's life, especially in an effort to "counteract the subjectively painful feeling of self fragmentation by a variety of forced actions, ranging from physical stimulation and athletic activities to excessive work in their profession or business" (p. 119).

Elsewhere I (Chessick, 1997a) have discussed "malignant eroticized countertransference" as a manifestation of fragmentation in technical detail, but keep in mind that female therapists are also vulnerable. For example, a female therapist may attempt to rescue a male patient:

> In such scenarios, the patient tends to be a young man with a personality disorder diagnosis characterized by impulsivity, action orientation, and substance abuse. Despite these characterological symptoms, however, the young man usually possesses considerable interpersonal charm and may have a knack for engaging females in a treatment capacity. A female clinician is often drawn to such men with an unconscious fantasy that her love and attention will somehow influence this essentially decent young man to give up his wayward tendencies. (Gabbard, 1994, p. 131)

This situation, a common one in movies and novels, inevitably leads to disaster.

Perspectivism

Nietzsche's (1882, 1887) *The Gay Science* comprises a series of aphorisms, poems, riddles, jokes, and songs in an attempt to overcome the dreary and systematic nature of traditional German philosophy. His central doctrine is usually labeled perspectivism, sometimes called perspectivalism. It holds that all our concepts, language, and culture represent perspectives that we impose on our experience to create a "world." This world picture currently takes the form of the materialism or scientific realism that dominates our age; Nietzsche claims this to be a "prejudice" that also underlies our internal sense of having a real essential self.

Nietzsche's title, *The Gay Science,* derives from the Provençal *gai saber,* referring to the poetic art of the medieval troubadours that was so admired by Ezra Pound and characterized by exuberance, lightness, and spirit. Cooper (1983) explained Nietzsche's point:

> The pursuit of truth should, in various regards, emulate this *gaya scienza*, whether at the global level of systematic philosophizing, or at the level of particular detailed enquiries. The spinning of new metaphors, the refusal to be opposed by the weight of tradition and orthodoxy: these are some of the ways truth should be pursued and educators should encourage. (p. 88)

Nietzsche (1882, 1887) introduced his epistemological orientation known as perspectivism in *The Gay Science*. Here he (1887) already described science as a "prejudice" (p. 334). By reducing everything to what can be measured, the natural scientist, wrote Nietzsche, divests existence of its "rich ambiguity" (p. 335). This permits counting, calculating, weighing, seeing, and touching, and nothing more" (p. 335). According to Nietzsche this "scientific" interpretation of the world might be one of the most stupid of all possible interpretations, "meaning that it would be one of the poorest in meaning" (p. 335). Nietzsche maintained that existence without interpretation is essentially nonsense because "the human intellect cannot avoid seeing itself in its own perspectives, and *only* in these" (p. 336).

In Nietzsche's view there are no self-evident first principles and no logically perfect rigor is possible. The decision among various philosophical systems, like the decision among various psychoanalytic systems (Chessick, 1992a) must be reached without the benefit of incorrigible facts or *a priori* and self-evident premises. Such questions can never be definitively settled and psychoanalytic theories, like philosophical systems, must be regarded as important perspectives. Above all, Nietzsche stressed that one cannot abstract any theory from its human settings, and that all mentalistic notions are artificial abstractions which Schacht (1983) pointed out "adversely affect the attempt to comprehend ourselves" (p. 268).

For Nietzsche, not only is God dead, but there is no human essence or soul; deep down we are all hollow and cover it with masks. As far as Nietzsche is concerned the ego does not exist at all; it is a fable, a fiction, a play on words, a conceptual synthesis.

The same is true for the notion of "I," a synthesis which is made by thinking, a word which we set up and which according to Nietzsche, is the point at which our ignorance begins.*

Nietzsche (1872), in *The Birth of Tragedy*, first said that the ancient Greeks and Wagner held the key to human living in this pessimistic Schopenhaurian world, finding creativity and vitality in human life through the arts. In *Untimely Meditations* (1873-1876) he expanded on this, but in the early 1880s he developed a new approach to value and meaning, leading eventually to *Thus Spoke Zarathustra,* an approach which he felt could fill the emptiness left by the death of God and the collapse of religion. Schacht (1993) believed that Nietzsche was against nihilism and radical relativism, and that his philosophy was an attempt to overcome these gloomy positions.

From Nietzsche one learns that looking at phenomena again and again in different ways is necessary for increasing comprehension, "if one agrees with Nietzsche that these phenomena are too complex and multiply conditioned to be adequately grasped by any single way of looking at them. This goal can be achieved only by taking collective interpretive account of what comes to light when phenomena are approached in many different ways, with eyes differently focused" (Schacht, 1996, p. 162). The starting point of my psychoanalytic approach also rests on this basic epistemological premise.

Interpreting Nietzsche

In their collection of essays, Magnus and Higgins (1996) emphasized that the interpretation of Nietzsche depends on the interests of the interpreter. They regarded Nietzsche's (1878) *Human All Too Human* as the first published work in which he discussed and defended perspectivism, the view that so-called "truths" are all interpretations formulated from particular perspectives. These authors

---

*The references for these phrases by Nietzsche are given by Schacht, (1983, p. 131), and are based on the assumption that Nietzsche's (1883-1888) unpublished *The Will to Power* is legitimate as a representation of Nietzsche's thought.

presented various positions regarding how radical Nietzsche's perspectivism actually is. Some scholars see it as a radical form of relativism and others see it more restrictedly as a kind of neo-Kantianism, reminding us that the world can only appear in the context of our particular human faculties. A common argument against Nietzsche's work is that if "perspectivism" in the radical sense is correct, then his views can also only be thought of as not preferable to any other views or perspectives. This would seem to undermine the force of his arguments, but other authors maintain that Nietzsche would be quite comfortable to have his arguments labeled as interpretations also. There are even some textual passages where Nietzsche himself seems to do that (see, for example, his *Beyond Good and Evil*, 1886, section 22, pp. 220-221).

Nietzsche's perspectivism immediately raises the question whether there is any way to judge among the various perspectives or rank them in some fashion with respect to their "true" value. Schacht (1996) maintained that, "at least in some kinds of cases and under certain conditions" (p. 167), some perspectives are privileged in relation to others, "making possible a comprehensive and more discerning view of the matters under consideration" (pp. 167–168). He claimed that perspectivism does not imply that nothing can be comprehended, and that perspectivism is linked to Nietzsche's doctrine that human life is a relational affair: "creatures come to exist and preserve themselves—and can develop and flourish—only by way of the establishment of relations with their environing world" (p. 171).

There are two sides to the crucial argument of whether or not Nietzsche was a total nihilist whose doctrine of perspectivism is a form of radical relativism. One group sees him as a radical nihilist, believing any proposition claimed to be truth is nothing but a fiction or an expedient expression of our needs and desires as groups or individuals. The other group of interpreters concentrates on his attempt to overcome nihilism by such methods, for example, as genealogical inquiry. Schacht (1993) discusses genealogical inquiry as an attempt to determine the evolution of the conditions of interpretation and evaluation that are generally accepted in a given historical period. Nietzsche, said Schacht, argued that although knowing is provisional and there is no such thing as absolute knowledge, it is still possible to obtain information that may be called knowledge. This is done by utilizing many perspectives, as in my (Chessick, 1992a) five-channel theory of psychoanalytic listening, allowing a kind of overall general comprehension, that of course may shift and change as more material is obtained and interpreted. It is also important to understand, as Schacht points out, that there cannot be one right way to interpret Nietzsche. This is demonstrated by the plethora of conflicting books on and interpretations of what Nietzsche was trying to communicate.

In summary, the more limited interpreters of perspectivism see it as a claim for tolerance of differing points of view presented by prestigious or otherwise qualified individuals, whereas the radical interpreters of perspectivism condemn it as encouraging a relativism in which one idea is as good as another, with devastating implications for both philosophical and ethical theory as well as psychoanalytic practice. This debate remains unresolved, as does the debate between the "hard" and "soft" interpreters of Nietzsche.

Constructivism

Introducing constructivism, Hoffman (1991) called attention to what he considered a new paradigm in the psychoanalytic field: "The general assumption in this model is that the analyst's understanding is always a function of his or her perspective at the moment" (p. 77). The emphasis in constructivism is on mutual influence and constructed meaning. Hoffman (1992a) insisted that analysts must now admit subjectivity can never be fully transcended; the analyst can never stand utterly outside of the interaction with the patient in order to generate hypotheses and judgments about the patient. He (Hoffman, 1992b) even tried to take constructivism a step past perspectivism:

> Whereas perspectivism merely promotes the idea that the patient's experience can be viewed in various plausible and compelling ways, none of which is comprehensive, constructivism also confronts the analyst and the patient with their responsibility for shaping the quality of their interaction through what they say and do, even through what interpretations they decide to pursue. (pp. 569-570)

Hoffman (1996) placed constructivism against self psychology, pointing out that in his paradigm "there is no objective interpretation and there is no affective attunement that is merely responsive to and reflective of what the patient brings to the situation" (p. 110).

Constructivism in psychoanalytic theory and practice, like Nietzsche's perspectivism, can be viewed either as a radical and nihilistic solipsistic relativism or a "critical constructivism." The latter simply recognizes the contribution of both a partially independent reality and the creative activity of the human subjects (patient and analyst). The constructivist Stern (1983) called attention to what he labeled the unformulated experience, a kind of confusion that arises in the patient who is finally able to think about a previously unaccepted part of his or her life. The construction of experience proceeds in levels of progressive articulation. The choice of words in which the experience is finally articulated is a function of the theory of the analyst, the personalities of the participants, and the current state of the interpersonal field.

Stern's (1992) perspective is that truth is a matter of creation or construction, not a slow accretion of "objective data." From his perspective, "the distribution of power in the analytic couple shifts to something closer to equality and balance; patient and analyst share in the creation of what they agree is true" (p. 322). Stern insisted that constructivism "does not require us to say that reality is an arbitrary or frivolous construction" (p. 333). This, he said, is because, as we saw in certain interpretations of Nietzsche's perspectivism, we are still able to choose a perspective that "works the best" and is "most complete and satisfying in its account of the phenomena in question" (p. 333). Here is a vital philosophical and psychoanalytic issue, because neither the interpreters of Nietzsche who insist that his perspectivism is not a radical nihilism nor the constructivists offer a clear view of exactly how one decides which particular construction may be labeled closer to the truth than another. I think this is what worried Bloom (1987) when he blamed Nietzsche for the moral relativism and indifference he claimed to be prevalent among contemporary college students, as discussed in Chapter 5. And indeed, Nietzsche rhetorically questions the value of truth altogether!

Stern (1996) asserted, "Constructivism, or perspectivism, is rooted in the premise that all experience is interpretation" (p. 260). He found it ridiculous to insist that all phenomena are constructions since some are so clearly and easily interpreted in the same way by everyone, although this is not true regarding the meaning of events in a person's past. The same remembered events can come to have different meanings in different interpersonal contexts, as is well known to any historian. Stern concluded, "Every perception and observation is simply one perspective on reality" (p. 264), a view that seems to come directly from Nietzsche.

From this Stern (1988) launched an attack on the self psychologists, who place empathy at the center of psychoanalytic healing. He argued,

> The empathizing analyst does more than simply resonate and record impressions. He actively constructs resonances and impressions. What is more, these constructions are not even articulations of the patient's unformulated experience—they are products of the *analyst's* unformulated material. Hypotheses based on empathic knowing, then, as crucial as they can be, are a less direct result of the patient's experience than the empathizing analyst may believe . . . interpretations based on empathic immersion do not only require the analyst to make sense of the patient's experience; they require the analyst to make experience for the patient. (p. 605)

He concluded, "We must cultivate a tolerance for the possibility of continuous unknown participation. . . . This perspective is incompatible with the view of most self psychologists, because they hold that, apart from the occasional and unavoidable failure, the analyst always assumes an empathic stance" (pp. 608-609). So Stern (1991) presented as a subtitle, "From Schleiermacher to Gadamer: Rejecting Empathic Knowing in Favor of Mutual Influence" (p. 56).

Stern (1994) insisted that empathy is not a privileged means of observation but rather a perspective, and observations made with empathic intent are interpretations like any other observations. What the analyst considers to be empathically derived knowledge, according to Stern, is partly a product of personal processes. Those relying on empathy as a privileged mode of perception assume that the experiences to be perceived are already there in the other person awaiting the analyst's empathic attunement or identification. This ignores what Stern considered to be "how fully the analyst and patient participate moment-to-moment in the construction of one another's experience, how they co-create everything that takes place in the analysis" (p. 443).

Kohut's Self Psychology: Empathy

Nietzsche (1886) said, "Gradually it has become clear to me what every great philosophy so far has been: namely, the personal confession of its author and a kind of involuntary and unconscious memoir" (p. 203). With this in mind consider the claim by Kohut (1978), the founder of self psychology:

> The father that I have set up in myself, that internal ally who helps me maintain the integrity of myself under psychologically trying circumstances, has taught me, from way back in my life, to turn to reflection, to the search for meanings and explanations. And I have learned that the enjoyment of these mental activities must often take the place of the direct gratifications that are hard to keep in bounds. And, increasingly, and with changing emphasis in the course of my life, these thoughts and reflections have become attempts to understand myself, to understand other individuals and also, most recently though tentatively and with great caution, to understand man as he feels, reacts, behaves in the arena of history. (p. 665)

Nietzsche's father died when he was five years old. Because of their personal psychodynamics, Nietzsche and Kohut come out with diametrically opposing solutions and, if one is willing to view Nietzsche's perspectivism as also a perspective, different perspectives.

Kohut (1978, p. 345) asked rhetorically some questions reminiscent of Nietzsche: Is the present world not different than the nineteenth century? Does it demand new values, new yardsticks, and new viewpoints by which to evaluate, measure, and understand it? Why did psychoanalysis appear at the end of the nineteenth century? Why is it isolated among the sciences? Why does it remain separated? Many people are not satisfied with Kohut's attempts to answer these questions, but he must be given credit for raising them in an interesting and stimulating fashion. I am sure that during his European education he studied Nietzsche, as did Freud (although Freud denied it).

It is assumed that the reader is familiar with at least the general aspects of Kohut's self psychology, which I (Chessick, 1993a) have described in detail elsewhere. Here I will concentrate on what Nietzsche would call Kohut's perspective: empathy. Does empathy have a healing power or is it simply a mode of observation? If a person feels understood empathically by another person, does this exert a healing effect? If so, is it possible to describe this healing effect in metapsychological terminology? When we take the position of another person, our imagination creatively moves from ourselves into the other person. To empathize does not mean that we must experience physical sensations; empathy can be physical, imaginative, or both. Fenichel (1945) quoted Reik, who maintained that empathy consists of two acts, "(a) an identification with the other person, and (b) an awareness of one's own feelings after the identification, and in this way an awareness of the object's feelings" (p. 511).

I (Chessick, 1965) called attention to the work of Katz (1963), who along with Reik (1949), presented some metapsychologically imprecise and intuitive definitions and discussions of empathy. Katz described the fielding of signals through "a kind of inner radar" that works from cues in the conversation or impressions we receive. Reik (1949) explained that "in order to comprehend the unconscious of another person, we must, at least for a moment, change ourselves into and become that person. We only comprehend the spirit whom we resemble" (p. 361).

No author before Kohut emphasized the importance of empathy as much as Harry Stack Sullivan. He never really defined the term, but spoke of empathy developing through "induction" and postulated that the tension or anxiety present in the mothering one "induces" anxiety in the infant. The process by which this induction takes place is referred to as a manifestation of an interpersonal process that Sullivan called empathy. Sullivan

(1953) also introduced the term "empathic linkage," meaning a situation in which two people are linked in such a way that one induces a feeling in the other.

Fromm-Reichmann (1950) insisted that empathy between the patient and therapist is crucial to psychotherapy. The use of empathy in psychotherapy calls for a pendulumlike action alternating between subjective involvement and objective detachment. Traditional analysts refer to this as regression in the service of the ego when it is used toward a specific goal. When the good empathizer regresses in the service of the ego, that person engages in a playful kind of creative activity, inwardly imitating events in the life of the patient. The activity is regressive only in the sense that it calls for a relaxed and unstructured experience usually associated with the fantasy of the child or the poetic license of the artist. The therapist must then be able to swing back to an objective and detached relationship in order to make clinical use of the information gained through the empathic process. However, in Chapter 15 I discussed the debate over whether "regression in the service of the ego" is a sufficient or appropriate explanation for the creative process, such as that involved in empathy.

Long before Kohut, Fliess (1942) explained that the skill of the therapist depends on the ability "to step into [the patient's] shoes, and to obtain in this way an inside knowledge that is almost firsthand. The common name for such a procedure is empathy" (pp. 212-213). Levine (1961) claimed that empathy, if handled correctly, leads to a type of immediate comprehension of the patient's problems, a comprehension superior to the intellectual variety of understanding. French and Fromm (1964) discussed "empathic thinking" in dream interpretation, stressing "empathic understanding" as a direct intuitive communication between the unconscious of the patient and that of the therapist. The patient evokes in the therapist an empathic sense of what is going on in the unconscious of the patient. Then must occur a translation from this empathic understanding into a language suitable for scientific analysis. This translation is called "conceptual analysis" by these authors, and we have again the pendulumlike action described earlier.

Kohut (1984) posited three functions for empathy: It is the indispensable tool of psychoanalytic fact finding; it expands the self to include the other, constituting a powerful psychological bond between individuals in order to counteract man's destructiveness against his fellows; and it arises out of the selfobject matrix, becoming the accepting, confirming, and understanding human echo evoked by and needed by the self as a psychological nutriment without which human life could not be sustained. In this shift from his primary definition of empathy as a mode of observation or psychoanalytic fact-finding to the other functions of empathy Kohut caused much controversy, especially because of its implications for psychoanalytic technique.

In a view similar to that of Nietzsche (see Chapter 5), Kohut (1971) recognized that the potential for empathic perception is acquired early in life. Empathic talent may arise paradoxically in the same situation that can present a danger to the formation of the nuclear self due to fear of archaic enmeshment with the parent. This may lead to a sensitive psychological apparatus with unusually great ability for the perception and elaboration of others' psychological processes. This skill may be employed later in a psychotherapeutic career, or it can be used for evil purposes.

Goldberg (1983) reviewed the division in the psychoanalytic literature on the role of empathy in psychoanalysis. One view, although agreeing that empathy may be desirable, sees it as a relatively rare and unreliable phenomenon fraught with the dangers of error due to countertransference. A sharply contrasting view sees empathy as a common and universal mode of communication between people. It distinguishes between two ways of knowing: "direct, outward, public observation or extraception, and inward, private observation or introspection. The combination of introspection and putting oneself in another's place is empathy" (Goldberg, 1983, p. 156). Hartmann (1927) earlier objected strongly to this approach in psychoanalytic work and claimed it was unscientific and unreliable. The situation was improved by Kohut's (1978) definition in 1959 of empathy as vicarious introspection, which proposed empathy as a method for finding out about another person's inner life. Like any scientific investigation, vicarious introspection must not be unnecessarily biased, and it must be subject to verifiability by further uses of the method, as we remain alert to the effects of our own observations and interventions. But Levy (1985) complained of the "multiple and different meanings" Kohut gave to empathy (p. 369).

The Self

The sense of self as originally used by Kohut refers to a subjective experience, grasped by the therapist through vicarious introspection or empathy with the patient. As such, it was not directly incompatible with Freud's structural theory and could have been thought of as based on certain sets of ego functions. However, as Kohut's theories developed, anthropomorphic language began to creep into the psychology of the self in a way similar to the way that the "ego" was anthropomorphized as "the little man within the man" by Freud in his final writings.

In the later publications of Kohut (1977, 1984), the self as a supraordinate concept becomes elaborated in its bipolar nature, showing itself primarily when self-cohesion is not firm. Metapsychological energic concepts are dropped, and the self is now seen to occupy "the central position" within the personality. This supraordinate self develops from a core self or nuclear self that does not begin (as Kohut thought earlier) as scattered nuclei that coalesce, but rather as a self which from the beginning of life constitutes a supraordinate configuration that is the basis "for our sense of being an independent center of initiative and perception, integrated with our most central ambitions and ideals and with our experience that our body and mind form a unit in space and a continuum in time" (Kohut, 1977, p. 177). The self is no longer a depth-psychological concept that can be metapsychologically defined using classical terminology, nor is the self thought of as an entity within the mental apparatus or even as a fourth "agency" of the mind. "The area of the self and its vicissitudes," as Kohut (1978, p. 753) called it, becomes separate from Freud's psychoanalysis; Kohut (1978) himself labeled it "the science of the self" (p. 752n).

Kohut's (1978) paper on "The Future of Psychoanalysis" (pp. 663-684), presented in 1973 on the anniversary of his sixtieth birthday, has a Nietzschean ring about it and could be subtitled "Revaluation of Values." He insisted that psychoanalysts must replace their archaic object (Freud) with a strong set of ideals and values that will lead to a new surge of independent initiative, for Freud was wrong on such subjects as religion and the psychoses. Kohut called for a shift of emphasis from a "truth-and-reality morality toward the idealization of empathy, from pride in clear vision and uncompromising rationality to pride in the scientifically controlled expansion of the self" (p. 676). He wanted an end to "tool-and-method pride" which leads to the wasteful isolation from one another of various branches of science. In addition to this, he offered a second way of coping with the world of tomorrow: "The expansion of the self, its increasing capacity to embrace a greater number and a greater variety of others through a consciously renewed and cultivated deepened empathy" (p. 682).

Empathy, for the aging Kohut, became a paramount issue, expanding beyond the status of a mode of observation to the "positively toned atmosphere" and emotional climate in which interactions between humans take place; empathy as a psychological bond and nutriment can produce "wholesome social effects" (p. 707). The importance of this empathic milieu in the psychotherapeutic situation, in the situation of every human being, and as a necessity for world peace became increasingly central to Kohut's thought.

Psychoanalyst as Creator

Although psychoanalysis clearly requires ongoing creative activity from the psychoanalyst, Gedo (1991) lamented that the psychoanalytic community no longer consists of scholars, scientists, humanists, or even the educated. There are no readers of serious literature, he complained, and only the earning of money becomes paramount: "The psychoanalytic world I aspired to join over forty years ago is entirely dead" (p. 168). Gedo was in his seventh decade of life when he wrote this.

Franz Brentano, whose courses in philosophical psychology Freud attended for about a year, believed that the mental differed from the physical by "intentional existence" or direction upon an object; mental phenomena as experienced always imply a stance toward the object and are not isolated "raw" or empirical data. The most extreme example of this comes from the work of Groddeck. This unusually intuitive internist, who labeled himself a wild analyst, engaged in a fantastic reverie process. When I as-

signed his *The Book of the It* (Groddeck, 1923) to residents in psychiatry, they reacted with anxiety and revulsion at the extremity
of his views, so I had to stop including this fascinating, provoca-
tive text in my courses. Groddeck attributed overwhelming power
to the "It," claiming that humans are lived by the It which shapes
our mental phenomena and our very lives. His crucial premise
was that humans seek pleasure first and foremost, and like Nietzsche who influenced him, he wrote, " 'I am I' is wrong. . . . I am
a continually changing form in which It displays itself. This is a
deception" (p. 233).

A great deal of work has been done in attempting to get at
deep structures underneath the phenomenology of human experience. Cultural phenomena are intrinsic to the creation of
language, and behind these, argued Lévi-Strauss (Kurzweil,
1980), are archetypal human structures. Lévi-Strauss analyzed
myths in order to find these structures in a way similar to psychoanalytic studies of the unconscious through the use of free association. Carrying this further, for Foucault (see Chessick,
1992b) history is not the continuity of the subject, but consists of
structural discontinuity in epistemological breaks. Each epoch
corresponds to the dominant structure. All structuralists extrap-
olate from rules/relations of grammar/speech to explore social
phenomena in terms of linguistic oppositions and transformations. This assumes the centrality of language to culture and culture to language. Structuralism is a systematic attempt to uncover
deep universal mental structures as they manifest themselves in
kinship and larger social structures, in philosophy, literature,
mathematics, and in unconscious psychological patterns that mo-
tivate human behavior. Piaget's structuralism even maintained
that structure and genesis are interdependent, so there is no
structure apart from creative construction, and underlying structure changes as the child's development proceeds.

Stein (1995) stressed the metaphor Lévi-Strauss used of the
craftsman as appropriate for our modern way of arranging knowledge. Every psychoanalyst carries a tool kit, whether he or she displays it or not, and Lévi-Strauss pointed out that the tool kit is for
the use of a *bricoleur,* a potter. The more tools in the analyst's kit,
the more sense the patient will make to him or her, a good argument for the five-channel theory of psychoanalytic listening I put
forth in Chapter 3.

One of Freud's original colleagues had a very bad reputation because he always made up a case that fit whatever was the main presentation topic during the meetings of Freud's Wednesday Evening Society. But Stekel (1950), for all his faults, was one of the first to recognize that the work of a psychoanalyst is the work of an artist. He wrote:

> The carrying out of real analysis is a work of art. The attitude which Freud has so stubbornly defended, namely, to analyze the patient without influencing him and to let him find his own way, is not worthy of a science which purports to be a form of psychotherapy. The physician must be his patient's teacher and guide him with gentle force out of the world of his fantasies onto the road of reality and work; again and again he must hold up to him the mirror of his inactivity, revealing to him his will to illness, and stimulating his constructive energies. (p. 206)

For a long time this attitude was ignored, but in recent years the truth of it has become increasingly apparent. The standard theory of psychoanalysis for many years emphasized insight into the developmental origins of psychopathology through analysis of the transference as the central mechanism of therapy. Transference was thought of as a unique opportunity to observe directly the past of the patient and thereby to understand the development of his or her conflicts. But the analyst today would be more likely to view the treatment process itself as central to psychoanalytic therapy, with a traditional Freudian theory of neurosis such as presented in the wonderful classic work by Fenichel (1945) used only as a guide to interpretation. Transference is now seen more as a jointly creative construction of the patient and the analyst, and the central mechanism of therapy is the exploration of the origins of transference as it appears in the therapeutic relationship. This is still analysis of the transference, but it includes attention to the analyst's contribution.

For Fenichel, psychoanalysis was about the infantile origins and dynamics of neuroses, and the current relationship between the analyst and the patient was ignored as a direct therapeutic factor. The analyst was supposed to be a blank screen, neutral and objective. Today psychoanalytic treatment is quite concerned about what transpires between the patient and the analyst rather than only about interpreting the infantile origins and adult dynamics of the neuroses. There is an additional focus on how that interaction can reshape the patient's character and life as part of the widening scope of psychoanalytic treatment. It involves what Freud (1940) called "after-education." As early as 1958, emphasis on after-education began to develop, focusing on getting the patient to live his or her life more with the matured ego in charge. Saul (1958) correctly insisted that the emotional attitude of the analyst to the patient was crucial.

An outstanding and even-handed view of this has recently been expressed by Jacobs (1997), who cautions us to be careful about so-called spontaneity and enactments on the part of the analyst: "Analysis is a discipline that requires containment, as well as the transformation of many of the analyst's inner experiences into useful interventions" (p. 1045). This is because "some behaviors on the part of the analyst are so hurtful, so wounding to the patient and destructive of the analytic process, that they cannot be affectively analysed" (pp. 1044-1045). In my experience with the re-analysis of patients who have failed in their previous treatment, I have learned that many impasses and failures can be traced to such behaviors on the part of the analyst or as misperceived by the patient, especially if they have not been frankly discussed in a co-operative spirit. Jacobs is correct when he writes, "Much of the analyst's art, in fact, consists in establishing a balance between restraint and the creative use of the self" (p.1045).

However, there are certain respected psychoanalysts who still follow Fenichel's classical approach. When I was in training in the 1950s, the "bible" for psychoanalysts and psychoanalytically oriented psychotherapists was Fenichel's (1945) textbook. This is ironic because Fenichel, a refugee from the Nazis, was ill treated in the United States. In order to practice psychoanalysis in California he was required to obtain a medical license although he was already a licensed physician in Europe. This entailed serving an internship, and produced the picture of an overweight, middle-aged man exhausting himself in a general medical internship that was terminated when he suffered a fatal coronary occlusion.

Recently, on the fiftieth anniversary of the publication of Fenichel's (1945) classic, the book was reissued with an introduction and epilogue by Leo Rangell (see Fenichel, 1996). Rangell still finds Fenichel's traditional Freudian formulations relevant to his contemporary psychoanalytic practice: "A small and seemingly dwindling minority has stayed with these general formulations throughout the last three decades, during which customs, numbers, trends, and popularity have led in other directions. I count myself among those few" (p. xii), and Rangell in his "epilogue" hoped that Fenichel's text would produce a return to "basic and enduring theory" (p. Ell), or "unified psychoanalytic theory" (p. E12).

The trend has actually been the other way. For example, Spence (1982) emphasized the creative aspect of the psychoanalyst's work. He believed that the reason interpretations work is due to their poetic value, because they help the patient "see" by the right words, they offer a coherent account, they remove a responsibility, and there is no evidence against them. Thus, an undocumented assertion can acquire a life of its own and in that sense all interpretations are "inexact," but, insisted Spence, some are more creative than others. He argued that in all of them we exchange narrative for historical truth. Each analyst "hears" material in his or her own way, making interpretation an aesthetic experience as well as useful for results.

Similarly, Schafer (1983) viewed psychoanalytic work as hermeneutic reconstruction, an interpretative discipline rather than a natural science, with various "story lines" (pp. 276-278) chosen by the analyst. The "truth" of a given analytic fact resides in fitting it into a system. This is a circular process wherein observations are influenced by interpretations, and it explains why there are different "schools" in the field. Schafer maintained that the analyst creatively constructs a "second reality" of the unconscious, which has nothing to do with empirical "truth," out of the narration. (For details of the hermeneutic approach to psychoanalytic data see Chessick, 1992b.)

Carrying this to an extreme, Frankl (1967) claimed that the ultimate meaning of a person's life is not found in the intellect but is found in that person's existential commitments. When there is a vacuum of existential commitments, the patient suffers from what Frankl called a noögenic neurosis. Like Sartre, he believed humans construct themselves and complained that psychoanalysis overlooked this freedom of the will, turning humans into objects. Horney (1937) was one of the first psychoanalysts to recognize the influence of the competitive, materialistic, and unbridled capitalistic nature of the society in which we live on the formation of neuroses. She believed a basic hostility resulted from living in such a society, and this hostility formed the main source of neurotic anxiety. In contemporary terms, Schlesinger (1997) declared, "Globalization is in the saddle and rides mankind, but at the same time drives people to seek refuge from its powerful forces beyond their control and comprehension. . . . The faster the world integrates, the more people will huddle in their religious or ethnic or tribal enclaves" (p. 10).

Every country creates the psychoanalysis that it needs (Kurzweil, 1989). Each psychoanalysis, or psychoanalytic listening channel as I have called it, operates with indigenous philosophical assumptions, intellectual controversies, journals and societies, and fashions of the culture in which it arises. A total muddle of theories results from this in international psychoanalysis, and in the spirit of Nietzsche, I (Chessick, 1997b) have called for a genealogical study of the various forms of psychoanalysis that have become established in different countries over the world.

Mathematicians speak of Cantor's law of conservation of ignorance (Klein, 1980). This law states that a false conclusion once arrived at and widely accepted is not easily dislodged, and the less it is understood the more tenaciously it is held. Max Plank pointed out that new scientific truth does not triumph by convincing its opponents and making them see the light, but rather because its opponents eventually die and a new generation grows up that is familiar with it.

But why does the abstract discipline of mathematics describe the working of nature with such accuracy? Why should long chains of reasoning produce remarkably applicable conclusions? For answers to questions like these one must turn to the glimpses of Truth that are inherent in the humanistic disciplines of artistic creativity and metaphysical speculation.

18 FAILURE

One of the remarkable things about the behaviour of the world is how it seems to be grounded in mathematics to a quite extraordinary degree of accuracy. The more we understand about the physical world, and the deeper we probe into the laws of nature, the more it seems as though the physical world almost evaporates and we are left only with mathematics. The deeper we understand the laws of physics, the more we are driven into this world of mathematics and of mathematical concepts. . . . Up to this point, I have talked about the Platonic world primarily in terms of mathematics, but there are other things which one might also include. Plato would certainly argue that not only the true, but also the good and the beautiful are absolute (Platonic) concepts. If there indeed exists some sort of contact with Platonic absolutes which our awareness enables us to achieve, and which cannot be explained in terms of computational behaviour, then that seems to me to be an important issue.
—*Roger Penrose,* The Large, the Small and the Human Mind

Hegel was a great visionary who presented a grand and all-inclusive picture of everything in the universe. He also reoriented the whole direction of philosophy by emphasizing the importance of growth, development, and change and the possibility that such change leads toward an intelligible goal. The problem he faced was how to determine the relationship of the finite to the infinite. The question was whether in some way through a study of the finite in a phenomenologic fashion one could get in touch with Being or the Infinite. His all-encompassing metaphysical system is hardly acceptable today, and it contains many arguments that, contrary to his belief, neither are convincing nor lead inevitably to the next phase of development as he thought they did. But his dialectical method has become an important tool for understanding matters that are beyond the scope of empirical science.

Hegel contrasted the fundamental activity of reason *(Vernunft)*, which functions to attain unified synthesis, to understanding *(Verstand)*, which tends to posit and perpetuate oppositions for the purpose of a dialectical approach to truth. One might say Hegel believed that through art, religion, and philosophy the human mind is led from Understanding to Reason, but there are as many interpretations of Hegel as there are readers of Hegel. This is because Hegel's entire system is very ambiguous, to say nothing of his tortuous writing style, and as a result many opposing explications of Hegel's work have arisen. But it is not the purpose of the present book to explore the many arguments about Hegel's philosophy; instead, I wish to simply list some of the features of it that are in my opinion useful and valuable in attaining an understanding of creativity and the creative mind from the point of view of phenomenology, in order to complement the psychoanalytic point of view. Of course my interpretation of Hegel, like all others, is open to the usual debate.

Hegel's Approach

Philosophy demands the elevation of Understanding through dialectical thinking to the level of Reason, so dialectical thought results in a deeper penetration of the nature of Being than Understanding in the narrow sense can possibly do. More importantly, as Copleston (1965) said, "For Hegel the infinite exists in and through the finite; the universal lives and has its being, as it were, in and through the particulars" (p. 238).

Hegel believed Christianity introduced the idea that the individual as such possesses an infinite value; he gave Christianity the credit for initiating the reverence for human life from birth to death that I have stressed in this book. Whether Christianity deserves this credit is a different issue; certainly the behavior of Christians throughout history is not consistent with such an accolade. At any rate, Hegel suggested that the poor, the sick, the mad, the ugliest human being, the criminal, the diseased, and the cripple—each of these individuals are still living human beings and deserving of our best efforts to help and to cure them.

That is to say, regardless of the privation (in Aristotle's sense), there is always a positive element in humans. Nobody who seriously attempts to do psychotherapy could believe otherwise; this is the physicianly vocation. How a society treats the poor, the sick, the weak, and the mad is the best measure of whether it is barbaric or civilized.

Hegel believed that it was the function of the philosopher to interpret the spirit of his or her time *(die Zeitgeist)*, as I have attempted to do in this book, and as both Barry and Ezra Pound also intuitively attempted to do. For Hegel this process would raise the consciousness of the society, but he believed that when that happens a form of life already has actualized itself and is ready to pass into or give way to another. I believe this is where we are now (also see Erickson, 1997).

For example, Copleston (1965) claimed Hegel's metaphysics imply that the ideal end of the whole movement of political history would be a world federation, since Hegel maintained world history is the process by which the universal Spirit actualizes itself in time. If this is true it seems logical that the goal of the process would be a universal world state, world society, or world federation that would maximize personal freedom. Hegel was not able to recognize the implication of his own point of view and remained immersed in the dialectic of national states. Perhaps if he were living today, he would reply that it proves his famous statement that no philosopher can rise above his time (Hegel, 1821, p. 11).

Hegel's teleology, as illustrated in his *Phenomenology of Spirit* (1807), is highly questionable, and I will not spend time arguing for or against his concept that the end point of the development of Spirit is that of Being actualizing itself through communal human spirit into self-thinking thought. For Hegel, Being objectifies itself in nature, the material world, and Being comes to exist as thought which thinks itself not through nature but as Spirit. This Spirit eventually manifests itself adequately only in and through the communal human spirit. It becomes Absolute Spirit when it knows itself as such, and according to Hegel it is in his philosophy that this finally occurs. Art, religion, and philosophy are the activities that represent the highest expression of Spirit (see Chapter 15). Art allows us to experience the immediacy of

Spirit as Beauty, and the same Absolute which is apprehended as Beauty by the aesthetic consciousness is apprehended as Truth in philosophy.

Copleston (1965) correctly pointed out how Hegel neglected natural beauty in his emphasis on artistic beauty and, of course, all of us have at times experienced ciphers toward transcendence in natural beauty. Hegel (1905) delineated the modes in which art manifests Being to us. In those modes of art where the sensuous element always predominates, the artist suggests rather than expresses his or her meaning, leaving ambiguity and mystery. Hegel called this mode symbolic art, and the example he gave is in the art of the ancient Egyptians, such as the Sphinx. There also is art that fuses the spiritual content into a harmonious unity; Hegel called this classical art, and his example is ancient Greek sculpture, which presents Spirit as the finite embodied human spirit.

In the highest mode of art for Hegel, spiritual content and sensuous embodiment are in perfect harmonious accord. By way of contrast, romantic art emphasizes an overflowing of finite sensuous embodiment, emphasizing interiority, moods, feelings, love, and the complications that arise from these, all of which was peripheral to classic art. But it is also concerned with the life of the Spirit, and Hegel argued that typical romantic art arose out of Christianity, although "no sensuous embodiment is felt to be adequate to the spiritual content" (Copleston, 1965, p. 278). The highest art for Hegel seems to have been poetry, sensuous images expressed in language; this was the art best suited for expressing the life of the Spirit. Much of the later writing of Heidegger also embraced this view.

The fact that Hegel had a limited view of what constitutes art does not negate the timeliness of his conception. He saw art as raising things out of their prosaic ordinariness in order to give us a sense of the wholeness and freedom of human life, to "afford us a breathing space in which to feel at one with ourselves and the world" (Houlgate, 1991, p. 137). Even twentieth-century painters like Francis Bacon or Lucien Freud who emphasize the frightening and the stark realism of human existence, as well as abstract expressionists and surrealists, or "confessional poets" and composers of atonal and cacophonous "modern" music, offer us many imaginative, new, and startling views of the human condition and environment. These art works also, in my opinion and in contrast to Hegel's emphasis on the traditional arts, accomplish the same sense of transcendence and the richness of human life, pointing to what the ancient Greeks referred to as τὰ ἐπέκεινα (see also Heidegger, 1997), that which is beyond. The difference of contemporary arts from traditional painting and the classical arts is that contemporary art reveals truths that are much harder to articulate and that are sometimes very unpleasant, but great art always offers an ineffable liberating and cipher (Jaspers, 1932c) experience, one that unites humans with each other and with the world. Hence the brilliance of Heidegger's (1971b) emphasis on the poet Hölderlin's concept of "the fourfold," the earth, the sky, the gods, and mortals, brought together for us and expressed over the centuries through great art works of architecture, sculpture, painting, music, and literature.

Hegel thought that romantic art inevitably led to a transition to the religious consciousness from the aesthetic consciousness. He believed religion was a form of pictorial thought and it actually was able to think the Absolute in its religious images. Finally, philosophy shifts the concentration on the Absolute from thinking of it in images as in religion, to thinking of it in pure conceptual thought: "Speculative philosophy, in other words, strips away the imaginative or pictorial element which is characteristic of religious thought and expresses the truth, the same truth, in purely conceptual form" (Copleston, 1965, p. 285).

For Hegel the history of philosophy is a very important part of his system because it demonstrates a similar necessary dialectical advance. Each philosopher looks "back on the past from the vantage-point of a system which he believes to be the highest expression of the truth up to date and seeing this system as the culmination of a process of reflection which, in spite of all contingent elements, has been in its essential outlines a necessary movement of Thought coming to think itself" (Copleston, 1965, p. 289).

The important focus of the Hegelian system is found in the *Phenomenology of Spirit*. Here Hegel (1807) put forward the view that there are a variety of types of consciousness, and each type of consciousness produces a different version of reality. His insistence there is a hierarchy of consciousness culminating in a special Absolute that for us consists of Truth, Reality, and Being, and his claim this can be reached by an inevitable unfolding of a dialectic are hard for most people to accept. This is not as important, however, as the notion that such a hierarchy is possible, and that it does culminate in something very special, perhaps in what Plato called the Form of the Good, or Heidegger called Being, and somehow glimpses or, as Jaspers (1932c) said, ciphers, of it can be reached through the glory of nature or the experience of myth, art, religion, and philosophy. Furthermore, "Hegel's recognition that each type of consciousness is reflected in the social, political, and economic institutions—as well as in the philosophy, science, art and religion—of a given epoch, has influenced men's thinking in profound ways and may be said to be one of the marks that distinguishes us and our time from every other" (Jones, 1975, p. 144).

Pound's Failure

If we look at the temporal unfolding of Barry's creativity and Ezra Pound's creativity we see a similarity in that neither represents Spirit unfolding itself but rather both display a kind of endless repetition of unresolved themes. It is as if both Barry and Pound got stuck in the dialectic and were unable to progress further to higher levels of intuition and understanding that would combine into what Hegel would call Reason. Why did this happen? I believe the psychopathology of these individuals constricted their intuitive and creative function, so that their epics became endlessly repetitive and the only Being they were able to express was being-towards-death. I have already illustrated this in Barry's case, and I now turn to what I call Pound's metaphysical failure.

The first interrogators of Ezra Pound when he was incarcerated in the United States formed the impression he was a crackpot. He was generally considered a vicious individual who should have been executed, and in many countries I think he would have been. Although he continued to flit from one idea to another and showed difficulty in concentration and signs of exhaustion, his speech seemed to be rational and there was little indication he was overtly psychotic. His clever attorney correctly decided that the best defense for him against the charge of treason would be the notorious insanity defense. Pound was now sixty years old.

Everyone agreed that Pound appeared egocentric and eccentric, and Dr. Winfred Overholser and his fellow psychiatrists agreed vaguely that his condition "resembled paranoia." This has led to a neverending dispute about whether or not Pound was really insane and whether his incarceration in St. Elizabeth's Hospital for almost thirteen years was justifiable or not; at any rate, it saved him from prosecution for treason and probable conviction. Commenting on Pound's unusual grandiosity, Carpenter (1988) wrote,

> Ezra's frequent and (in his early life) self-confessed use of different masks and personae as a way of making contact with the exterior world, and his fondness for private systems of esoteric knowledge, are both classic symptoms of the "schizoid" or potentially schizophrenic personality, the type of withdrawn and "split" character whose mental breakdown (if it happens) usually takes the form of paranoia (p. 732)

Apparently, although exhausted and depressed, Pound did not show overt paranoid schizophrenia, but it was observed that he had noticeable swings of mood that today would suggest placing him in the bipolar category. The *DSM-IV* diagnosis of schizoaffective disorder that I have suggested previously could be reasonably applied to Pound at that point or, alternatively, the diagnosis is a mixed personality disorder with schizotypal, paranoid, and narcissistic features. His mood swings became worse, although at the same time he reviewed the typescript of *The Pisan Cantos*. He remained thoroughly fascist and anti-Semitic even during his early legal hearings, and continued to display a grandiosity beyond any reality testing, for example, announcing his plan to learn Georgian so he could be sent to talk to Stalin. There is no question about what Stalin would have done with Ezra Pound.

After his incarceration in St. Elizabeth's Hospital, Pound began an extensive correspondence with all sorts of fanatics and well-wishers, but none of the correspondence showed the faintest trace of regret for his previous actions. The words and ideas expressed in his correspondence remain extremely obscure. About a year after he had been in the hospital, he was given his own room in this crowded place, which, by the standards of that hospital at that time, constituted special treatment. He was eventually allowed to spend time on the grounds outside of the hospital building with Dorothy Shakespear and other visitors, and he could even play tennis on the hospital tennis court. He expressed concern about being assassinated and viewed himself as the target of some international group of Jewish bankers or warmongers. He continued to maintain the same ideas about economics, Roosevelt, and the Jews as before. He was given no psychiatric treatment of any kind at St. Elizabeth's Hospital, and there was no further development of his mental illness than what has already been described.

A *festschrift* was organized to mark his sixty-fifth birthday, and *The Pisan Cantos* were published in 1948, bringing him a one thousand dollar Bollingen Prize. An enormous stream of visitors began appearing at the hospital, including young writers and academics as well as fascists and other extreme right-wingers; again, a circle of admiring listeners formed around him! One of these disciples was Eustace Mullins, who has been quoted in the present book. According to Carpenter, Mullins "called himself Director of the Aryan League of America, and had a letterhead printed with the slogan 'Jews are betraying us!'" (Carpenter, 1988, p. 801).

Carpenter (1988) described the scene:

> "Granpaw" was the persona he now invariably adopted in the presence of visitors. He had developed a special costume for the role. The summer version consisted of "floppy sandals, walking shorts several sizes too large, gathered at the waist with a belt, his shirt thrown off to take in more sun.". . . On less warm days he might be found in "a loose sweatshirt, an old GI overcoat, baggy trousers, heavy white socks, bedroom slippers, long underwear showing at his ankles." It was a great contrast to . . . earlier costumes. (p. 802)

He continued work on *The Cantos*, and *Section: Rock-Drill De Los Cantares LXXXV-XCV* appeared in 1955, but these cantos did not receive critical acclaim. Pound's creative capacities were burning out by the time he was approaching seventy. *The Cantos* had become almost incomprehensible even to the reader with the best of intentions. Around that time Noel Stock, whose text has also been quoted in the present book, became at least temporarily under the influence of Pound's ideas and arranged for some of his material to be published in Australian journals, attempting to form an international organization dedicated to Pound's work and beliefs.

On his tenth anniversary at St. Elizabeth's and around the time of his seventieth birthday, his various friends in the literary world began making serious attempts to get him released. Pound commented, "Obviously it is kikes keeping me in here" (Carpenter, 1988, p. 820).

After twelve years in St. Elizabeth's, Pound was released in 1958 when the treason indictment was dropped and he was permitted to return to Italy. In parting he allegedly said, "I do not know how it would be possible to live in America outside a madhouse." When the ship carrying Pound arrived in Italy, he was surrounded by Italian reporters and photographers and raised his arm in the Fascist salute. He lived another fourteen years in Italy, and denied until his death that he was a traitor, nor did he see anything wrong with his radio broadcasts during World War II or with his ideas about economics and Jews. He prepared for publication another batch of cantos that had been composed at St. Elizabeth's, entitled *Thrones de los Cantares XCVI-CIX*. These seemed little different from the previous batch of cantos. The impression even of his followers was that he was getting bored with the cantos and beginning to have a gnawing feeling that they were a failure.

At first he lived with his daughter and then he moved with his wife to Rapallo. When he was with his wife in Italy he proposed marriage to Marcella Spann, a woman from Texas who had joined Pound's circle of admirers at St. Elizabeth's in 1957 and accompanied him to Italy, Dorothy Shakespear sent Marcella Spann back to America, and Pound at that point had lapsed into depression, hypochondria, and self-pity, and it seemed that his creative capacities had ended. This is consistent with what I have discussed previously from the self psychology channel regarding the outbreak of lust and falling in love as the self attempts to maintain its integrity in the face of inevitable decay and dissolution. Marcella was an important source of narcissistic stimulation for him.

By the time he was seventy-five he began to complain that he had made many mistakes, never made anybody happy, and spoiled whatever came into contact with him, and he found it impossible to concentrate. He lapsed into self-imposed silence which had its own dramatic effect, as, for example, on an interviewer from the *Paris Review:* "Again I saw vigor and energy drain out of him, like air from a pricked balloon. The strong body visibly sagged into old age; he disintegrated in front of me, smashed into a thousand unconnected and disorderly pieces" (Carpenter, 1988, p. 867). *Drafts and Fragments of Cantos CX-CXVIII* was published in 1969, the self-proclaimed poetry of his old age. In them Pound (1950, later editions in 1969, 1972) said, "I lost my center fighting the world. The dreams clash and are shattered—in that I tried to make a paradiso terrestre. . . . Let those I love try to forgive what I have made" (pp. 802-803).

All attempts to settle down seemed to fail, and Pound began to refuse food and remained motionless for hours at a time, becoming bent and shrunken. He was filled with all sorts of self-reproach and regrets, expressing suicidal ideation. He ended up living with Olga Rudge in almost total silence, probably as a consequence of his depression. Because of his occasional unexpected, weird, furious lapses from silence, it is also possible to believe that some sort of catatonic state had set in. But there was another *festschrift* on his eightieth birthday, and he visited Paris and other European cities. The administration of amitryptiline did not help. A remarkable waffling statement was made by a professor who examined him at the University of Genoa:

> It seemed as if the personality of the patient had always been on the autistic side, with prevailing phantastic attitudes and insufficient contact with reality, inadequacy of associative structures of thinking. . . so that a psychotic-like situation came out ("borderline patient"), permitting, however, and perhaps encouraging, poetic activity. (Carpenter, 1988, p. 892)

He admitted that *The Cantos* were a failure, and that it would be better to know something about a few things rather than picking out all varieties of topics that interested him and jumbling them into a bag, which was not the way to make a work of art. *The Cantos* ended in disarray, with three available editions each with a different ending. Living in Venice with Olga Rudge, he was annoyed again and again by intrusions of visitors of all kinds. He told the Jewish poet Alan Ginsberg when he was eighty-two years old, "Any good I've done has been spoiled by bad intentions—the preoccupation with irrelevant stupid things. . . . But the worst mistake I made was that stupid, suburban prejudice of anti-Semitism" (Carpenter, 1988, p. 899). At eighty-four he revisited the United States. When he was eighty-five, some praise of *Drafts and Fragments of Cantos CX-CXVIII* by certain critics appeared, but at the same time his daughter published a memoir of her childhood that was most disparaging of Ezra Pound and Olga Rudge. He died November 1, 1972, at eighty-seven and was buried in Venice.

Carpenter (1988) concluded of Pound's achievements that, "The *Cantos* are a botch, but they do have unity and coherence, for they are autobiography. . . . Not as complete an autobiography as they might have been. It is a pity that the Pisan Cantos were not followed by a section inspired by life in Howard Hall and Chestnut Ward" (p. 912), where Pound resided in St. Elizabeth's Hospital.

His disciple Mullins, of course, viewed Pound as a martyr, ill-treated by the liberal community in the United States government. Stock (1970) wrote that in Pound,

> there was much to admire, not least a generosity of spirit which caused him to yearn for beauty and justice and to dream of a realm in which perfect beauty might be fused with perfect justice . . . . a man of sixty in a prison-camp dreaming of a celestial city "now in the mind indestructible" or a penniless young man, with no future, sitting on the steps of the customs house in Venice in 1908 gazing at the palaces and towers, the changing light and colour, and in his notebook writing poems to "Venice of dreams." (pp. 460-461).

Rather favorably inclined toward Pound, Stock believed that the broadcasts and the economics of Pound will be forgotten. But it should be remembered, as Ackroyd (1987) reported, "Although Pound could be witty and disarmingly candid in conversation about literary matters, in his political diatribes he was wilful, suspicious, and still virulently anti-Semitic" (p. 95). There were certainly signs of incipient and sometimes manifest paranoia. Note how this dissociation could serve as evidence for the "dissociative function of the ego" in the creative person, described by Weissman (1967) and discussed in Chapter 15.

Pound never adequately learned to understand or control the mass of his disturbed emotions: "His own abandoned self was continually haunting him, pushing him from pose to pose until it becomes unclear where the mask ends and the man begins" (Ackroyd, 1987, p. 98). This description is consistent with Nietzsche's position about the self discussed in Chapters 15 and 17.

Ackroyd had good things to say about the "Rock-Drill" section of *The Cantos,* that are reprieved by "passages of brilliant lyric and observation" (Ackroyd, 1987, p. 98). He also contrasted what appeared to be Pound's schizophrenic-like depression (schizoaffective disorder?) at the end of his life with the lightness and disciplined attention in the vision of the last drafts and fragments of the cantos. This debate over *The Cantos* (see Wilhelm, 1977) will probably be an interminable argument among literary experts; what is clear is that the genius of Pound was heavily weighted down by his psychopathology and could only appear, if at all, in bits, snatches, and flashes, and less and less of these as he grew older:

> Pound had always been invaded by such contradictions, and was sometimes impaled upon them. . . . It was also this mangled and difficult identity which gave his poetry its powerful and complex shape. Pound lived during a period when there was no significant context for his intuitions and his sometimes wayward perceptions; and so he set out, single-handed, to create one. (Ackroyd, 1987, pp. 115-116)

Stock (1970) believed *The Cantos* do not really constitute a poem but are notes toward a poem. For him *The Cantos* are a collection of fragments, some of which are extraordinarily beautiful and powerful as poetry, but with a quality that varies overall and certainly does not form anything like a unified work of art. Pound's metaphysical striving was clear; he was trying to describe and create in the most grandiose possible manner a paradise here on earth, a kind of Platonic Form of the Good. His model was Dante, but he was incapable of the sustained concentration and poetic power of Dante's *Divine Comedy,* all three books of which deserve careful reading and rereading and gain depth with increasing acquaintance. This aesthetic experience is not achieved by Pound's cantos in any sort of fashion.

I agree with Tytell (1987) that Pound's renewed energy when he returned to Italy "may have been related to the attentions of Marcella Spann, but it also was a response to the task of finishing *The Cantos* with a 'Paradiso' section which could make the entire work more coherent" (p. 329). However, although there was a final upsurge of creativity, Pound was only able to suggest the possibilities of a terrestrial paradise in bits and short passages of splendid poetry surrounded by much obscure and vapid writing. Tytell claimed that the "Thrones" cantos, mostly written at St. Elizabeth's, "invoked a wide range of mythical, divine, and fabulous entities, almost as a form of entreaty, a plea to unseen powers to give him the energy and imagination to complete what he had begun forty years earlier" (p. 329), but clearly the "Thrones" failed to move Pound out of his narcissism and psychopathology and restore order to his fragmented self. His metaphysical quest failed. *The Cantos* as a whole represent a glorious failure, and the reader is not, except for brief moments, transported into the realm of Truth and Beauty as he or she would be, for example, by the whole of Dante's *Divine Comedy* or Proust's *Remembrance of Things Past.*

Porteus (1950), like Pound, maintained, "All the urgent problems of our time are, after all, in some sense, communication problems" (p. 217). Brook-Rose (1971) opposed the critical work of Kenner (1971), who described Pound as maintaining a Cartesian point of view. Brook-Rose argued that Pound is closer to Husserl's phenomenology (see Chapter 1 in the present book) that "eliminated the old dichotomy between realism and idealism by reducing a world, once regarded as transcendental, to its manifestations within the consciousness" (pp. 123-124). Pound, like Jaspers (and like Barry), was concerned with the presentation of ciphers toward transcendence that would lead to a fusion of the finite with the infinite, fundamentally an Hegelian quest.

Artistic endeavors over the centuries have attempted to communicate the eternal world of Truth and Beauty as it is allowed to unfold itself in artistic productions; the greater the artist, the more successfully Truth and Beauty can shine forth in his or her finite and substantive artistic products. The argument of this book is that the psychopathology of the artist, while on the one hand rendering the artist alienated and uncomfortable with the prevailing mythology of the civilization and filling him or her with the motive to express either this mythology or a new mythology in some artistic form, at the same time mars the product due to either the intrusion of the artist's delusions and/or obsessional preoccupations into the creative endeavor or the constriction of that endeavor by the artist's impaired ego functioning and fragmented sense of self, for example, Pound's paranoid crystallization. Although, as Ernest Jones is reputed to have said, neurotics are the torchbearers of civilization, psychopathology can steer their artistic endeavors into a dead end, an Hegelian bad infinity, as illustrated in the work of Ezra Pound and Barry.

Stock (1966) explained how what he called Pound's "personal work" interferes with communication in Pound's *Cantos*. Pound

> takes it for granted that the rest of the world somehow shares his own knowledge of his own life and experiences. It does not occur to him that his own views of his own encounters, especially mere passing incidents in far-off times and places, are not available to the world unless he recreates them. . . .
> It is Pound's peculiarity to think that because he knows something *therefore* we know it too." (pp. 4-5)

This kind of blurring of ego boundaries is typical, in my clinical experience, of seriously emotionally disturbed patients. As they move to the left on the ego axis, they next expect you to know their thoughts, and at the extreme they are convinced you or some demonical force controls their thoughts (see also Chapter 19).

Rosenthal (1966) maintained that *The Cantos* descend from the Enlightenment: "They conceive of a world creatively ordered to serve human needs, a largely rationalist conception. . . . Pound's conclusion must be introduced as emergent from the midst of things, still struggling from all in life and consciousness that make for disorder" (pp. 50-51). As McDougal (1985) put it,

"Pound never ceased to 'refine' the materials of his art in the model of Dante, and that image remains a central one in his verse" (p. 79). Pound thought of Dante as a "donative artist" who could draw from the air around him; Pound dreamed of a Renaissance but he was unable to actualize it, nor was he able to communicate it to us or allow it to shine through to us except in brief moments of unforgettable beauty.

My edition of *The Cantos of Ezra Pound* (1950) is published by New Directions Books for Mr. James Laughlin, a supporter of Pound. Curiously, it leaves out *Canto LXXII* and *Canto LXXIII* which, I am told, contains praise of the Nazi war efforts. Many have criticized Pound's language, terse and harsh syntax, abrupt and fractured rhythms, and indecipherable idioms as not simply representing a failure but actually constituting a disintegration of poetry entirely. So in spite of his hunger for certainties in the aesthetic and political sphere and his "beauty spots," as he called them, referring to the flashes of brilliant poetry in *The Cantos*, Pound's psychopathology destroyed what was meant to be the major artistic product of his life.

Barry's Last Letter

Pound's life ended in muteness and despair, but he had the genius to actualize some of his aspirations. Barry died a premature death but with a more hopeful attitude, even though he did not have either the luck or the ability to actualize his narcissistic blossom dreams.

One morning not long after the collapse of the Soviet Union, Barry got up earlier than usual and composed a letter to his daughter in response to her question "What is the point of life?" He dictated this into a tape recorder for his secretary and then went down to his car preparing to drive to the office. Before he had a chance to start the car he had a massive coronary occlusion and died immediately. The letter was transcribed and sent to his daughter, and she has been kind enough to allow me to reproduce it here in full as a sort of counterweight to Barry's tortured imagination. It is Barry's last written statement.

Dear B,

It is 5 a.m. on Saturday morning and I have been troubled by your question, "What is the point of life?", one that I have heard many times over during my own long and difficult lifetime, and which has been asked by individuals in many situations since the beginning of recorded history. The question is asked by lonely and depressed people, by religiously inclined people, by philosophers, and by many brilliant novelists.

It is especially a question that troubles people like us who work in the medical profession and encounter suffering, pain, senescence, and death every day; in my lifetime there was the added horror of World War II, which took 40 million lives, and the Holocaust. So in addition to all the suffering that is imposed on us by external forces of nature such as sickness and death, we have to deal with the amazing cruelty of some people who have the need to inflict pain and suffering on us even when we approach them with friendliness, openness, and love. This is certainly the entire point of the Christian religion, which bases its gospels on the fate of Jesus, who was rewarded for his doctrine of love with being nailed to a board. But the issue was raised much earlier by the Jews in *The Book of Job*. Actually this work, which was probably written about 500 B.C.E., ends with the statement from God to shut up and mind your own business; in essence the Lord asks, Who do you think you are to ask Me to justify to you what I have imposed on the human race? There is no doubt that every person must learn to deal with bitter disappointment and with the arbitrary meanness and the downright cruelty of others, sometimes even coming from those whom they love the most.

Freud said the point of life is to follow the program of the pleasure principle. By this he meant that we all try to find some way of shaping a gratifying existence for ourselves within the limitations that nature and fate have given to us. Each person has to find their own way, often with much suffering, and this way invariably involves compromises, substitutions, and negotiation with what Sartre (you remember—you took a course from Hazel Barnes on Sartre's *Being and Nothingness*) called the "practico-inert," a kind of viscous gluey force against which all of us have to push in order to carve out our existence. This includes bureaucracies, scarcity of what we need, and a whole variety of impediments to our leading a decent existence. You may remember that Sartre had to spend some time in a German prison camp as a prisoner of war and managed to escape. So this brilliant man with an ugly face and an aberrant eye did not have a soft existence, either; his life was lived in a series of rented rooms in which he kept all his possessions, and he gave his money away about as fast as he made it.

In the Middle Ages tradition and religion dictated the point of life and people were diverted from your question, but for some people since then the point of life is to find the answer to "What is the point of life?' There is no one answer to this question, which is consistent with my argument that each person has to find his or her own way. In general I have discovered that if you are dedicated to a purpose greater than yourself, it helps. The best way to find happiness is not to look for happiness directly, but to immerse yourself in whatever your interests may be. For some people that greater purpose is scientific discovery or artistic achievement; for others it is helping the unfortunate, or political action. For some people like yourself, it is the enjoyment of the outdoors and nature, in which consciously or unconsciously you can feel a part of a greater whole. The philosopher Heidegger [1971b] talked of the "resonance of the fourfold," in which the gods, the earth, mortals, and the sky blended together in a harmonious One. This always struck me as a brilliant idea, and although it is very flowery, it expresses the sense that we *can* develop, that there is more to life than just the accumulation of material goods or technical gadgets. I think your enjoyment of nature and the outdoors is one of your strongest assets and I am happy that you have it.

Some people spend their life pursuing their various ambitions for money, power, and sexual gratification. Others, who do not, immerse themselves in aspects of ordinary life greater than they are, such as community service, or immerse themselves in music or the arts. There is no reason that a person cannot combine many of these solutions in one lifetime and sometimes all at once.

But the central issue about the point of life is the issue of love. If one has people and animals in one's life that one loves, life has a meaning. The lives of these others become as vital to one as one's own existence. But it is not easy to find love in life, especially in our current civilization, the "culture of narcissism" [Lasch, 1978]. The only way to find people to love is to go out and look for them. You have your parents and your sisters and brothers and now your children and your adorable nieces and nephews, all of whom will need you in the future, and you have your pets. But of course you need more, and it is part of the struggle of life to find more, to establish an empathic network of human relationships. Here is where the most painful disappointments take place, but this is not an indication that life has no point but only that it is a hard struggle for everybody. I do not know how to help you in this struggle, except to stand behind you and assure you that whenever you stumble your mother and I will be there and will be happy to be in your corner. What happens to you, happens to us, even if we no longer live together.

As I sit in this house which is now on the market, it is natural to reminisce on the past since we raised our family here, and to wonder what mistakes we have made. There are of course certain major, gross errors parents make that injure their children, but even if parents make no minor mistakes at all, this is no guarantee that an individual will grow up with any kind of happiness or good luck in life. In fact it is possible that the parents' minor mistakes, that we all make, strengthen the child because it helps the child to learn to deal with disappointments and failures of other people to come through as they should.

So if you want to find more love in your life you will have to get up in the morning and seek it out. You will have to suffer and struggle and endure many disappointments, and that is our universal fate. But this does not mean there is no point in life; it only means that life is a struggle. This struggle can make a person or break a person, depending on genetic inheritances and inner determination. It is very hard to face loneliness and disappointment, and in the teeth of all this one must creatively carve out one's own existence and give a meaning to one's own individual life, a meaning that no one else can develop for you. Being young, healthy, and attractive, you have many options in front of you and we are always available to help in any way that we can. But the hard truth is that each of us must behave as if we are the master

of our own ship and must steer in our own direction, *au fond*
making the voyage of life alone.

This is true whether one is married or not married,
and it has been my experience that marriage does not automatically bring happiness; it simply replaces one set of problems with another set of problems. It is a great mistake to
think that finding a spouse will solve one's problems. Of
course, marriage and children can bring happiness, and fortunately we are living in a culture where it is even possible to
have children or foster children, or to adopt children,
without the necessity of having a mate. Some people choose
that solution as the point of their life. What I am trying to say
is that nobody can answer your question about the point of
life for you; you will have to create the answer to it for yourself in your own way. All I can tell you is that life does have a
point and it is up to each of us to find it.

Love,
Dad

With this chapter I conclude my examination of the personal and artistic failures of Ezra Pound and Barry. Perhaps the
metaphysical failures of these men so dedicated to writing and literature could be attributed to their not heeding Plato's famous
warning, "No intelligent man will ever be so bold as to put into
language those things which his reason has contemplated, especially not into a form that is unalterable—which must be the case
with what is expressed in written symbols" (Hamilton and Cairns,
1973, p. 1590).

I saw a ladder rising up so high
that it could not be followed by my sight:
Its color gold, when gold is struck by sunlight.
(Dante, 1986, *Paradiso*, Canto xxi; ll. 28-30)

19 METAPHYSICS AS ARTISTIC CREATIVITY

Speculative philosophy is the endeavour to frame a coherent, logical, necessary system of general ideas in terms of which every element of our experience can be interpreted. . . . Philosophers can never hope finally to formulate these metaphysical first principles. Weakness of insight and deficiencies of language stand in the way inexorably. Words and phrases must be stretched towards a generality foreign to their ordinary usage; and however such elements of language be stabilized as technicalities, they remain metaphors, mutely appealing for an imaginative leap. . . one aim of philosophy is to challenge the half-truths constituting the scientific first principles.

—Alfred North Whitehead, Process and Reality

The classical philosopher is a devotee of the contemplative life and asks such questions as, "What is the most profound experience a person can have?. . . Love?. . . Art?. . . Natural Beauty?" Philosophy is an attitude of the mind, an irrepressible impulse toward inquiry, an itch to probe the meaning of things (Tomlin, 1952) through the application of reason, even though Abelard in the twelfth century warned that through rationalism lies the way to atheism. But belief in acquiring knowledge as the supreme ideal in human life runs like a red thread throughout the work of Maimonides (1952); this twelfth century Jewish philosopher already claimed that science describes but does not explain. Explanation, he argued, comes from religious truths, and these must come from the heart. In a modern version of this, Niebuhr argued that intellectuals *must* supply myths and *must* give meaning to our lives, not by presenting objective truth but by offering a sort of personally useful knowledge (Fox,

379

1985), what I would call a mythology created by artists. He pointed out that a form of faith underlies even science. All systems of belief give meaning to life. They are all in that sense what he would call religious beliefs and what, following Plato, I would call artistic myths. All the arts are vehicles for such mythology and for ciphers indicating something beyond us and beyond the artwork itself.

In historical development, myths lead to metaphysics, metaphysics leads to science, and science generates new myths that found new metaphysics; this circle is beautifully described by Langer (1942). She claimed that the contemplation of an unspoken idea gives aesthetic pleasure. Art is the symbolic expression of the artist's knowledge of his or her inner feeling; music conveys forms which language cannot articulate, also a central theme of the opera *Ariadne auf Naxos,* by Richard Strauss. Art, said Langer, attempts to overcome the barrier of word-bound thought; deep feeling leads to images, which lead to language, sometimes all expressed only in a dream. This is very important to understand if one is to get beyond naive nineteenth-century positivism.

Cultural background skills are so pervasive it is almost impossible to specify all of them. They form our primordial truths. Our cultural backgrounds are not beliefs but habits and customs, what Foucault called micro-practices (Hollinger, 1985). Heidegger deserves credit for calling our attention to these primordial, noncognitive, nonlinguistic preconditions of understanding. Gadamer's (1985) "prejudices" (see Chapter 20) represent the preunderstanding (not individual personal prejudices) that people in a given culture have, a somewhat different and more cognitive concept than that of Heidegger. One of the most crucial functions of art is to express these ineffable preunderstandings, background practices, and culturally assumed feelings and emotions which yield to us the intuitive conviction that we are part of something greater than our individual selves. It helps to understand these intuitive convictions or prejudices by examining pathological distortions of them, as I will now proceed to do by presenting an even more extreme example than that of Ezra Pound.

The Being-Question Creatively Answered

A patient claimed to have solved the Being-question for once and for all. He was a middle-aged philosophy professor who came to see me after what appeared at first to be a standard midlife crisis; his children were grown and married and his wife, as in Barry's situation, was getting tired of the role of housewife and nuturant supporter of her husband. She was beginning to indicate that she wished to have a life and career and self of her own, thus disrupting a rather long-standing gratifying arrangement and a cozy empathic support matrix for my patient.

About half a year ago, he noted certain peculiar sensations suggesting an inner change inside of him that he had difficulty in actually explaining to himself. These feelings of an inner change especially occurred when he was in a small office at the university with two or three of his male colleagues working closely together on some philosophical project. After a while it seemed to him these changes, which led to a puzzling sense of estrangement of various parts of his body, did indeed have an identifiable source. He felt their origin was from certain electric currents that were emanating from a specific focus in his body, which he gradually recognized to be his right testicle.

As these sensations continued he became convinced this focus in his testicle was not really a part of himself but was a source within him that was not actually him, a source which he eventually identified as some kind of radioactive material that had been placed there in some mysterious fashion, perhaps while he slept.

The feeling of inner change began to continue even at night. As he would fall asleep he began to see images in front of him in which the world took on a kind of distorted appearance; vague shadows flitted across his visual field. He dimly became aware of the fact that the focus of radiation was not, after all, an original or autochthonous focus but was receiving messages sent from outside of himself. The way these messages were transmitted to the focus in his testicle he at first vaguely thought was through some sort of gas, electron beams, X-rays, or cosmic radiation from an unidentified source. Eventually, as he reflected on his experiences, it became clear to him that this unidentified external source exerting such influence on him was not a friendly source. It was also apparently making changes in his wife and children without their awareness of it. This unidentified source was revealing itself to him but also concealing itself from him (notice the parallel to Heidegger's, 1962, concept of Truth) in that it was vague and mysterious; to his wife and children it was completely concealed, so that he was in the privileged position of having stumbled into a clearing in which he could get a glimpse of a cosmic process that seemed more and more to him to pervade the entire being of himself and his family.

Gradually a certain clarification took place regarding the nature of this cosmic process. He realized that everything being done to him, and that even accounted for his very existence and life experiences, was transmitted and regulated by this unseen influencing apparatus, a machine of obscure construction containing large and unimaginable parts and incredibly complicated, far beyond the grasp of any normal mortal to understand. As time passed it became apparent that this remarkable machine served as the ground of the Being of all the entities with which the patient had to interact and determined the very mode of their existence and the way in which they experienced the world and communicated these experiences to him.

The final revelation came to my philosopher-patient when in a lightning flash, a moment of vision (*Augenblick;* see Chapter 15), he realized that behind this enormous machine was a group of unidentifiable enemies, all men, perhaps male demons, who were operating the machine. The impression grew stronger and stronger that these male demons bore a suspicious resemblance to the very men he was working closely with in his university office. In a way, these male colleagues of his seemed to him to have been created in the image of the male demons.

Interestingly, the details of my patient's influencing machine have been described before (Tausk, 1933). Since it was capable of producing the world of visual reality for the patient, everything he saw was generated by the machine. It could produce as well as remove moods, thoughts, and feelings by means of waves or rays or mysterious forces that the sophisticated philosopher with all his knowledge of modern physics was unable to explain. It produced all the motor phenomena of his body, including erections and other body movements, through the use of air currents, electricity, magnets, or X-rays. It also created indescribable sensations, sometimes ecstatic, that were even strange to the patient himself and which he had never felt before, and it was definitely responsible for all physical occurrences in the patient's body, such as skin eruptions, abscesses, and various diseases. A constant concern of the patient in talking with me was that as his therapist I also was under the influence of the apparatus, although it was not clear whether I was allied with the conspiracy of demonic enemies who were driving this apparatus or was simply another victim of it, like the patient and his family. Obsessed with his discovery, our philosopher reminded me that Nietzsche (1886) was right when he wrote,

> A philosopher—is a human being who constantly experiences, sees, hears, suspects, hopes, and dreams extraordinary things; who is struck by his own thoughts as from outside, as from above and below, as by *his* type of experiences and lightning bolts; who is perhaps himself a storm pregnant with new lightnings; a fatal human being around whom there are constant rumblings and growlings, crevices, and uncanny doings. A philosopher—alas, a being that often runs away from itself, often is afraid of itself—but too inquisitive not to "come to" again—always back to himself. (p. 420)

Absurd, you say? Poor sick schizophrenic man? Is this really any more absurd than Leibniz's (1714) windowless monads having an unconscious knowledge of each other, or Whitehead's (1929b) nexuses of actual entities, inorganic, having a "prehension" of each other, or Aristotle's Unmoved Mover contemplating only itself while the planets revolve around it in absolute circular motion because they love it so much? Heidegger pejoratively derided all this as metaphysics, but what is the φύσις (*phusis*) before which, according to Heidegger, the pre-Socratic Greeks stood in awe and wonder? Is his notion of φύσις? any different or any less absurd? If so, why? Or what about the quarreling pantheon of Greek gods, or Heidegger's (1971b) "fourfold"—earth, sky, gods, and mortals—that he borrowed from Hölderlin, a schizophrenic poet? Why is the careful ontological analysis of my unfortunate patient not entitled to an equal hearing? How do we differentiate it from artistic creative philosophical systems—metaphysical or postmetaphysical—that have been taken seriously by scores of highly educated scholars over the centuries? Why do we keep asking this question about Being altogether? Where does the foreknowledge of it—a necessary precondition for asking *any* question—come from?

The Limits of Language

Infant researchers and neurophysiologists today generally agree, contrary to Freud, that from birth the human brain is a stimulus-seeking organ; it is challenged by stimuli to creatively find orders and patterns. This activity, which at first consists of the establishment of sensorimotor expectations and is prelinguistic, develops by late adolescence into what Kant called the regulative principle of pure reason. The establishment of orderly background activity patterns and expectations is shared among all the species of hunting animals because it has a high adaptational value in terms of finding and killing the prey.

Whenever we are confronted with the flow of perceptual data that constitutes human consciousness there is an innate tendency to "see" in this flow and to seek in it repetitive patterns and orders in a hierarchical arrangement. When order cannot be found there is stress and renewed activity; if such activity fails, in some situations it leads to a bizarre fragmentation of thought and even hallucinations and delusions. Here lies the explanation of "brainwashing," because under conditions where one's treatment from moment to moment is unpredictable, there occurs a regression and an eager grasping at any technique or belief system that will promise the establishment of some kind of reliable pattern in order to allow a set of expectations to develop. This is also the reason humans are always seeking a fixed transcendent world and the reason for their never-ending effort to find a ground and meaning to the flow of perceptual data, obstinately ignoring those philosophers who insist the Being-question has no meaning! Solutions vary from epoch to epoch, but the effort to find an ultimate grounding to existence is another version on an intellectual level of our primordial requirement to produce an order in the chaos.

Dreyfus and Rabinow (1982) described an essential contribution of Foucault's work; he explained that language cannot be known objectively because it is already a kind of know-how: "Man can never get behind his language to frame an objective account of how it began or how it works" (p. 38), they wrote, paraphrasing Foucault's (1973b, p. 331) discussion in *The Order of Things*. We can never reach a clear understanding of the very language we are trying to use to articulate and answer the Being-question and furthermore, we cannot pinpoint the background practices or know-how that constitute language and begin our history, because as we study these practices we find them retreating further and further into the distant past until they become what Heidegger called "the essential mystery." Foucault emphasized there is always a darkness at our borders. Psychoanalysis above all points to this—to the unconscious and to the human being's finitude, death, and desire, always lurking in the shadow-world at the edge of consciousness. But it does not follow, as Heidegger claimed, that concealment is built into the very nature of Being itself; this concealment could simply be a function of the limitations of human understanding and language. After all, our brains evolved for the purposes of hunting and gathering, not for understanding the universe.

Even Plato repeatedly stressed the inadequacy of language in trying to grasp essential reality; Plato (Hamilton and Cairns, 1973) claimed, in his famous *Seventh Letter*, that written work cannot be the most serious concern of a serious person. In *The Republic*, Plato refused to give either a clear definition of dialectic or a description of the metaphysical visions of the Form of the Good that he claimed are possible to attain. Later, especially in the *Sophist* and the *Statesman*, he tried to demonstrate the method of dialectic. Only a special elite, according to Plato, who have had a long and meticulous education, can eventually reach such metaphysical visions. This elite is driven by a passion (*éros*) which leads the human from beautiful objects in the natural world of appearances to beautiful thoughts and thence to the very essence of Beauty or Good that is experienced in an ecstasy of joy. Philosophers who have climbed their way up the ladder of the tedious education in "mathematica" eventually reach a sense of transcendent vision that illuminates their lives and renders matters in the world of appearances irrelevant and unimportant.

Visionary thinkers like Plato, who emphasize the "higher regions" of thought, tend to arrive at a two-world theory in which a superior world of Eternal Forms presides and is grasped through an inferior world of apparent experience and constantly changing chaos. But philosophers like Aristotle try to reduce the two worlds to one by making the productions of reason and the mind simply abstractions creatively derived from sensory experiences, such abstractions as the laws of science. Yet Aristotle insisted on the paradoxical (in his own system) concept of reason alone having a partly divine or eternal nature as an immaterial thinking substance. He did not escape the metaphysical question of the relationship of mentation to matter, and he floundered inconsistently on the metaphysical concept of substance. Like Plato, he emphasized intuitive thought as an important procedure by which first principles are directly grasped, and separated this from deliberative reason which aims at practical wisdom, and even from the process of inductive generalization, another function of the highest form of reason according to Aristotle.

It is easy to see how metaphysical thinking conceived of as "intuitive grasping" can quickly lead to autism, mysticism, and ecstatic religious experiences. Therefore, Freud (1927b) said, "I not only have no talent for it [metaphysics] but no respect for it, either. In secret—one cannot say such things aloud—I believe that one day metaphysics will be condemned as a nuisance, as an abuse of thinking, as a survival from the period of the religious *Weltanschauung*" (p. 228).

Freud (1914b) argued that metaphysical speculation was based on self-observation, which he also regarded as the basis of the self-criticism of conscience. He called self-observation a kind of "internal research, which furnishes philosophy with the material for its intellectual operations" (p. 96). In paranoid patients such as the one described in this chapter, this self-critical function becomes projected, and their delusions of being watched, manipulated, and criticized by external "voices" or demons have the same psychodynamic root as their "characteristic tendency. . . . to construct speculative systems" (p. 96). He viewed the heightening of the activity of this critically observing agency as the basis of both conscience and philosophic introspection.

Toward a Methodology

Kant (1781), although he was not always consistent in his use of the terms, established the important distinction between scientific understanding *(Verstand),* and *Vernunft,* a human faculty or higher sort of reason that seeks out transcendental ideas of unity. He characterized this seeking as a natural tendency of the human mind to exercise what he called a regulative function. For Kant the only science of metaphysics possible is the investigation of the boundaries or limits of human reason; speculative metaphysics, seeking out the transcendental, is similar to artistic or religious mythological visions, which may even come from a variety of sources, sometimes including psychopathology. Kant did not deny the natural impulse of the reflective mind to strive after unified conceptual syntheses—to think obstinately beyond the limits of reason—and indeed in his own lifetime there appeared the first great German idealist constructions, which rested on what some call the fundamental error of claiming that metaphysical speculation could reach knowledge of a *cognitive* nature on a par with or even higher than the knowledge of science.

The quest for meaning, as Arendt (1977) defined metaphysical thinking, must contain within it some possible criteria for distinguishing between the "meaning" assigned to the world by a paranoid schizophrenic, by a religious mystic, and by a "normal" philosopher attempting to employ his or her rational capacities in finding the answers to certain fundamental questions of our common experience. The only possible method of validation that we know to protect us from autism is some form of debate or dialectic or consensual conversation with its mutually enhancing and intrinsically correcting values. This requires that metaphysical propositions be put in communicable form—into a logical, consistent, and coherent language. Here again, we run into the limits of language. Or we could conclude with Freud (1927a), as he wrote in his old age: "The moment a man questions the meaning and value of life, he is sick, since objectively neither has any existence; by asking this question one is merely admitting to a store of unsatisfied libido to which something else must have happened, a kind of fermentation leading to sadness and depression" (p. 436).

Metaphysics represents an ongoing debate in the history of humans regarding the validity of certain fundamental premises that allegedly have been grasped by Aristotle's intuitive reason, or transcendental reflection (Kant's *Vernunft*, as defined earlier), or perhaps by the later Heidegger's poetic thinking, as opposed to calculative thinking. When generally accepted by a given culture, metaphysical systems or their offspring called ideologies have led to the flowering of various cultures and the explosion of science. Metaphysics differs from autism, religion, art, or mysticism essentially because it ultimately demands the application of the rules of reason to its speculative findings. Metaphysics differs from science because metaphysical propositions cannot be demonstrated by standard scientific methodology; in fact, when certain metaphysical propositions become demonstrable by scientific methodology, this leads to the establishment of a new science and the issues involved are no longer labeled as metaphysics.

The problem of methodology in metaphysics falls within the realm of Dilthey's (Ermarth, 1978) *Geisteswissenschaften*, the human sciences, which attempt to reach the inward spiritual structure by empathic identification (see Chapter 17), moving from the external phenomena to operative inward purposes and ideals that are expressed in them. This is consistent with Bergson's (1950a) *Introduction to Metaphysics*, rarely cited these days, which opens by contrasting the two ways of knowing anything. When our intellect approaches phenomena externally from some point of view alien to it, we develop Dilthey's "natural sciences," in which allegedly independent observers study objects from without. The second way of knowing is through a process Bergson called intuition, whereby we "enter into" phenomena and identify ourselves with them by a kind of "intellectual sympathy" or the art of "intellectual auscultation." This is comparable to identifying ourselves with a figure in a novel we are reading, and results in a "knowledge" of "reality" that the method of empirical science can never yield. Similarly, phenomenologic psychiatrists have pointed out how a direct phenomenologic (see Chapter 1) grasp of the patient at hand provides important complementary and vital information about the being-in-the-world of that person.

The prime example of this, with which we are all familiar, is our sense of self. The existence we know best is unquestionably our own, as pointed out by Descartes, Bergson, and even Husserl, regardless of all the disagreement over what they went on to develop from this fact. Our sense of self, as apprehended directly by "intellectual auscultation," or Freud's introspective self-observation, gives us a clue to the methodology necessary to grasp the truths of metaphysics. The translation of truths grasped in such a manner from what Arendt (1977) called "ineffable metaphors" into communicable language represents the greatest challenge to the metaphysician but is an absolute necessity in order to establish consensual validation and distinguish the fruits of intellectual auscultation from the delusions of autistic reverie (Chessick, 1982a). This translation is primarily a creative, artistic activity.

We have come a long distance in metaphysics from the naive subject-object distinction of Descartes and the scientific positivism based on it. We now know that our mind and our sense of self are inextricably mixed into our perceptions of "facts" or "empirical reality." Recently, idealism has been given a rebirth as Rescher's (1973) "conceptual idealism," in which he contended that our ordinary conceptions of things in nature involve concepts whose adequate explication always makes reference to minds and their activities and capacities, that is, mind-involving concepts. I will discuss this in more detail later in this chapter. The dependence of "reality" on mind is not ontological in Hegel's sense but is conceptual, with the mind contributing such concepts as "possibility," "law of nature," "space," "time," and "empirical properties," the ordinary concepts that frame our experience of everyday life. This kind of ontological thinking, conceptual idealism, has important ramifications for the field of psychotherapy and for science in general, as it brings into question the adequacy for answering human existence issues of using the traditional scientific methodology of establishing empirical verification of hypotheses. Our answer to the Being-question will in turn affect our notions of Truth and how to obtain it and, in my opinion (but not in Heidegger's view), will also affect our values and behavior toward each other.

I discussed in Chapter 11 the possible effect of our social, cultural, and economic milieu on what constitutes the prevailing ideology or philosophical points of view. Without some form of communicable language and dialectical interchange, we are left with either Schelling's important assertion that art is an alternative way of disclosing Being (Lawrence, 1988); or the obscurantism of the late Heidegger, whose writing sometimes degenerates into highly idiosyncratic translations, empty incantations, and a withdrawal into magic and preoccupation with the sound of words (Bruns, 1989); or what I believe to be Derrida's (1980) satirical deconstruction and attack on "the metaphysics of presence"; or a pessimistic nihilism and hopeless relativism. I agree with the argument of Castoriadis (1989) that philosophy is not "over"; it consists of a questioning that has to go on and is absolutely vital to the flourishing of a democratic society, to supporting the refusal of dogmatic closure, and to preserving humane values and reverence for human life from birth to death.

The Search for Transcendence

Wittgenstein (1961), in his *Tractatus* 5.6, said, *"The limits of my language mean the limits of my world"* (p. 115). In the last work Wittgenstein (1972) produced, *On Certainty,* he explained that, for each of us, our world picture is a system of not easily removed or replaced convictions. It is a framework that we use for all discussions and proofs. Our world picture is tied to the practices we are taught as children when our parents say, "This is the way we do it." Our actions lie at the basis of our language games, and we rely on a memory bank of examples taught by our parents. Our world picture therefore rests neither on empirical knowledge nor on the scientific verification of hypotheses, for any sort of testing has to stop at or be based upon some underlying points of belief, axioms, or so-called self-evident premises. Where do these come from? What we are taught as children we take on faith, and in so doing we form an organized structure, a world picture, a web of belief. The conclusions and premises from this structure give each other mutual support.

Our world picture is not easily shaken by conflicting empirical propositions; it is an important function of art in each culture to shape and communicate this world picture directly and to announce when it is changing or fragmenting! Our world picture is more like a methodology that one decides to adopt while ignoring conflicting evidence. The changeover to another system represents a conversion, and it is a shift moved more by loss of a war, persuasion, and dramatic unexpected aesthetic or spiritual experiences than by reason. Wittgenstein (1972) wrote, "When two principles really do meet which can not be reconciled with one another, then each man declares the other a fool and heretic" (p. 81e).

Wittgenstein explained that at the foundation of every apparently well-founded belief lies a belief that is not founded. Belief systems are acquired by observation and instruction; they are acquired, not learned. We teach a child when we point and say, "This is your hand," not by asking the child if this is really a hand or by getting the child to learn to know that he or she has a hand. Certainty, claimed Wittgenstein, becomes a matter of attitude. Along with the learning of language games also comes the learning of what is acceptable to be investigated in a given culture and what is not to be investigated.

Heidegger (1961) pointed out that the Europeanization of the earth took place because the classical Greek concepts are unrivaled as instruments of power, since they allow things or beings to become objects for manipulation and control. At the same time there is a nebulousness in Heidegger's concept of Being that is understandable, because thinking for Heidegger was a wayfaring with continuous transformation. Heidegger returned to the pre-Socratic thinkers; he maintained they were closer to Being and were eclipsed by Plato, whose metaphysical system that founded Western philosophy actually served to conceal Being. But Rescher (1993) complained that, "the large ongoing response to writers such as Heidegger, Derrida, and their epigones clearly shows that there is more academic hay to be made nowadays by debunking metaphysics and epistemology as traditionally conceived than by practicing them" (p. 737). He attributed this "widespread assault by a disaffected avant-garde" against the usual practice of academic philosophy to an expression of a *fin de siécle* disillusionment with traditional philosophy and perhaps our entry into "a postphilosophical era, where philosophy as traditionally conceived is no longer viable" (p. 737).

Lindley (1993) described the same kind of situation in modern Western physics, pointing out there can be no "real world" as assumed in classical physics and no such thing as an "objective world":

Where the classical physicist assumed that measurements could in principle be made both infinitely precise and perfectly unobtrusive, the quantum physicist knows that the thing measured is influenced by the measurement, and will act quite differently when measured than if it had never been measured at all. It makes no good sense to talk of an objective world of real facts if those facts cannot be apprehended without altering them in the process. There is no longer any meaning to be attached to the idea of real, objective world; what is measured, and therefore known, depends on the nature of the measurement. (p. 63)

Reason and Truth

There has even been a change in the concept of reason itself in the Western world; it is now recognized that "reason" is culturally mediated and interwoven with social practices. It seems to me best, as Rorty (1991) suggested, to think of Heidegger and Derrida simply as post-Nietzschean philosophers and to assign them into the conventionally described great conversation sequence running from the pre-Socratics to the present time, rather than to view them as initiating or manifesting a radical departure. I believe that the originator of the new postmetaphysical mode of Western thinking was actually that archmetaphysician Hegel, who pointed out how a personality and its consciousness develops through action and interaction that alter the self in unforseen ways. Rather than an essential human core, there is a lifelong dialectic between self-knowledge, self-actualization, and praxis. Striving for a set of goals founded on knowledge of one's self, often enhanced and further expressed by artistic experience, leads to new self-knowledge, new goals, altered strivings, and so forth, in a dialectical upward spiral. Beiser (1993) added that in Hegel's framework the historically prevailing self-conception of the human being indicates where a given culture stands in its level of spiritual expression. For Hegel, Truth is eternal, universal, and permanent, but for Hegel "thought" is historical and all philosophy can do is raise the self-consciousness of each culture about its spirit, values, and beliefs. Philosophy, according to Hegel, can never be separated from its social context, and so the subject matter of philosophy or speculative metaphysics is constantly transforming.

Whitehead (1933) wrote that philosophy is a survey of possibilities and their comparison with actualities. He did not want philosophy to be a ferocious debate between professors, but rather to constitute a never-ending attempt to clarify the fundamental beliefs that finally determine the areas of emphasis and of attention lying at that base of each of our characters. In his (Whitehead, 1929a) magnificent essay, "The Function of Reason," he divided reason into "the reason of Ulysses" and the "reason of Plato." The "reason of Ulysses" is the reason of so-called professionals in various clinical fields, and is characterized by a lack of vision, and, I might add, by technical jargon and an absence of artistic communication. It seeks an immediate method of action; science directs us to things rather than values. But Whitehead reminded us of the consequences of basing life only on this; Ulysses had no use for Plato, and as a result the bones of his companions were strewn on many a reef and many an isle.

The "reason of Plato" seeks a complete understanding of "the universal scope of things." It is continuously opposed by common sense and the apparent chaos of everyday experience, and it is on this basis that scientists have attacked and devalued it. The problem of speculative reason, or poetic metaphysics, two of the many names for the "reason of Plato," is that we must find a method that on the one hand keeps it from being anarchic or, as psychiatrists would say, autistic, and that on the other hand enables it to exercise its function of reaching beyond all set bounds. Only too often, as is apparent in *The Cantos,* the poetry of Ezra Pound was typically autistic, and the metaphysics of the patient presented in this chapter was even more so.

In metaphysics, Whitehead suggested, the Greeks made important advances in defining the rational method, setting off speculative reason from idiosyncratic "inspiration" or "autistic reveries." The Greeks insisted that speculative reason must conform to intuitive experience, have clarity of propositional content, have internal and external logical consistency, and present a logical scheme with widespread conformity to experience, coherence among its categorical notions, and methodological consequences for further expansion and progress. This Greek orientation from the time of Plato leads us from the lower to the higher world, from the world of senses to the world of ideas. Whether or not this higher world has a separate "existence" is irrelevant. The point is that the Greek orientation contains an implicit and sometimes explicit hope that we can abide in this higher world as much as possible, a world of concepts, or "ideas" and permanent eternal Truths and Forms. So although we all lie in the gutter and slime of everyday life, we can, if we will, fix our gaze as much as possible on the stars.

The classic exposition of this Greek orientation is to be found in Plato's *Republic, Book VI* (Hamilton and Cairns, 1973), containing the famous "divided line" analogy, in which Plato attempts to reach the Ultimate (Absolute, Being, Reality, Form of the Good) through the use of more and more abstract reason. But Hegel realized that what the West thought was eternal was only historical, and that so-called innate ideas are predominantly cultural. Reified values of the West turn out to be products of the human unconscious, and reason alone cannot create a presuppositionless philosophy. A similar crisis arose in the greatest area of Western purely rational accomplishment, mathematics. Gödel proved that a mathematical system containing no unfounded propositions was impossible (Nagel and Newman, 1974), so every mathematical system is essentially incomplete.

From Hegel, traditional Western philosophy has gone off in two directions. Russell attempted to produce a form of "Platonic atomism" when he abandoned Hegelian philosophy, establishing his system on so-called "atomic facts" upon which everything could be grounded. This reached its fruition in the founding of "analytic philosophy," which until recently unfortunately dominated the British and United States academic departments of philosophy. These philosophers adopted a quasi-scientific model of philosophizing and employed detailed investigation by logico-linguistic methods of analysis, producing many sterile, jargon-laden publications.

As described in Chapter 1, an entirely different style of philosophizing was developed by Husserl, who attempted to move in the direction of a transcendental absolute through the employment of phenomenology. For him this led to a transcendental ego that intuited the essences of objects. His student Heidegger attempted to use phenomenology in studying those aspects of Being that could be approached through hermeneutic analysis, ferreted out from the phenomenology of the being of humans, but he gave up these earlier efforts and ended his career with nonmetaphysical thought more akin to the mysticism of Meister Ekhart.

A similar debate goes on today among psychoanalysts regarding the role of their creative processes. For example, Fajardo (1993) outlined the varieties of epistemologic perspectives employed in contemporary psychoanalysis. Some analysts think clinical inquiry to be a form of empirical investigation "that positions the neutral analyst-observer on the edge of the psychoanalytic situation, watching the patient's psyche at work" (p. 978). Others, still with an empirical stance, study the patients' intrapsychic structures as they manifest themselves in the patients' behavior and communications, and distinguish this from the interpersonal process between the patient and the therapist. The meaning of "truth" in this context is still that of correspondence to that remembered past.

What Fajardo (1993) calls the "hermeneutic constructivist" clinical psychoanalytic position, on the other hand, "positions the analyst as emotionally and subjectively involved, if not embedded, with the patient, immersed in a reciprocal process, and watching and responding to both her own and the patient's experience" (p. 979). I have discussed this form of psychoanalytic creativity in Chapter 17. Such a dyadic process teaches us about how the patient organizes experience and makes it meaningful, a creative activity. This kind of postmodern explication of the psychoanalytic process can be more or less radical; "truth" here is seen as emerging out of the particular patient-analyst dyad, with mutual agreement and coherence of their webs of belief rather than correspondence to the past as the determinant, that is, "narrative truth" rather than "historical truth" (Spence, 1982), as I have reviewed it in Chapter 17. Emphasis may be strictly on the "here-and-now" or "intersubjective" aspects of the dyadic situation (Stolorow and Atwood, 1992) or on a combination of the "here-and-now" and "transference" aspects of the dyadic situation (Gill, 1982).

The diversity of psychoanalytic approaches leaves the postmodern era in psychoanalysis in a situation similar to that of philosophy and the arts, characterized by positions ranging from the traditional to the radical. Kohut's self psychology is somewhere in between. The Lacanians want to throw out Freud's structural theory altogether. In psychoanalysis as well as in Western philosophy there are conflicting conceptions of "meaning" and "truth," and disagreement as to how these arise, how they are established, and whether they are specific to each dyad or culture or have some transcendent or repeatable quality. The problem is that "no one can claim to occupy an Archimedean point from which all theories can be objectively studied and a judgement rendered as to which is *the* correct theory" (Phillips, 1991, p. 408).

Are we in the West to retain some sense of eternal or transcendental truths about "reality" and about "the self" of individuals, or are we to accept the notion that everything is radically contingent and historical, and that even our method of reason itself, which lies at the basis of all Western thinking, is a product of a learned language game and background cultural practices? In the face of this dilemma it is no surprise therefore that Nietzsche the artist, coming at the end of traditional metaphysics, perhaps ironically suggested there was nothing left for Western man to do but to laugh and to dance.

Postfoundationalist Art and Thought

Hegel began the attempt to make the irrational rational. He tried to unite the working days of the week, the profane life, with the Sunday of existence, the time of sacred and poetic exultation. As the young Marx saw it, truth emerges from a dialectic in which meaning spontaneously appears at the intersection of the very actions by which humans organize themselves with respect to nature and others (Descombes, 1980). For Foucault our entire postmodern epoch of philosophy is an attempt to struggle free from Hegel; the Other of reason is unreason or madness, and a continuous dialectic occurs between the rational and the irrational. But Desmond (1995) turned this argument completely around by insisting that determinate scientific intelligibility is not the ultimate horizon of intelligibility: "Hence in the measure that metaphysics extends mindfulness to the ultimate sources of intelligibility, its thinking is at the edge of, if not beyond, the border of determinate intelligibilities" (p. 764). He insisted there are modes of mindfulness that are not scientific but seek to understand the meaning of ultimate horizons and sources, the meaning of Being, topics that are not reducible to scientific objectification and, "At this boundary the affiliation of metaphysical thinking with art and religion becomes more evident. . . . Art and religion are speakers of transcendence, and to their voices the philosopher must listen" (pp. 764-765).

Desmond (1995) rejected Hegel's insistence that there is a rigid, inevitable dialectical self-determination in which Absolute Spirit expresses itself first in art, then in religion, and then in philosophy, a view I share. Instead, Desmond argued, there is an ongoing, open intermediation between art and religion that forms a fertile challenge to philosophy, not the challenge Hegel saw, namely, how to incorporate their otherness into the dialectically higher philosophical concept, but "rather, just their otherness serves as reminder that a sense of transcendence might be manifest that is not at all reducible to the self-determination of dialectical thinking. . . . Consider how we find something inexhaustible about a great work of art, and this is not entirely determinable by any finite analysis" (pp. 765-766). Hegel's contemporary, Schelling, put art and creativity at the apex of human endeavors, perhaps the first in the nineteenth century to do so (Stambaugh, 1994), and Nietzsche even viewed art as the activity most crucial to human life. For him, creating art is affirming the world by transforming it.

Lyotard (1984) set the theme of postmodernism as the rejection of all metanarratives, or "incredulity toward metanarratives" (p. xxiv), meaning by "metanarrative" any theory about Reality that is supposed to be true for all time and from all points of view. This is similar to the arguments of Rorty (1979), who essentially reduced metaphysics to pragmatism and Wittgensteinian language games. Since all observation is theory-laden there can be no Reality that is objectively there for all knowers, argue the postmodernists, and they reject even partial or contingent "truth," claiming that "truth" is "hegemonic," "logocentric," "phallocentric," and so forth (Himmelfarb, 1994). It follows from their contentions, as Kane (1993) claimed, "Any attempt to show that one point of view is objectively right and all others wrong would have to appeal to the presuppositions and standards of rationality of one among other points of view and could not therefore either claim certainty or objective truth" (p. 414). Since all knowing and understanding involve interpretation in terms of some conceptual scheme or linguistic framework, or some language game or form of life local and particular to the knower or inquirer, postmodernists argue that human inquirers are embedded in historical and cultural traditions that they cannot transcend in order to attain a neutral or objective point of view. Kane called this, "A pervasive image (perhaps *the* dominant image) of the modern intellectual landscape" (p. 414). He continued, "The claim that human inquirers are embedded in historical traditions and cultural frameworks from which they cannot escape to a 'neutral' or 'absolute' perspective eventually threaten the ideal of objective explanation as well as that of objective worth" (p. 417).

I agree with Kane's (1993) answer to this dilemma. We are not actually trapped between a Platonic realism and a postmodernist nihilism: "For the way the world is may simply be all the different ways the world is, described in different vocabularies" (p. 418). For example, the history of a city could be simply the *summation* of what the weatherman, the economist, the social historian, the geographer, and others correctly say—which means that to describe fully the way that the world is would require broad learning, using many vocabularies, paying attention on many listening channels, and phenomenologically allowing that which will manifest itself to appear to us or, in Bion's (1967) terms, place itself in our psyche. Kane concluded, "If some of these ways are incommensurable with, or irreducible to, others (if they cannot be wholly translated into or reduced to, some one level of description) so be it" (p. 419). This is the point of view I have also advocated (see Chapter 3).

In metaphysical speculation, I have found the work of Rescher (1973, 1991, 1992) especially sensible. He and I both believe there is an empirical Reality "out there" that can be approached by our study of it. Rescher (1992) defined his position of conceptual idealism or pragmatic idealism as: "Any fully adequate descriptive characterization of the nature of physical ('material') reality must make reference to mental operations: some recourse to verbal characteristics or operations; is required within the substantive content of an adequate account of what it is to be real" (p. 305). Like Rescher, I agree with the postmodern claim that the activity of the knower permeates what we know, not only in the constituting but also in the constitution of what is known. But our point of view is a guarded notion of scientific realism which at the same time concedes that both constitutive and regulative principles are applied by the mind. This represents a sort of half-way point of view between classical scientific naive empiricism as advocated by the contemporaries of Freud, and the postmodern approach. Rescher (1973) wrote, "Descriptive information about the empirical features of things is always in part a product of mental contrivance" (p. 9). What I wish to emphasize here is the phrase "in part." Even if our conceptual machinery is not innate and is a cultural artifact socially formed and transmitted, there remains the possibility of a hermeneutic study to tease out these artifacts and supply us with an approximation of a residue that may be called objective Reality. Another way we can reach this approximation is through the use of ciphers, as presented to us directly in our phenomenologic experiences of natural beauty, ecstatic love, boundary situations that involve basic existential choices and call our attention to our Being-towards-death, and aesthetic experiences.

There is at least a minimal core of epistemologic agreement in this debate. Most thinkers accept the postfoundationalist viewpoint that reason is inextricably rooted in history and that there is no intuitive grasp of truth that would not be mediated by social and linguistic structures, bringing an inevitable essential element of ambiguity or undecidability to what we call Truth. This is not a defeat for reason, but a renewed call to a more critical and hermeneutic use of reason as well as a renewed motivation to focus on ciphers and aesthetic experiences in an attempt to thematize and articulate unformulated and even unthought presuppositions and critically assess their cogency. Indeed, there are many unthought and impossible-to-articulate presuppositions of our experience that can *only* be expressed through the artistic medium! An example of this is the second act of Wagner's *Tristan und Isolde,* a representation of the fusion of individual ego boundaries in ecstatic love, as I have discussed it in Chapters 7 and 9. An allusion to this inexpressibility is also found in one of the poems in Barry's play, presented in Chapter 16. Even in psychoanalytic treatment, as Ingram (1994) suggested, "I believe that what actually occurs in good therapy is unavailable for discussion and review because there is no legitimate discourse for reporting it. I

warrant that experienced and successful therapists know precisely what I mean and will join me in acknowledging how much
this is so, even if they scowl at other opinions expressed in this
essay" (p. 184).

This suggestion contains an echo of Wittgenstein's (1961)
Tractatus. Originally published in 1921, Wittgenstein's seminal
work ends with a nihilistic and famous sentence: "What we
cannot speak about we must pass over in silence" (p. 151).
Wittgenstein should have considered at this point the capacity of
the arts to express Truths that we cannot otherwise articulate, or
to convey Truth, especially humanistic truth, in a more direct
and distinctive manner. What psychologist or psychiatrist in the
traditional sciences could ever compare with Shakespeare or Nietzsche. . . or Proust, who replaced the one human relationship
that was his sustaining selfobject, his mother, with a creative masterpiece he produced after she died? Wilson (1931) described
the "chief exemplification" of Proust's central idea, the tragedy of
Albertine, as

> the tragedy of the little we know and the little we are able to
> care about those persons whom we know best and for whom
> we care most; and the pages which tell how Albertine's lover
> forgot her after she was dead, by reason of their very depar-
> ture from any other treatment of death that we remember in
> fiction, give us that impression of a bolder honesty, of a
> closer approach to reality, which we get only from deep and
> original genius. (p. 154)

This brings me to the concluding topic in the present book,
the expression of Truth, Beauty, and Reality in art, with emphasis
on the inhibition or destruction of this expression by the personal psychopathology of the artist.

20 TRUTH IN ART

Plato had, of course, dealt with many definitely artistic subjects, such as the importance of unity in a work of art, the necessity for tone and harmony, the aesthetic value of appearances, the relation of the visible arts to the external world, and the relation of fiction to fact. He first perhaps stirred in the soul of man that desire which we have not yet satisfied, the desire to know the connection between Beauty and Truth, and the place of Beauty in the moral and intellectual order of the Kosmos. The problems of idealism and realism, as he sets them forth, may seem to many to be somewhat barren of results in the metaphysical sphere of abstract being in which he places them, but transfer them to the sphere of art, and you will find that they are still vital and full of meaning.
—Oscar Wilde, The Artist as Critic

In the middle of his life Dante seems to have abandoned the notion that reason was enough to understand the universe; perhaps this is the secret of why his poem had such great appeal to Ezra Pound and Barry. In youth he was in love with love, and in his maturity he was in love with reason, but a new and astonishing Dante emerged with the appearance of *The Divine Comedy* around his fortieth year of life. The proper way to read *The Divine Comedy* is to linger over each canto until one imaginatively sees its unique action and it comes to life in every detail (Fergusson, 1966) but, as in Barry's complaint, who has time to do this in our hurried civilization? So, as already mentioned in Chapter 11, Oscar Wilde (1982) said, "we live in the age of the overworked and the undereducated; the age in which people are so industrious that they become absolutely stupid" (p. 385).

Science is always based on a picture or a model created by the mind, often with the utmost daring and freedom, as in the great systems of Galileo, Newton, Darwin, Einstein, and Freud.

But different fundamental hypotheses, called networks by Wittgenstein (McGuinness, 1988), might equally fit the world. Modernity is now ending. It began between 1600 and 1656, especially around 1630 with Galileo and Descartes. It was a response to the crisis of 1600, with the end of the domination of Spain; the explosion of genius in the seventeenth century moved from Italy (Galileo, Bernini, Caravaggio) to Holland (Descartes, Huygens, the great Dutch painters) to England (Hobbes, Dryden, Purcell, Wren, Milton, Newton, Locke). The poet John Donne (1572-1631) expressed the frailty and decay in the foundational framework of his contemporary world, a situation also sadly characteristic of our time, for since the 1980s it has become clear that *all* the sciences are context-dependent, and no science is an abstract enterprise entirely free of subjectivity. Descartes's foundational hopes are gone and we are back to the premodern sixteenth-century skepticism of Montaigne. We have lost what was believed to be the authoritative underpinnings of conceptual structures constituting the foundation of rational or scientific knowledge; the dream of foundationalism is just a dream (Toulmin, 1990). More urgently, God is dead as a communally recognized indisputable source of biblical morality, and Western civilization verges on moral anarchy. As the nineteenth century French philosopher Charles Renouvier already sadly observed, the world is suffering from a lack of faith in transcendental truth.

What Will Replace Foundationalism?

Does the way out of this disappointing dilemma lie in the arts? Proust, as I have repeatedly pointed out, was a great observer and psychologist; his character Vinteuil claimed that art is not only real, it is even more real than life! For Proust a fleeting sensation liberates the timeless essence of things and simultaneously reawakens our true self. He attempted to immobilize these moments in literature; art becomes the spiritual equivalent of them, the true reality. Proust believed and tried to demonstrate that art, not intellect, rediscovers lost time. The taste of the madeleine, the clink of a spoon, he maintained, helped him to escape death and recapture time. Underneath it all lies Being-towards-death, as I wrote in the first sentence of the present book. For Proust, the writer is a painter, and dreams are also a mode of rediscovery but not good enough by themselves; associations are necessary.

Humans are an accident, a late and opportunistic predatory newcomer species whose life in Sartre's view is governed by contingency and the practico-inert, as I have illustrated by the case histories in the present book. Humans as thinkers are a byproduct, a nonessential component of reality; humans and all their works (Popper's "world 3"— see Chapter 15) cling to existence with a hold that is tenuous and feeble. Sartre believed that the so-called justifications for existence, such as science, bourgeois values, and even humanism are all false, no more than self-delusions. The possibility for salvation, he (1938) said in an early work, is through art, what I would call temporary contemplation of the Form of Beauty (and, I would add, Truth) expressed in artworks. Similarly, he believed experiencing the pure form of melodies and mathematical figures, even though these are humanmade, paradoxically makes sense of life in the course of our fundamentally absurd existence.

That unsavory character (Chessick, 1995a) Martin Heidegger began his lectures at 7 A.M., four days a week, a behavior more characteristic of professors in my medical school days than of philosophers. I once assigned Heidegger's (1954) *What Is Called Thinking?* to a group of psychiatric residents and found myself with a revolution on my hands. Overwhelmed by the struggle of having to learn how to satisfy the bureaucrats of managed care with enough redundant paperwork to eke out some payment for their services, they were unwilling to put in the effort necessary to understand Heidegger's concepts, expressed in a book where he cleverly points out that science does not think and poetry summons us. For Heidegger (1977), art or poetic revealing is the necessary remedy to technology; otherwise the frenziedness of technology will entrench itself everywhere. Of course this has already happened!

Heidegger complained that mortals no longer dwell poetically on the earth under the heavens. He insisted, although for different reasons than Hegel, that great art is a thing of the past. Heidegger believed in his later years that Truth comes to pass while it is being poetized (Kockelmans, 1984). *Art breaks open a clearing in whose openness everything is suddenly other than usual.* He reminded us how for Parmenides, one of the great original pre-Socratic philosophers, thinking and poetizing are inseparable. Heidegger (Kockelmans, 1984) claimed that the poetizing of poets and the meditative thinking of thinkers are expressions of a primordial form of thinking involving both Being and humans. He called this "primordial poetizing" (p. 150) or "originating thinking" (pp. 199-200), having to do with a docile listening to Being.

In authentic poetizing one shows a world not yet shown; then authentic thinking makes the unsaid come to light in the said. It is a great mistake, he thought, to believe that science or technicity (technology) can put the world in order, for technology submits all to the uniformity of production and everything in the world becomes an object of calculation. Humans become encircled and enchained by forces of quantifiable "energy," an extreme version of what Sartre later called the practico-inert. Heidegger argued that meditative thinking must be placed resolutely against calculative thinking. We must use but not be enslaved by technology, something easy to say but in the current era almost impossible to avoid. Meditative thinking of the sort defined by Heidegger never reaches an end; there is never a time when the true thinker no longer has to learn. For Heidegger, the origin of the artist, of his or her creative truth, and of a work of art, are all in the phenomenology of the work of art itself, if we will just take the time and patience to immerse ourselves in it.

Before they rejected the totality of Heidegger's conceptions as mystical gobbledegook, I asked my psychiatric residents to remember Oscar Wilde's (1982) statement that "each form of Art with which we come in contact dominates us for the moment to the exclusion of every other form. We must surrender ourselves absolutely to the work in question, whatever it may be, if we wish to gain its secret. For the time, we must think of nothing else, can think of nothing else, indeed" (p. 392). They were not impressed and I learned not to assign Heidegger to contemporary residents in psychiatry. Unfortunately, as they say, only a fool makes the same mistake twice; I subsequently assigned *The Ambassadors* by Henry James to a group of psychiatry residents, giving them all summer to read it. The intent was to utilize James's masterpiece in an effort to demonstrate the effect of the sociocultural milieu

(New England vs. Paris) on the formation of the self, a current postmodern conception. The result was another revolution. *O tempore, O mores*, as that great teacher Cicero complained!

What Is Art?

One of the biggest problems that face us when we talk about "art" is the contemporary issue of what constitutes art, a philosophical problem that has been tackled, for example, by Danto (1997). He came close to saying that artworks are whatever artists make; as for critical standards, he urged people to look as much as possible and to judge for themselves. In our era, he argued, there is no standard about how a work of art should look, nor does it have to have any political or social message. I agree with the opposing view to this, as represented for example by Wolheim (1993), who claimed that art is not just anything at all. Art embodies values—Beauty, Reality, Truth, all phenomenologically directly given to us by that unique vehicle of aesthetic communication; otherwise art would be pointless. . .and it is not. Artistic and creative endeavors are found in all cultures and all eras, evidence for the universal need of humans even in the gutter to try to make contact with the stars. Consider, for example, the anguish of Joan Miró, who evolved "from an artist closely attached to peasant origins, seeking to represent nature with an almost pedestrian realism, to a seer whose aim is a transcendental escape" (Penrose, 1992, p. 198). This evolution parallels that of another significant contemporary artist of his, Piet Mondrian, and alongside of it Miró suffered from chronic depression that he had to balance against his creative drive. Like Hegel, "Miró shows us at every turn that it is not the sublime that leads to the transcendental; the reality of material things can provide the starting-point for our voyage of escape—a voyage which is essentially creative and valid as an experience, because it is spiritually and materially the ultimate symbol of life" (Penrose, 1992, p. 198). Musical composition, poetry, and art even emerged out of the living hell of Auschwitz or the Warsaw ghetto.

All his life Marcel Duchamp struggled with the question of what constitutes art (Tomkins, 1996). He felt one must approach art with an aesthetic emotion, one must experience the aesthetic echoes if one can, and not just utilize words or understanding. Like Heidegger, he argued that the work of art is independent of the artist and has a life of itself, defining the artist as the way a picture gets itself painted. So for Duchamp, art becomes an opening toward transcendent regions, outside space and time. There is an aesthetic osmosis from the artist to the audience, and the audience must complete the process of the creation of the artwork. So, over the proscenium of the famous Goodman Theatre in Chicago there is written, "You yourself must inflame the faggots you have brought."

Controversy continues regarding the role of museums and the reproduction of art in our contemporary era, as I have pointed out in previous chapters. In Chicago and other United States cities, and also as I have experienced it in France and Japan, art museums stage "blockbuster exhibits" with much advertising and featuring a famous artist and a very expensive catalog for sale along with innumerable trinkets and souvenirs. These draw huge crowds. The paintings can barely be seen and most of the viewing is of the back of the heads of people in front of the viewer, pushing and shoving. These exhibits generate enormous publicity and much revenue for the museum.

I have already mentioned Benjamin's (1968) complaint, "Even the most perfect reproduction of a work of art is lacking in one element; its presence in time and space, its unique existence at the place where it happens to be" (p. 220). What is eliminated in the age of mechanical reproduction is the aura of the work of art, for the technique of reproduction, he said, detaches the reproduced object from the domain of tradition. Making many reproductions substitutes a plurality of copies for a unique existence. Benjamin further complained that permitting the reproduction to meet the beholder or listener in his or her own particular situation reactivates the object reproduced, leading to a tremendous shattering of tradition, a process unfortunately intimately connected with contemporary mass movements. Benjamin insisted,

> The uniqueness of a work of art is inseparable from its being
> imbedded in the fabric of tradition. This tradition itself is

thoroughly alive and extremely changeable. An ancient statue of Venus, for example, stood in a different traditional context with the Greeks, who made it an object of veneration, than with the clerics of the Middle Ages, who viewed it as an ominous idol. Both of them, however, were equally confronted with its uniqueness, that is, its aura. (p. 223).

Detaching the work of art from the domain of its tradition results in the withering of the aura of the artwork. The Art Institute of Chicago had on temporary display the magnificent little fifteenth-century Van Eyck painting *The Annunciation*, which they massively advertised as "The Meeting of Heaven and Earth." I made a special trip through all the usual summer highway construction from Evanston to the Chicago Loop just to see this one painting. When I arrived I found it in a small hall, hanging at about chest height. A huge mob of people filled the hall and a little man stood before it, giving a lecture on the theological details in the painting. The lecture was not mentioned in the advertisement and could easily have been given using slides in the auditorium. One could not get anywhere near the painting; only a glimpse of it was available through the space between the backs of many people's heads. Yet in the brilliant colors and composition even at a distance one could sense the aura which must have existed in this painting at one time, the transcendent Truth expressed through its creator. It was like catching fleeting glimpses of the sunset through the trees, just as Heidegger said of Truth, both revealing and concealing itself. But it was as though the Chicago museum, by a series of blunders and mercenary greed, had done all it could to eliminate the aura of the work of art and convert it into a "thing,' a vehicle for drawing a crowd.

Grotjahn (1957) attempted to distinguish between art and entertainment. Art is a rebellion against the dominance of repression and keeps us to the task of working through our unconscious conflicts. Art lifts repression temporarily and makes us healthier and stronger, whereas entertainment is the submission to a life of shallow contentment. Entertainment reassures and substitutes, thereby avoiding anxiety and working through, and it is automatic and stereotyped. For Steiner (1995), experiencing the variety of meanings in a work of art helps to make us tolerant and mentally lithe. Art is a realm of thought experiments that quicken, sharpen, and sweeten our being-in-the-world. Art is inherently paradoxical in its meaning, always open to various interpretations. Although these interpretations are socially and historically grounded, they are personal. Steiner called for more tolerance of contemporary art and claimed, as did Hegel, that art shows us what we respond to and what we are. For Steiner, if something is in an art museum and labeled as art, it is art.

Mahler believed that what moves us in a work of art is precisely its mysterious and unfathomable elements. Feeling incapable of explaining his musical intention in words, "He was nevertheless conscious of expressing in his music, powerful truths which reached far beyond the realm of art" (LaGrange, 1995, p. 522). Mahler believed his music expressed his whole self and changed continuously as his self developed, but that it also went much farther. He said creative artists are the people least able to answer the question of what is creative activity, and insisted he could not even explain his compositions to himself, let alone obtain an explanation for others.

Although some thinkers are convinced that Truth and Beauty express themselves in art in a unique manner, the famous critic Walter Pater (see Donoghue, 1995), in contrast to the views of Ruskin and Arnold, implied in his work that there were no fixed principles of philosophy or religion and no such concept as Beauty in the abstract. He believed the merit of artistic labor is relief from the pressure of the world and that art contains no moral design or message but simply offers release to a distressed soul, soothing someone with mental illness or temporary emotional chaos. He described art as artistic labor, performing what today we would call an important selfobject function to improve the cohesion of the self. For Pater, when one studies a series of works by an artist a distinctive mode of feeling is revealed, and that is the meaning of the art. His thought resembles Nietzsche's denial of the intellect, arguing that life in the world is justified only by aesthetics.

Pater had a distaste for bourgeois values and exhibited a quiet refusal to live by the rhythms of public life, commerce, and technology. Such individuals also exist today, actualizing Barry's continual yearning for leisure as he defined it, but they rarely can publish books, as they did in the nineteenth century. This is partly because book publishers are becoming increasingly swallowed up by corporate conglomerates that are interdigitated with huge retail book outlets. Working together, these behemoths determine statistically what will sell the most and the fastest, and eliminate the production of anything that will not bring the largest possible profits. This represents an acute exacerbation of the same publishing situation that Pound confronted in Europe (see Chapter 10) and fought so hard against. Another reason is the continually diminishing audience of individuals with the prerequisites for (e.g., ability or training to read carefully) and willingness to take the time for and pay serious attention to the arts. Similarly, the demise of classical music, as manifest in both the diminishing size of concert audiences, falling sales of classical recordings, and the stubborn resistance to serious contemporary compositions, has reached a point of crisis at this time, another example of uninformed turning away from what the arts have to offer in our spiritually devoid era.

Although Pater stressed the power of art to deepen our consciousness of life, and Tolstoy (along with Marxists) claimed that the value of art lies in its social use for us and not revelation of Beauty or Truth, Matthew Arnold argued that poetry is the most perfect speech of humans and the nearest to Truth. Edgar Allen Poe insisted that Beauty is different from Truth, and that poetry is the rhythmical creation of Beauty. We are faced with many conflicting points of view from many brilliant critics and artists.

For Santayana, as Pound discovered to his dismay (see Chapter 12), the joy of life is in contemplation rather than in overt activity, and Beauty is more important than Truth (Arnett, 1955). Aesthetic value, he said, is the criterion that really determines the choice of one's philosophy, and for him only an inner harmony makes life worth living, primarily an attitude toward life developed by philosophy. In his twenties he already informed William James that he had no interest in philosophy that sets out to solve problems. For him philosophy was the same as art; both "attempt to express a half discovered reality" (Epstein, 1987) and they add to each other's values. Santayana (1896) seemed to think that the misery of humans cannot be alleviated so we might as well contemplate the imaginary rather than take social action. Obviously, he did not recognize the consequences that would follow if everyone heeded such advice, and the importance of unconscious forces in determining personal choices.

In a kind of muddled philosophy that is totally out of fashion these days, Santayana (1955) claimed that without animal faith we cannot find evidence of any existence of Reality purely through the use of intuition. The discovery of "essence" is the discovery of the quality of something which it inherently, logically and inalienably is, and for Santayana "essences" are as close as we can get to Reality. Santayana did not believe that the recognition of "essences" in the data of experience as existing in the world of matter can be accomplished in a mystical way; it is more a matter of animal faith. He argued that all the insecurity of knowledge is irrelevant to the inherent and determined effort of the mind to describe natural things. Animal faith posits existence where existence is: "the existence of things is assumed by animals in action and expectation before intuition supplies any description of what the thing is that confronts them in a certain quarter" (Santayana, 1955, p. 133). Belief in matter (substance), he said, is the most irrational, animal, and primitive of beliefs. "It is the voice of hunger" (p. 191).

Carrying this hopeless antifoundationalism to an extreme, *The Myth of Sisyphus* (Camus, 1955) began with the famous lucid invitation to live and to create in the very midst of a desert, and posed the idea that there is only one crucial philosophical problem, whether or not to commit suicide. Camus of course concentrated on the absurdity of the human condition; he was very pessimistic and negative, claiming that a dull resonance vibrates throughout these days and that today's thoughtless human cannot enter into art, as he or she must hasten off to chase some ambitious, materialistic, or sexual hope. Only the absurd human can enter art today, wrote Camus. He agreed with Nietzsche that humans and the universe are absurd since every arrogant rationalism must founder on irrational premises; for Camus there is art and nothing but art to save us from withering under the cold gaze of nihilistic truth.

Emotional Illness and Creativity

We are left with many mysteries. A variety of great and not so great artists have suffered from mental illness (but not all of them). For example, Paddy Chayefsky, probably one of the best writers describing the contemporary American scene in the middle of the twentieth century and a powerful creative force in television and the movies (author of *Marty*, one of the first classic works written for television), devolved from hopeful optimism in the 1950s to a depressed skeptical view of contemporary life. He was never able to understand himself in spite of a great deal of desultory psychotherapy, and he suffered from chronic depression. His son described him as being absolutely gloomy a lot of the time, miserable and dispirited from morning to night with an underlying dysthymic disorder. His life was characterized by an unrelenting chronic rage that he sublimated into his work with great skill (Considine, 1994).

This is not an uncommon story. The capacity for sublimation seems to be a critical issue in understanding the relationship between mental illness and creativity. If an artist can wall off his or her psychopathology (see Chapter 15), and somehow sublimate or transform his or her emotional conflicts and personal passions into creative work, these conflicts and passions can serve as a motor that drives the work forward, along with the selfobject function of the artwork or of the creative process itself. When coupled with talent, what emerges is a genuine work of art that speaks directly to the audience, is capable of many interpretations because it is multiply determined, and withstands subsequent generations of critics and variegated critical approaches. When this capacity for sublimation is not present, the mental illness of the artist encloses his or her talent in a sort of straightjacket, restricting the creativity and, in the worst cases, disrupting it with obsessions and delusions. From a psychoanalytic point of view it is usually not very difficult to recognize when such disruption has taken place, as in the instance of Ezra Pound.

A careful study of the complete artworks of the artist usually reveals areas of constriction due to emotional difficulties. Within the areas that are not constricted, however, the artist may produce reputable work. For example, the poetry of Emily Dickinson, a reclusive, self-effacing woman who wrote many of her poems on little scraps of waste paper, still has a lasting and universal appeal. I must conclude that mental illness per se does not prevent the production of good art; it simply may constrict or disrupt it even to the point where, as in *The Cantos* of Ezra Pound, the whole work becomes a botched failure with spots of beauty in it. It follows that the removal of mental illness in such cases would enormously enhance the creative product of the artist, allowing his or her talent to expand and flourish.

The question of whether Reality, Truth, and Beauty shine forth and are presented in art is one of the central issues of the great human conversation from the time of Plato to the present. It is probably unanswerable because there are not enough ciphers, or individuals who can experience these ciphers, or appearances of ciphers to groups so they may be experienced in a consensual fashion, to produce agreement on the topic. My view is that the phenomenology of natural beauty, artistic experiences, and intense love are the most reliable ciphers indicating that human life has transcendent meaning and is connected to something outside of ourselves. What constitutes that meaning and that Being outside of ourselves is a matter each person in their unique curve of life must determine for himself or herself. The ciphers only give us a chance to produce or choose what mythology appeals directly to us; the arts create the alternatives or communicate the possibilities that speak through the artist, many of which cannot be articulated or expressed any other way.

Hermeneutics

Hermeneutics goes beyond the limits that traditional scientific method sets. But science is only one mode of experience, one way to organize the phenomena. Other modes, for example, are philosophy, art, and history; the arts and the so-called human sciences go beyond the range of scientific method. Philosophy today differs from classical philosophy and is not a continuation of it because historical consciousness has emerged, at least from the time of Hegel, leading to new understanding of old philosophical issues that were not solvable by science. Art presents humans with themselves and at times directly expresses moral ideas; I have already mentioned as examples the poetry of Adrienne Rich and the writings of Paddy Chayefsky. Even indirectly, as a consequence of its cipher function, art can affect one's morality and behavior. A famous recent example of this is Rilke's (1984b) demand that contemplating the "archaic torso of Apollo" (p. 61) should change a person's life. Barnes (1997), the well-known translator of Sartre's *Being and Nothingness*, reported how her first reading of Plato's magnificent *Symposium* in a beautiful natural setting had a dramatic effect on her entire life outlook, an unforgettable experience I also derived from my first introduction to Plato's inimitable poetic dialogues (as I am sure many others have had also over the centuries):

> On a warm spring day, I carried the book to a secluded grassy spot on the edge of campus. Lying on my stomach, in the sun, flowers and birds pouring their scent and song into the air around me, in this idyllic setting I perused what must surely be the most poetic of all philosophical works. I could scarcely credit what I was reading. So this, too, was philosophy—this drama, half comic, half tragic, wholly poetic, with its psychologically penetrating insight into love's universal yearning. The fusion of emotion and intellect overwhelmed me. Diotima's description of the ascent from the first impulses of erotic love for another's bodily beauty to the vision of eternal and absolute beauty and truth commanded all the powers of my imagination. I was dazzled, half-blinded. (p. 93)

The self-encounter of humans as embedded in nature and in the human historical world is presented in art; literature is where art and science merge, and hermeneutics as an approach to it involves a coming into being of meaning. Art does not entirely lose its meaning when it is removed from its original location, for works of art reveal essences if one has the time and determination to immerse one's self in them. My favorite example is Dante's *Divine Comedy*. Given the proper complete focus and total attention, this poem from the beginning of the fourteenth century, seven hundred years ago, speaks out to us as a contemporary, expressing more and more as we study and restudy it. No wonder it fascinated and preoccupied Ezra Pound and T. S. Eliot! It is true that the cipher evidence of art is too weak in the sense that the artwork withholds the very truth that it embodies and prevents it from becoming conceptually precise. But we must remember that the tranquil distance from art engendered by the usual middle-class education "does not take into account *how much of ourselves* must come into play and is at stake when we encounter works of art and studies of history" (Gadamer, 1997, p. 27).

I never realized how much I have been influenced by the work of Gadamer (1991), whose picture along with Proust's hangs on the wall of my consulting room under that of Freud, until I wrote this book (see also Chessick, 1992b, for a report of my brief discussion with him). For Gadamer, dialectic is the art of having a conversation, including having a conversation with one's self, seriously questioning what one really means. He thinks there is a natural disposition of humans toward philosophy, and that our thinking is intrinsically never satisfied. He echoed Heidegger's teaching that truth is an unconcealing and a concealing at the same time: "The concepts in which thinking is formulated stand silhouetted like dark shadows on a wall. They work in a one-sided way, predetermining and prejudging" (Gadamer, 1997, pp. 35–36).

Heidegger interpreted the work of art as the primordial showing forth of Truth, even though, as I have explained, for Hegel art was dialectically destined to be inevitably supplanted by higher forms. But Gadamer objected to the rigid fixing of hierarchies and terminology in philosophical thought, although it is sometimes appropriate in the realm of modern science. He claimed one never completely understands an artwork; there is no final interpretation and, "This is what moves us to tarry with a work of art, of whatever kind it may be. To be tarrying (*Verweilen*) is clearly the distinguishing mark of the experience of art. An artwork is never exhausted. It never becomes empty . . . No work of art addresses us always in the same way. The result is that we must answer differently each time we encounter it" (Gadamer, 1997, p. 44).

The concept of aesthetic consciousness makes art very subjective and is associated with the work of Kant and Schiller, who maintained that the significance of the work of art for the human subject is entirely an inner or subjective experience. Schiller hoped to restore harmony into a civilization that he claimed had separated emotion from intellect and was cut off from nature by the advance of technology through what he labeled the aesthetic education of mankind. In this process the prolonged comparing and contrasting of works of art adds immeasurably to our understanding of our position in human history and where we are headed, and re-injects a sensuous immediacy into humans living in the age of science.

Schiller presupposed a basically harmonious human nature; the encounter with art for Schiller is an empirical stimulant to the awakening of categories of aestheticism, making art an inner experience that creates a certain kind of consciousness. Gadamer correctly attacked this, claiming that the experience of art is neither subjective nor objective but rather a dialectical interchange between the object of art and the subjective viewer. What transpires is a fusion of horizons that changes both the work of art and the viewer. I (Chessick, 1992a) believe this creative fusion of horizons occurs also in psychoanalysis, changing both the patient and the analyst. It follows there is no such thing as a "correct" interpretation of a work of art, nor is there a completely free subjectivity. The viewer completes the work of art by his or her interpretation, but at the same time the work of art completes the subject by helping to realize or actualize his or her potential.

There is Truth appropriate to the humanities that is not of the same order as the Truth appropriate to the natural sciences. I have in Chapter 13 discussed both how Schiller articulated this in his essay on aesthetic education, and how Hegel in *The Phenomenology of Spirit* brought it to the level of philosophy. These thinkers insisted it was not correct to say that beyond the natural sciences exists only irrationality, undecidabilty, and mysticism characterizing the humanities. The correlate and justification for "tarrying" in Gadamer's context in front of a work of art is the permanence of the artwork. Gadamer makes tarrying a distinguishing mark of the experience of art (analogous to Benjamin's [1968; see Chapter 14 in the present book] *flâneur* who wanders aimlessly through the hurrying crowds of a metropolis), and this phenomenologic approach to art also applies to religious experiences, indigenous folk festivals, and myths.

Perhaps it also ought to be appropriate to philosophy. I think so. Heidegger explained that each great philosopher in his or her complete works expresses one central vision of Being. It was this insight that enabled Heidegger to be a great teacher of philosophy and make the neglected ancient texts come alive to offer us an event of contemporary importance. To experience this central vision of a great philosopher, or of philosophical psychiatrists like Freud or Jaspers, or of artists like Shakespeare and many others, we have to tarry over their complete works. This takes proper preparation, much time, and serious dedication to the task. But the result is well worth it, serving a cipher function as their various central visions of Being or Reality or Spirit finally shine forth. As is true of the artist and the artwork, this central vision seems to have a life of its own, and the writer or artist may be only subliminally aware of it, if at all. In this sense it uses the creative product and the creator to express itself, just as Hegel's "cunning of reason" used human history to reach expression of Absolute Spirit. Is all this just our imagination or is it a variety of opportunities given to us, who are inevitably immersed in being-towards-death, to experience phenomenologically the Being of beings, to stand in awe before φύσις, as did, according to Heidegger, the pre-Socratic Greek philosophers . . . or perhaps as Moses did before the burning bush?

What we do not have and probably never will have is a consensually agreed-upon definition of Truth. If one understands the artistic writing produced by the genius of Nietzsche, one realizes this is not so important as was once believed. The truth of an artwork cannot be differentiated from the work itself; it is experienced directly, and such a truth is not what we encounter in a technical philosophical or scientific theory. Truth expressed in art ties Truth directly to Being, akin to the Aristotelian bond of Truth with Being in *Metaphysics*, Book Theta, Section 10. Hermeneutics disavows the foundationalism of traditional philosophy but maintains that an overcoming of metaphysics does not necessarily entail the end of philosophy, nor does it require us to retreat to a position of localism. There is still the possibility for universal validity even though every author is positioned in the midst of a culture and tradition, and so is every interpreter of a work of philosophy or a work of art. A great work of art always communicates at many levels and conveys more than the artist intends. As Plato said in the *Phaedrus*, words, once written, drift all over the place.

Heidegger's (1971a) essay on the origin of a work of art began as a single lecture in 1935 and expanded to a group of three lectures in 1936. They produced a similar effect to the explosion in philosophy when Heidegger's *Being and Time* (1962) appeared, a philosophical sensation. Heidegger was attempting to bring the truth of art onto a par with the truth of science; earlier aesthetic theories did not do this. For example, Kantian aesthetics makes aesthetic judgments purely subjective, and although Hegel took both art and nature to be objectifications of Absolute Spirit, it was at the expense of the truth of art being treated as an inferior expression of philosophical truth. The neo-Kantians also diminished the status of art because art had to be literally viewed or experienced for its truth to be identified, and any aesthetic qualities attributed to it were considered purely subjective. This was an attempt to apply the scientific method to understanding art.

For Heidegger, the truth of a work of art comes directly from the work of art itself, and I believe this to be correct. This means it is also accurate to say that the Being of the work we experience when we encounter a work of art does not solely depend on our experiencing of it. Heidegger claimed that the work of art opens up not only its own Being, but the Being of a new world. It does not simply appear as a thing within our local world or an object hanging in a museum to be contemplated for its beauty. This certainly is a re-presentation of what Jaspers (1932c) meant by a cipher. Gadamer added that the truth *of* the work of art is the truth that *is* the work of art itself. In addition, following Heidegger, the work of art always holds something back in reserve, so there is always a surprise in the effect of a work of art no matter how many times one goes back to a great masterpiece.

There may even be the experience of a shock; as an example, coming suddenly and unexpectedly upon Renoir's magnificent 1881 painting, "The Luncheon of the Boating Party," hanging on a wall by itself, in the Phillips collection in Washington, D.C., had an extremely direct, indescribable intense effect on me that I will never forget. The same is true for one's first encounter with the Elgin Marbles or the Pergamum temple, and so on. Gadamer adds that an artwork is a challenge and carries a demand that is ethical, because the increase in Being that the work of art represents disturbs the feeling of compatibility that one generally has with life itself and exposes one to questions like *"What is there in life that is truly valuable?" "Where am I headed?" "What is it that I ought to be doing?"* (Michelfelder, 1997, p. 447). Forced to deal with questions like this, we are presented with the problem of self-interpretation, and this is the activity involved in recognizing the meaning of a work of art, an activity that is fundamentally different from getting a clear picture of what was originally intended by the artist. Thus, great art speaks to us at a very personal level. As an example, Gadamer recommended Cubist paintings, where a contribution is absolutely required on the part of the observer in order to bring the work together into a whole. But even traditional portraits, if they are great works, need to be "filled out" by the observer. In this manner, Gadamer found a way of unifying the art of our times and the art of the past.

One needs to move into the world of the work of art rather than the other way around, and this takes time, tarrying, being a *flâneur*. As Barry recognized, tarrying creates a break with the continuity of daily everyday temporal events and draws one into another aspect of time that forms as a result of one's interaction with the artwork, requiring one to spend considerable effort on and time with a given masterpiece. Gadamer, in a view that I have also advocated in the present book, is against Hegel's judgment that art is a thing of the past and irrelevant to our own times because its truth is better represented by philosophy. Even Heidegger tried to combat Hegel's view by insisting that art sets up a new beginning for history and therefore cannot be thought of as solely a thing of the past (for more details, see Gadamer, 1987).

Conclusion

Mental illness, unless it can be effectively dissociated or walled off, complicates and obscures the Truth that attempts to communicate itself through a work of art. First, it interferes with and constricts the creative process of the artist in many ways, sometimes even causing the artist to destroy his or her own work entirely. Second, because of the defective aspects of the artwork mental illness engenders, it discourages us from tarrying before the work and interferes with our focus and capacity to directly experience the aesthetic phenomena expressed to us through the artist.

It is a great amateur mistake to think that psychopathology is necessary for and always a motivation for the production of great art. Creativity requires a relatively intact ego; when the individual slides onto the unhealthy side of the ego axis, artistic production deteriorates. Inherent genius along with the capacity for sublimation through artistic creativity is required for the production of great artworks that are not flawed. The driving force to creativity may be thought of as the universal human need to resolve intrapsychic conflicts (which is the driving force of *all* solutions, neurotic or healthy) or the universal human need to provide one's self with enhancing selfobjects as a "glue" to ensure cohesion of the self, or both. The artwork itself may form such a selfobject, or the mirroring appreciation of the audience may perform this function. But in the creation of a great artwork there is something more we experience, the shining forth of Truth, Beauty, and Being in new and unique modes of expression.

In the wonderful Freud-Pfister correspondence (Meng and Freud, 1963), Freud said humans are trash; Pfister insisted one must love mankind or get an ugly distorted picture of the calculating machine man. Freud said there was no synthesis in psychoanalysis; Pfister insisted there was and it led to the will to be moral. Freud demanded pure empiricism; Pfister responded that we differ in philosophy, music, and religion. Freud maintained science solves everything; Pfister said it does not solve problems of human happiness or aspiration. Freud claimed psychoanalysis was self-contained; Pfister said it was a practice within a plan of life that must be in accord with the nature of humans and the world. Freud emphasized the isolation of humans; Pfister insisted the adult needs an inner spirit, religion, and philosophy. Freud maintained that morals were developed due to exigencies; Pfister maintained there is a moral world order outside humans. For Freud religion and God represented merely sublimated infantilism; Pfister insisted this was not entirely so. Freud admitted he was pessimistic, depressed, and less pleasant as a person; Pfister put up with the unfairness of life better and was more pleasant and tolerant. Freud predicted that civilization was going nowhere; Pfister believed, *contra* Spengler, through evolution it is getting better and higher. Freud maintained the mind was insignificant in nature; Pfister thought the development of mind was an extremely significant step. For Freud the ego ideal is just the introjected parents; Pfister agreed the ego ideal begins there but added that the ego ideal has a lot more to it. Freud claimed there was no innate human aspiration; Pfister insisted that humans differ from animals because we aspire to climb higher and over the dead images of our parents, and he suggested Freud was an example of this. Freud argued that his pessimism was a conclusion from the empirical study of reality, not some emotional hangup. But was Freud's willingness to maintain a friendly correspondence of this nature, with a Swiss Protestant clergyman over a 28-year period of time, because in spite of himself he sensed a cipher in what Pfister said and how Pfister conducted himself? . . . Freud perhaps also sensed a cipher when he remarked at the age of eighty, "spring is beautiful and so is love" (Schur, 1972, p. 480). And so the great civilized conversation continues to the present day.

> "What's this? Am I falling? My legs are giving way," thought he, and fell on his back. . . . Above him there was now nothing but the sky—the lofty sky, not clear yet still immeasurably lofty, with gray clouds gliding slowly across it. "How quiet, peaceful, and solemn; not at all as I ran," thought Prince Andrew—"not as we ran shouting and fighting. . .how differently do those clouds glide across that lofty infinite sky! How was it I did not see that lofty sky before? And how happy I am to have found at last! Yes! All is vanity, all falsehood, except that infinite sky."
>
> (Tolstoy, 1868, *War and Peace*, pp. 301-302)

REFERENCES

Achebe, C. (1961), *Things Fall Apart*. New York: Astor-Honor.

Ackroyd, P. (1984), *T. S. Eliot: A Life*. New York: Simon & Schuster.

——— (1987), *Ezra Pound*. New York: Thames & Hudson.

——— (1990), *Dickens*. New York: HarperCollins.

Alberoni, F. (1983), *Falling in Love*. New York: Random House.

Alexander, F. (1951), *Our Age of Unreason*. New York: Lippincott.

——— (1960), *The Western Mind in Transition*. New York: Random House.

Allan, D. (1952), *The Philosophy of Aristotle*. New York: Oxford University Press.

Allison, E., Ed. (1985), *The New Nietzsche: Contemporary Styles of Interpretation*. Cambridge, Mass.: MIT Press.

Altman, L. (1977), Some vicissitudes of love. *J. Amer. Psychoanal. Assn.*, 25:35-52.

Alvarez, A. (1971), *The Savage God*. New York: Bantam Books.

American Psychiatric Association (1994), *Diagnostic and Statistical Manual of Mental Disorders* (4th ed). Washington, D.C.: American Psychiatric Association.

Appleby, J., Hunt, L., & Jacob, M. (1994), *Telling the Truth about History*. New York: Norton.

Arendt, H. (1977), *The Life of the Mind* (Vol. 1). New York: Harcourt Brace Jovanovich.

Aries, P. (1962), *Centuries of Childhood: A Social History of Family Life*, trans. R. Baltic. New York: Vintage.

Arlow, J. (1980), Object concept and object choice. *Psychoanal. Quart.*, 49:109-133.

——— (1985), The concept of psychic reality and related problems. *J. Amer. Psychoanal. Assn.*, 33:521-535.

Arnett, W. (1955), *Santayana and the Sense of Beauty*. Bloomington, Ind.: Indiana University Press.

421

Aronson, M., & Scharfman, M. (1992), *Psychotherapy: The Analytic Approach*. Northvale, N.J.: Aronson.

Ashmore, H. (1989), *Unreasonable Truths: The Life of Robert Maynard Hutchins*. Boston: Little, Brown.

Atlas, J. (1992), *The Battle of the Books: The Curriculum Debate in America*. New York: Norton.

Bair, D. (1978), *Samuel Beckett: A Biography*. New York: Harcourt Brace Jovanovich.

Bak, R. (1973), Being in love and object loss. *Internat. J. Psycho-Anal.*, 54:1-8.

Balint, M. (1953), *Primary Love and Psychoanalytic Technique*. New York: Liveright.

Balzac, H. (1837-1843), *Lost Illusions*, trans. H. Hunt. New York: Penguin, 1976.

Barnes, H. (1981), *Sartre and Flaubert*. Chicago: University of Chicago Press.

——— (1997), *The Story I Tell Myself*. Chicago: University of Chicago Press.

Basch, M. (1980), *Doing Psychotherapy*. New York: Basic Books.

Bataille, G. (1988), *Inner Experience*, trans. L. Boldt. Albany, N.Y.: State University of New York Press.

Baudrillard, J. (1988), *Jean Baudrillard: Selected Writings*, ed. M. Poster. Cambridge. Mass.: Polity Press.

Becker, G. (1994), Unity and university: The neo-humanist perspective in the age of post-modernism. *Internat. Philo. Quart.*, 34:177-189.

Beckett, S. (1960), *Krapp's Last Tape and Other Dramatic Pieces*. New York: Grove Press.

Beiser, F., Ed. (1993), *The Cambridge Companion to Hegel*. New York: Cambridge University Press.

Bellow, S. (1994), The distracted public. In: *It All Adds Up: From the Dim Past to the Uncertain Future*. New York: Viking, pp. 153-169.

——— (1997), *The Actual: A Novella*. New York: Viking.

Benedek, T. (1977), Ambivalence, passion and love. *J. Amer. Psychoanal. Assn.*, 25:53-80.

Benjamin, W. (1968), *Illuminations*, trans. H. Zohn. New York: Schocken Books.

——— (1994), *The Correspondence of Walter Benjamin*, ed. G. Scholem & T. Adorno. Chicago: University of Chicago Press.

Benner, A. (1931), *Selections From Homer's Illiad*. New York: Appleton-Century-Crofts.

Berger, P., & Luckmann, T. (1967), *The Social Construction of Reality: A Treatise on the Sociology of Knowledge*. Garden City, N.Y.: Doubleday.

Bergmann, M. (1980), On the intrapyschic function of falling in love. *Psychoanal. Quart.*, 49:56-77.

———— (1982), Platonic love, transference love, and love in real life. *J. Amer. Psychoanal. Assn.*, 30:87-112.

———— (1988), Freud's three theories of love in the light of later developments. *J. Amer. Psychoanal. Assn.*, 36:653-672.

Bergson, H. (1950a), *Introduction to Metaphysics*, trans. T. Hulme. New York: Liberal Arts Press.

———— (1950b), *Time and Free Will: An Essay on the Immediate Data of Consciousness*. New York: Macmillan.

Berman, E. (1986), *In Africa with Schweitzer*. Far Hills, N.J.: New Horizon Press.

Berne, E. (1964), *Games People Play: The Psychology of Human Relationships*. New York: Grove Press.

Bettelheim, B. (1950), *Love Is Not Enough*. Glencoe, Ill.: Free Press.

Binswanger, L. (1963), *Being-in-the-World: Selected Papers of Ludwig Binswanger*, trans. J. Needleman. New York: Basic Books.

Bion, W. (1963), *Elements of Psycho-Analysis*. New York: Basic Books.

———— (1967), *Second Thoughts*. New York: Aronson.

Blake, W. (1974a), The book of Ahania. In: *The Portable Blake*, ed. A. Kazin. New York: Penguin Books, pp. 348-356.

———— (1974b), Enion and Tharmas. In: *The Portable Blake*, ed. A. Kazin. New York: Penguin Books, pp. 370-371.

———— (1974c), The song of Los. In: *The Portable Blake*, ed. A. Kazin. New York: Penguin Books, pp. 364-368.

Bloom, A. (1987), *The Closing of the American Mind*. New York: Simon & Schuster.

———— (1993), *Love and Friendship*. New York: Simon & Schuster.

Bloom, H. (1994), *The Western Canon: The Books and Schools of the Ages*. New York: Harcourt Brace.

Blos, P. (1962), *On Adolescence*. New York: Free Press.

Boss, M. (1963), *Psychoanalysis and Daseinanalysis*, trans. L. Lefebre. New York: Basic Books.

Brent, J. (1993), *Charles Sanders Peirce: A Life*. Bloomington, Ind.: Indiana University Press.

Breslin, J. (1993), *Mark Rothko: A Biography*. Chicago: University of Chicago Press.

Brookner, A. (1994), *A Private View.* New York: Random House.

Brook-Rose, C. (1971), *A ZBC of Ezra Pound.* Berkeley, Calif.: University of California Press.

Bruns, G. (1989), *Heidegger's Estrangements: Language, Truth, and Poetry in the Later Writings.* New Haven, Conn.: Yale University Press.

Bryan, D. (1996), *Einstein: A Life.* New York: Wiley.

Bush, M. (1969), Psychoanalysis and scientific creativity: With special reference to regression in the service of the ego. *J. Amer. Psychoanal. Assn.*, 17:136-190.

Callinicos, A. (1990), *Against Postmodernism: A Marxist Critique.* New York: St. Martin's Press.

Camus, A. (1955), *The Myth of Sisyphus.* New York: Knopf.

Carpenter, H. (1988), *A Serious Character: The Life of Ezra Pound.* New York: Houghton Mifflin.

Castoriadis, C. (1989), The "end of philosophy"? *Salmagundi*, 82(3):3-30.

Chasseguet-Smirgel, J. (1970), *Female Sexuality.* Ann Arbor: University of Michigan Press.

———— (1985), *The Ego Ideal: A Psychoanalytic Essay on the Malady of the Ideal,* trans. P. Barrows. London: Free Association Books.

Chessick, R. (1965), Empathy and love in psychotherapy. *Amer. J. Psychother.*, 19:205-219.

———— (1974), *The Technique and Practice of Intensive Psychotherapy.* New York: Aronson.

———— (1977a), *Great Ideas in Psychotherapy.* New York: Aronson.

———— (1977b), *Intensive Psychotherapy of the Borderline Patient.* New York: Aronson.

———— (1980), *Freud Teaches Psychotherapy.* Indianapolis, Ind.: Hackett.

———— (1981), The relevance of Nietzsche to the study of Freud and Kohut. *Amer. J. Psychother.*, 17:359-373.

———— (1982a), Metaphysics or autistic reverie? *Contemp. Psychoanal.*, 18:160-172.

———— (1982b), Psychoanalytic listening: With special reference to the views of Langs. *Contemp. Psychoanal.*, 18:613-634.

———— (1983), *A Brief Introduction to the Genius of Nietzsche.* Washington, D.C.: University Press of America.

———— (1986), Heidegger for psychotherapists. *Amer. J. Psychother.*, 40:83-95.

———— (1987), Lacan's practice of psychoanalytic psychotherapy. *Amer. J. Psychother.*, 42:571-579.

———— (1989), On falling in love II: The two-woman phenomenon revisited. *J. Amer. Acad. Psychoanal.*, 17(2):293-304.

———— (1990), In the clutches of the devil. *Psychoanal. Psychother.*, 7:142-151.

———— (1991), The unbearable obscurity of being. *Amer. J. Psychother.*, 45:576-593.

———— (1992a), *The Technique and Practice of Listening in Intensive Psychotherapy.* Northvale, N.J.: Aronson.

———— (1992b), *What Constitutes the Patient in Psychotherapy?* Northvale, N. J.: Aronson.

———— (1993a), *The Psychology of the Self and the Treatment of Narcissism.* Northvale, N.J.: Aronson.

———— (1993b), *A Dictionary for Psychotherapists: Dynamic Concepts in Psychotherapy.* Northvale, N.J.: Aronson.

———— (1995a), The effect of Heidegger's pathological narcissism on the development of his philosophy. In: *Mimetic Desire: Essays in German Literature from Romanticism to Post Modernism*, ed. J. Adams & E. Williams. Columbia, S.C.: Camden House, 1995.

———— (1995b), Postmodern psychoanalysis or wild psychoanalysis? *J. Amer. Acad. Psychoanal.*, 23:47-62.

———— (1996a), Franz Alexander and the development of psychoanalysis in the United States. In: *Psychoanalysis Today and 70 Years Ago*, ed. H. Weiss & J. Lang. Tubingen, Germany: Edition Discord, pp. 196-211.

———— (1996b), Impasse and failure in psychoanalytic treatment *J. Amer. Acad. Psychoanal.*, 24:193-216.

———— (1996c), Mired in melancholy. *Readings: Amer. Orthopsychiatr. Assn.*, 11:8-13.

———— (1996d), Nothingness, meaninglessness, chaos, and the black hole revisited. *J. Amer. Acad. Psychoanal.*, 23:581-601.

———— (1996e), The application of postmodern thought to the clinical practice of psychoanalytic psychotherapy. *J. Amer. Acad. Psychoanal.*, 24:385-407.

———— (1997a), Malignant erotic countertransference. *J. Amer. Acad. Psychoanal.*, 25:219-236.

———— (1997b), Perspectivism, constructivism, and empathy in psychoanalysis: Nietzsche and Kohut. *J. Amer. Acad. Psychoanal.*, 25:373-398.

———— (1997c), Psychoanalytic treatment of the borderline patient. *J. Amer. Acad. Psychoanal.*, 25:91-109.

———— (1999), The phenomenology of Erwin Straus and the epistemology of Psychoanalysis. *Amer. J. Psychother.*, 53: 82–95.

Clark, K. (1969), *Civilization.* New York: Harper & Row.

Clower, V. (1992), Aging in a mirror. In: *How Psychiatrists Look at Aging,* ed. G. Pollock. Madison, Conn.: International Universities Press, pp. 69-84.

Cohen, M. (1997), Why I'm still left. *Dissent,* 44(2):43-50.

Confucius (1997), *The Analects of Confucius,* trans. S. Leys. New York: Norton.

Considine, S. (1994), *Mad as Hell: The Life and Work of Paddy Chayefsky.* New York: Random House.

Cook, D. (1996), *The Culture Industry Revisited: Theodore W. Adorno on Mass Culture.* Boston: Roman & Littlefield.

Cooper, D. (1983), *Authenticity and Learning: Nietzsche's Educational Philosophy.* London: Routledge & Kegan Paul.

Copleston, F. (1964), *A History of Philosophy:* Vol. 6. Part II. Garden City, N.Y.: Doubleday.

—— (1965), *A History of Philosophy:* Vol. 7. Part I: *Fichte to Hegel.* Garden City, N.Y.: Doubleday.

Cornford, F. (1975), *The Republic of Plato.* New York: Oxford University Press.

Cronin, A. (1997), *Samuel Beckett: The Last Modernist.* New York: Harper-Collins.

Dahlberg, C. (1970), Sexual contact between patient and therapist. *Contemp. Psychoanal.,* 6:107-124.

Dante Alighieri (1980), *The Divine Comedy of Dante Alighieri: Inferno,* trans. A. Mandelbaum. New York: Bantam.

—— (1984), *The Divine Comedy of Dante Alighieri: Purgatorio,* trans. A. Mandelbaum. New York: Bantam.

—— (1986), *The Divine Comedy of Dante Alighieri: Paradiso,* trans. A. Mandelbaum. New York: Bantam.

Danto, A. (1997), *After the End of Art.* Princeton, N.J.: Princeton University Press.

Davies, R. (1988), *The Lyre of Orpheus.* New York: Penguin.

—— (1990), *The Deptford Trilogy.* New York: Penguin.

Davis, M., & Wallbridge, D. (1981), *Boundary and Space.* New York: Brunner/Mazel.

De Botton, A. (1997), *How Proust Can Change Your Life: Not A Novel.* New York: Pantheon.

De Grazia, S. (1962), *Of Time, Work and Leisure.* New York: Twentieth Century Fund.

De Rougemont, D. (1983), *Love in the Western World*. Princeton, N. J.: Princeton University Press.

Derrida, J. (1980), *Of Grammatology*, trans. G. Spivak. Baltimore: Johns Hopkins University Press.

——— (1981), *Dissemination*, trans. B. Johnson. Chicago: University of Chicago Press.

——— (1994), Deconstruction and the other. In: *Contemporary Approaches to Philosophy*, ed. P. Mosaer & D. Mulder. New York: Macmillan, pp. 368-382.

Descombes, V. (1980), *Modern French Philosophy*. New York: Cambridge University Press.

Desmond, W. (1995), Being, determination and dialectic: On the sources of metaphysical thinking. *Rev. Metaphysics*, 48:731-769.

Diggins, J. (1996), *Max Weber: Politics and the Spirit of Tragedy*. New York: Basic Books.

Donald, D. (1987), *Look Homeward: A Life of Thomas Wolf*. Boston: Little, Brown.

Donoghue, D. (1995), *Walter Pater: Lover of Strange Souls*. New York: Knopf.

Doob, L., Ed. (1952), *"Ezra Pound Speaking": Radio Speeches of World War II*. New York: Greenwood Press.

Dostoevsky, F. (1864), *Notes from Underground*, trans. C. Garnett. New York: Dell, 1960.

——— (1872), *The Demons*, trans. R. Pevear & L. Volokhonsky. New York: Knopf, 1994.

Dreiser, T. (1989), *Jennie Gerhardt*. New York: Penguin.

Dreyfus, H., & Rabinow, P. (1982), *Michel Foucault: Beyond Structuralism and Hermeneutics*. Chicago: University of Chicago Press.

Durant, W., & Durant, A. (1968), *The Lessons of History*. New York: Simon & Schuster.

Eagleton, T. (1993), *The Significance of Theory*. Cambridge, Mass.: Blackwell.

Edwards, J., & Vasse, W. (1957), *Annotated Index to the Cantos of Ezra Pound*. Berkeley, Calif.: University of California Press.

Eksteins, M. (1989), *Rites of Spring: The Great War and the Modern Age*. Boston: Houghton Mifflin.

Eliot, V., Ed. (1971), *T. S. Eliot: The Wasteland: A Facsimile and Transcript of the Original Drafts*. New York: Harcourt Brace.

Epstein, J. (1987, June), George Santayana and the consolations of philosophy. *New Criterion*, 5:15-28.

Erenreich, B. (1989), *Fear of Falling: The Inner Life of the Middle Class.* New York: Pantheon.

Erikson, E. (1950), *Childhood and Society.* New York: Norton.

———— (1959), *Identity and the Life Cycle.* New York: International Universities Press.

Erickson, S. (1997), Philosophy in the age of thresholding. *Internat. Philos. Quart.,* 37:263-276.

Ermarth, M. (1978), *Wilhelm Dilthey: The Critique of Historical Reason.* Chicago, Ill.: University of Chicago Press.

Espey, J. (1974), *Ezra Pound's Mauberly.* Berkeley, Calif.: University of California Press.

Fairbairn, W. (1994), *From Instinct to Self: Selected Papers of W. R. D. Fairbairn* (2 vols.), ed. D. Scharff & E. Birtles. Northvale, N.J: Aronson.

Fajardo, B. (1993), Conditions for the relevance of infant research to clinical psychoanalysis. *Internat. J. Psycho-Anal.,* 74:975-991.

Federn, P. (1952), *Ego Psychology and the Psychoses.* New York: Basic Books.

Feibleman, J. (1982), *Conversations: A Kind of Fiction.* New York: Horizon Press.

Fenichel, O. (1945), *The Psychoanalytic Theory of Neurosis.* New York: Norton.

———— (1996), *The Psychoanalytic Theory of Neurosis: 50th Anniversary Edition.* New York: Norton.

Ferenczi, S. (1988), *The Clinical Diary of Sandor Ferenczi,* trans. M. Balint & N. Jackson. Cambridge, Mass.: Harvard University Press.

Fergusson, F. (1966), *Dante.* New York: Macmillan-Collier.

Fitzgerald, R., trans. (1961), *Homer: The Odyssey.* Garden City, N.J.: Anchor.

Flax, J. (1990), *Thinking Fragments: Psychoanalysis, Feminism, and Postmodernism in the Contemporary West.* Berkeley, Calif.: University of California Press.

Fliess, R. (1942), The metapsychology of the analyst. *Psychoanal. Quart.,* 2:211-227.

Flory, W. (1989), *The American Ezra Pound.* New Haven, Conn.: Yale University Press.

Fölsing, A. (1997), *Albert Einstein: A Biography,* trans. E. Osers. New York: Viking.

Foucault, M. (1973a), *Madness and Civilization,* trans. A. Smith. New York: Vintage.

———— (1973b), *The Order of Things.* New York: Viking.

————— (1984), What is an author? In: *The Foucault Reader*, ed. P. Drabinow. New York: Pantheon, pp. 101-120.

Fox, R. (1985), *Reinhold Niebuhr: A Biography*. New York: Pantheon.

Frankl, V. (1967), *Psychotherapy and Existentialism*. New York: Simon & Schuster.

Freedman, R. (1996), *Life of a Poet: Rainer Maria Rilke*. New York: Farrar, Straus & Giroux.

French, T., & Fromm, E. (1964), *Dream Interpretation*. New York: Basic Books.

Freud, E., Ed. (1960), *Letters of Sigmund Freud*. New York: Basic Books.

Freud, S. (1905a), Fragments of an analysis of a case of hysteria. *Standard Edition*, 7:3-124. London: Hogarth Press, 1953.

————— (1905b), Three essays on sexuality. *Standard Edition*, 7:125-243. London: Hogarth Press, 1953.

————— (1912a), On the universal tendency to debasement in the sphere of love. *Standard Edition*, 11:177-190. London: Hogarth Press, 1957.

————— (1912b), Recommendations to physicians practicing psychoanalysis. *Standard Edition*, 12:109-120. London: Hogarth Press, 1958.

————— (1913), On beginning the treatment. *Standard Edition*, 12:121-144. London: Hogarth Press, 1958.

————— (1914a), The Moses of Michelangelo. *Standard Edition*, 14:211-236. London: Hogarth Press, 1957.

————— (1914b), On narcissism: An introduction. *Standard Edition*, 14:67-104. London: Hogarth Press, 1957.

————— (1914c), Remembering, repeating, and working through. *Standard Edition*, 12:145-156. London: Hogarth Press, 1958.

————— (1915a), Instincts and their vicissitudes. *Standard Edition*, 14:109-140. London: Hogarth Press, 1957.

————— (1915b), Observations on transference love. *Standard Edition*, 12:157-171. London: Hogarth Press, 1958.

————— (1916), On transience. *Standard Edition*, 14:305-307. London: Hogarth Press, 1957.

————— (1917), Mourning and melancholia. *Standard Edition*, 14:239-258. London: Hogarth Press, 1957.

————— (1921), Group psychology and the analysis of the ego. *Standard Edition*, 18:67-144. London: Hogarth Press, 1955.

————— (1924), An autobiographical study. *Standard Edition*, 20:7-74. London: Hogarth Press, 1959.

———— (1927a), The future of an illusion. *Standard Edition*, 21:5-58. London: Hogarth Press, 1961.

———— (1927b), Letter to Werner Achelis (1927). In: *Letters of Sigmund Freud*, ed. E. Freud. New York: Basic Books, pp. 374-375.

———— (1928), Dostoevsky and parricide. *Standard Edition*, 21:177-194. London: Hogarth Press, 1961.

———— (1930a), Civilization and Its Discontents. *Standard Edition*, 21:64-148. London: Hogarth Press, 1961.

———— (1930b), The Goethe prize. *Standard Edition*, 21:206-212. London: Hogarth Press, 1961.

———— (1931), Female sexuality. *Standard Edition*, 21:225-246. London: Hogarth Press, 1961.

———— (1940), An outline of psychoanalysis. *Standard Edition*, 23:144-173. London: Hogarth Press, 1964.

Fromm, E. (1941), *Escape from Freedom*. New York: Rinehart.

———— (1955), *The Sane Society*. New York: Rinehart.

———— (1962), *Beyond the Chains of Illusion: My Encounter with Marx and Freud*. New York: Simon & Schuster.

Fromm-Reichmann, F. (1950), *Principles of Intensive Psychotherapy*. Chicago: University of Chicago Press.

Froula, C. (1983), *A Guide to Ezra Pound's Selected Poems*. New York: New Directions.

Fukuyama, F. (1992), *The End of History and the Last Man*. New York: Free Press.

Gabbard, G. (1982), The exit line: Heightened transference-counter-transference manifestations at the end of the hour. *J. Amer. Psychoanal. Assn.*, 30:579-598.

———— Ed. (1989), *Sexual Exploitation in Professional Relationships*. Washington, D.C.: American Psychiatric Press.

———— (1994), Psychotherapists who transgress sexual boundaries with patients. *Bull. Menn. Clin.*, 58:124-135.

———— Lester, E. (1996), *Boundaries and Boundary Violations in Psychoanalysis*. New York: Basic Books.

Gadamer, H. (1985), *Philosophical Apprenticeship*. Cambridge, Mass.: MIT Press.

———— (1987), *The Relevance of the Beautiful and Other Essays*, trans. N. Walker. Cambridge: Cambridge University Press.

———— (1991), *Truth and Method* (2nd ed.), translation revised J. Weinsheimer & D. Marshall. New York: Crossroad.

—— (1997), Reflections on my philosophical journey. In: *The Philosophy of Hans-Georg Gadamer*, ed. L. Hahn. Chicago: Open Court, pp. 3-63.

Galatzer-Levy, R., & Cohler, B. (1993), *The Essential Other: A Developmental Psychology of the Self.* New York: Basic Books.

Galbraith, J. (1958), *The Affluent Society* . New York: Mentor.

García Márquez, G. (1988), *Love in the Time of Cholera.* New York: Knopf.

Gay, P. (1988), *Freud: A Life for Our Time.* New York: Norton.

Gaylin, W., & Person, E. (1988), *Passionate Attachments: Thinking about Love.* New York: Free Press.

Gediman, H. (1975), Reflections on romanticism, narcissism, and creativity. *J. Amer. Psychoanal. Assn.*, 23:407-423.

—— (1981), On love, dying together, and libestod fantasies. *J. Amer. Psychoanal. Assn.*, 29:607-630.

Gedo, J. (1977), Notes on the psychoanalytic management of archaic transferences. *J. Amer. Psychoanal. Assn.*, 25:787-803.

—— (1979), *Beyond Interpretation.* New York: International Universities Press.

—— (1983), *Portraits of the Artist.* New York: Guilford Press.

—— (1984), *Psychoanalysis and Its Discontents.* New York: Guilford Press.

—— (1988), *The Mind in Disorder: Psychoanalytic Models of Pathology.* Hillsdale, N.J.: Analytic Press.

—— (1991), *The Biology of Clinical Encounters: Psychoanalysis as a Science of Mind.* Hillsdale, N.J.: Analytic Press.

—— (1996a), Creativity: The burdens of talents. *Annual Psychoanal.*, 24: 103-112.

—— (1996b), *The Artist and the Emotional World.* New York: Columbia University Press.

—— & Gehrie, M., Eds. (1993), *Impasse and Innovation in psychoanalysis: Clinical Case Seminars.* Hillsdale, N.J.: Analytic Press.

—— & Goldberg, A. (1973), *Models of the Mind: A Psychoanalytic Theory.* Chicago: University of Chicago Presss.

George, M. (1986), *The Autobiography of Henry VIII.* New York: St. Martin's Press.

Ghiselin, E., Ed. (1952), *The Creative Process.* New York: Mentor.

Gill, M. (1982), *Analysis of the Transfererence: Vol. 1. Theory and Technique.* New York: International Universities Press.

Ginsberg, M. (1973), Nietzschian psychiatry. In: *Nietzsche: A Collection of Critical Essays*, ed. R. Solomon. Garden City, N.Y.: Anchor, pp. 293-315.

Giovacchini, P. (1968), Characterological faculties and the creative personality. *J. Amer. Psychoanal. Assn.*, 19:524-542.

Goethe, J. (1774), *The Sufferings of Young Werther*, trans. B. Morgan. New York: Ungar, 1954.

Goldberg, A. (1983), On the scientific status of empathy. *Annual Psychoanal.*, 11:155-159.

———— (1995), *The Problem of Perversion: The View from Self Psychology.* New Haven, Conn: Yale University Press.

Goldstein, R. (1989), *The Late-Summer Passion of a Woman of Mind.* New York: Anchor.

Golomb, J. (1989), *Nietzsche's Enticing Psychology of Power.* Ames, Iowa: Iowa State University Press.

———— (1995), *In Search of Authenticity: From Kierkegaard to Camus.* London: Routledge.

Gramsci, A. (1985), *Selections from the Prison Notebooks of Antonio Gramsci,* trans. Q. Hore & G. Smith. New York: International Publishers.

Gray, W. (1985), *Homer to Joyce.* New York: Macmillan.

Greenacre, P. (1953), *Affective Disorders.* New York: International Universities Press.

Greenberg, J., & Mitchell, S. (1983), *Object Relations in Psychoanalytic Theory.* Cambridge, Mass.: Harvard University Press.

Greene, G. (1956), *The Last Angry Man.* New York: Scribner.

Greenson, R. (1992), *On Loving, Hating and Living Well: The Public Psychoanalytic Lectures of Ralph R. Greenson, M.D.,* ed. R. Neminoff, A. Sugarman, & A. Robbins. Madison, Conn.: International Universities Press.

Grene, D., & Lattimore, R. (1959), *The Complete Greek Tragedies: Vol. II. Sophocles.* Chicago: University of Chicago Press.

Groddeck, G. (1923), *The Book of the It.* New York: Mentor Books, 1961.

Grotjahn, M. (1957), *Beyond Laughter.* New York: McGraw-Hill.

Gunther, M. (1976), The endangered self: A contribution to the understanding of narcissistic determinants of countertransference. *Annual Psychoanal.*, 4:201-224.

Gutheil, T. (1989), Borderline personality disorder, boundary violations and patient-therapist sex: Medical legal pitfalls. *Amer. J. Psychiatry,* 146:597-602.

Habermas, J. (1971), *Knowledge and Human Interest.* Boston: Beacon Press.

———— (1973), *Theory and Practice.* Boston: Beacon Press.

———— (1975), *Legitimation Crisis.* Boston: Beacon Press.

Hamilton, E., & Cairns, H., Eds. (1973), *The Collected Dialogues of Plato: Including the Letters.* Princeton, N.J.: Princeton University Press.

Hanly, C. (1986), Psychoanalytic aesthetics: A defense and an elaboration. *Psychoanal. Quart.*, 55:1-22.

Hardy, T. (1897), *The Well-Beloved.* London: Macmillan, 1985.

Harrington, M. (1989), *Socialism: Past and Future.* New York: Little, Brown.

Harris, H. (1995), *Hegel: Phenomenology and System.* Indianapolis, Ind.: Hackett.

Harrison, I. (1979), On Freud's view of the infant-mother relationship and of the oceanic feeling—some subjective influences. *J. Amer. Psychoanal. Assn.*, 27:399-422.

Harrison, J. (1967), *The Reactionaries: A Study of the Anti-Democratic Intelligentsia.* New York: Schocken Books.

Hartmann, H. (1927), Understanding and explanation. In: *Essays on Ego Psychology.* New York: International Universities Press.

——— (1958), *Ego Psychology and the Problem of Adaptation,* trans. D. Rapaport. New York: International Universities Press.

Hatttingberg, M., Ed. (1987), *Rilke and Benvenuta: An Intimate Correspondence.* New York: Fromm International Publishing.

Hawking, S. (1993), *Black Holes and Baby Universes and Other Essays.* New York: Bantam Books.

Hayman, R. (1980), *Nietzsche: A Critical Life.* New York: Oxford University Press.

——— (1990), *Proust: A Biography.* New York: HarperCollins.

Hegel, G. (1807), *Phenomenology of Spirit,* trans. A. Miller. Oxford, England: Clarendon Press.

——— (1821), *Hegel's Philosophy of Right,* trans. T. Knox. New York: Oxford University Press, 1976.

——— (1833), Lectures on the history of philosophy. In: *Hegel's Introduction to the Lectures on the History of Philosophy,* trans. T. Knox & A. Miller. Oxford: Clarendon Press, 1985.

——— (1905), Lectures on aesthetics. In: *G. W. F. Hegel on Art, Religion, Philosophy,* ed. J. Gray. New York: Harper & Row, 1970, pp. 22-127.

Heidegger, M. (1954), *What Is Called Thinking?* trans. F. Wieck & J. Gray. New York: Harper & Row, 1968.

——— (1961), The fundamental question of metaphysics. In: *An Introduction to Metaphysics,* trans. R. Manheim. Garden City, N.Y.: Anchor Books, pp. 1-42.

—— (1962), *Being and Time,* trans. J. Macquarrie & E. Robinson. New York: Harper & Row.

—— (1971a), The origin of the work of art. In: *Poetry, Language, Thought,* trans. A. Hofstadter. New York: Harper & Row, pp. 1-88.

—— (1971b), The thing. In: *Poetry, Language, Thought,* trans. A. Hofstadter. New York: Harper & Row, pp. 163-186.

—— (1977), *The Question Concerning Technology and Other Essays.* New York: Harper & Row.

—— (1979), *Nietzsche: Vol. 1: The Will to Power as Art,* trans. D. Krell. New York: Harper & Row.

—— (1982), *Nietzsche: Vol. 4: Nihilism,* trans. F. Capuzzi & D. Krell. San Francisco: Harper & Row.

—— (1984), *Nietzsche: Vol. 2: The Eternal Recurrence of the Same,* trans. D. Krell. New York: Harper & Row.

—— (1987), *Nietzsche: Vol. 3: The Will to Power as Knowledge and as Metaphysics,* trans. J. Stambaugh, D. Krell, & F. Capuzzi. San Francisco: Harper & Row.

—— (1993), *Basic Concepts.* Indianapolis, Ind.: Indiana University Press.

—— (1994), *Basic Questions of Philosophy: Selected "Problems" of "Logic,"* trans. R. Rojcewicz & A. Schuwer. Bloomington, Ind.: Indiana University Press.

—— (1997), *Plato's Sophist,* trans. R. Rojcewicz & A. Schuwer. Bloomington, Ind.: Indiana University Press.

Heymann, C. (1976), *Ezra Pound: The Last Rower.* New York: Viking.

Hiller, E., Ed. (1979), *The Basic Kafka.* New York: Pocket Books.

Himmelfarb, G. (1994), *On Looking into the Abyss.* New York: Knopf.

Hitschmann, E. (1952), Freud's conception of love. *Internat. J. Psycho-Anal.,* 33:421-428.

Hobsbawm, E. (1997), *On History.* London: Weidenfeld & Nicolson.

Hoffman, I. (1991), Discussion: Toward a social-constructivistic view of the psychoanalytic situation. *Psychoanal. Dial.,* 1:74-105.

—— (1992a), Some practical implications of a social-constructivist view of the psychoanalytic situation. *Psychoanal. Dial.,* 2:287-304.

—— (1992b), Reply to Orange. *Psychoanal. Dial.,* 2:567-570.

—— (1996), The intimate and ironic authority of the psychoanalyst's presence. *Psychoanal. Quart.,* 65:102-136.

Hölderlin, F. (1965), *Hyperion or The Hermit in Greece,* trans. W. Trask. New York: Ungar.

Hollinger, R., Ed. (1985), *Hermeneutics and Praxis*. Notre Dame, Ind.: University of Notre Dame Press.

Holt, R. (1975), *Abstracts of the Standard Edition of the Complete Psychological Works of Sigmund Freud*. New York: Aronson.

Horney, K. (1937), *The Neurotic Personality of Our Time*. New York: Norton.

———— (1939), *New Ways in Psychoanalysis*. New York: Norton.

Houlgate, S. (1991), *Freedom, Truth and History: An Introduction to Hegel's Philosophy*. New York: Routledge, Chapman & Hall.

Huizinga, J. (1924), *The Waning of the Middle Ages*. London: Edward Arnold.

Huntington, S. (1996), *The Clash of Civilizations and the Remaking of World Order.* New York: Simon & Schuster.

Husserl, E. (1913), *Ideas: General Introduction to Pure Phenomenology*, trans. W. G. Gibson. New York: Macmillan, 1952.

———— (1970), *The Crisis of European Sciences and Transcendental Phenomenology*, trans. D. Carr. Evanston, Ill.: Northwestern University Press.

———— (1989), *Ideas Pertaining to a Pure Phenomenology and to a Phenomenological Philosophy: Second Book, Studies in the Phenomenology of Constitution*, trans. R. Ojcewicz & A. Schuwer. Dordrecht, Netherlands: Kluwer.

Hutchins, R. (1935), To the graduating class, 1935. In: *No Friendly Voice*. New York: Greenwood Press, 1968.

———— (1936), *The Higher Learning in America*. New Haven, Conn.: Yale University Press.

———— (1948), The arts of freedom [Speech in Rockefeller Chapel September 21, 1948]. Chicago: University of Chicago Alumni Association.

———— (1968), *The Learning Society*. New York: Praeger.

Huxley, A. (1936), *Eyeless in Gaza*. New York: Harper.

Hyman, T. (1998), *Bonnard*. London: Thames and Hudson.

Ingram, D. (1994), Poststructuralist interpretation of the psychoanalytic relationship. *J. Amer. Acad. Psychoanal.*, 22:175-193.

Inwood, M. (1983), *Hegel*. London: Routledge & Kegan Paul.

Jacobs, T. (1997), In search of the mind of the analyst: A progress report. *J. Amer. Psychoanal. Assn.*, 45:1035-1059.

Jacoby, R. (1987), *The Last Intellectuals: American Culture in the Age of Academe*. New York: Basic Books.

———— (1994), *Dogmatic Wisdom: How the Culture Wars Divert Education and Distract America*. New York: Doubleday.

Jaspers, K. (1932a), *Philosophy* (Vol. 1). Chicago: University of Chicago Press, 1969.

――― (1932b), *Philosophy* (Vol. 2). Chicago: University of Chicago Press, 1970.

――― (1932c), *Philosophy* (Vol. 3). Chicago: University of Chicago Press, 1971.

――― (1972), *General Psychopathology*. Chicago: University of Chicago Press.

Johnson, P. (1991), *The Birth of the Modern: World Society 1815-1830*. New York: HarperCollins.

Jones, M. (1991), *Gaston Bachelard, Subversive Humanist: Text and Readings*. Madison, Wis.: University of Wisconsin Press.

Jones, W. (1969), *A History of Western Philosophy IV*. New York: Harcourt Brace.

――― (1975), *Kant and the 19th Century* (2nd Ed.). *A History of Western Philosophy*. New York: Harcourt Brace Jovanovich.

Joyce, J. (1947), *The Portable James Joyce*. New York: Viking.

――― (1961), *Ulysses*. New York: Random House.

Kafka, F. (1973), *Letters to Felice*. New York: Schoken Books.

Kakutani, M. (1997, April 25), [Review of *The Actual*, by Saul Bellow.] *New York Times*, p. 28.

Kane, R. (1993), The ends of metaphysics. *Internat. Philos. Quart.*, 33:413-428.

Kant, E. (1781), *Critique of Pure Reason*, trans. N. Smith. New York: St. Martin's Press, 1965.

Kaplan, F. (1988), *Dickens*. New York: William Morrow.

Katz, R. (1963), *Empathy, Its Nature and Uses*. New York: Glencoe Free Press.

Kellner, D. (1988), Postmodernism as social theory: Some challenges and problems. *Theory, Culture & Society*, 5:239-269.

Kenner, H. (1971), *The Pound Era*. Berkeley, Calif: University of California Press.

――― (1993, November 9), Pound and Eliot in Academe. *Times Literary Supplement*, pp. 13-14.

Kenyatta, J. (1938), *Facing Mount Kenya*. London: Secker & Warburg.

Kernberg, O. (1975), *Borderline Conditions and Pathological Narcissism*. New York: Aronson.

――― (1976), *Object Relations Theory in Clinical Psychoanalysis*. New York: Aronson.

———— (1980), *Internal World and External Reality: Object Relations Theory Applied*. New York: Aronson.

King, H. (1657), The exequy. In: *Oxford Book of Seventeenth Century Verse,* ed. H. Grierson & G. Bullough. Oxford: Clarendon Press, 1934, p. 355-359.

Klein, M. (1929), Infantile anxiety—situations reflected in a work of art and in the creative impulse. In: *Love, Guilt and Reparation and Other Works 1921-1945*. New York: Free Press, 1975.

———— (1958), On the development of mental functioning. In: *Envy and Gratitude and Other Works 1946-1963*. New York: Free Press, 1975.

———— (1975), *Envy and Gratitude and Other Works 1946-1963*. New York: Delta Books.

Klein, Morris (1980), *Mathematics: The Loss of Certainty*. New York: Oxford University Press.

Klíma, I. (1993), *Judge on Trial*, trans. A. Brain. New York: Knopf.

Knowlson, J. (1996), *Damned to Fame: The Life of Samuel Beckett*. New York: Simon & Schuster.

Kockelmans, J. (1984), *On the Truth of Being: Reflections on Heidegger's Later Philosophy*. Bloomington, Ind.: Indiana University Press.

Kohut, H. (1966), Forms and transformations of narcissism. *J. Amer. Psychoanal. Assn.,* 145:243-272.

———— (1971), *The Analysis of the Self*. New York: International Universities Press.

———— (1977), *The Restoration of the Self*. New York: International Universities Press.

———— (1978), *The Search for the Self*. New York: International Universities Press.

———— (1984), *How Does Analysis Cure?* Chicago: University of Chicago Press.

———— (1991), *The Search for the Self* (Vol. 4), ed. P. Ornstein. Madison, Conn.: International Universities Press.

———— (1994), *The Curve of Life: Correspondence of Heinz Kohut 1923-1981,* ed. G. Cocks. Chicago: University of Chicago Press.

———— (1996), *The Chicago Institute Lectures*. Hillsdale, N.J.: Analytic Press.

Kojève, A. (1980), *Introduction to the Reading of Hegel*. Ithaca, N.Y.: Cornell University Press.

Körner, S. (1970), *Kant*. Baltimore, Md.: Penguin Books.

Krarl, F. (1991), *Franz Kafka: Prague, Germans, Jews, and the Crisis of Modernism*. New York: Ticknor & Fields.

Kris, E. (1952), *Psychoanalytic Explorations in Art.* New York: International Universities Press.

Kubie, L. (1958), *Neurotic Distortion of the Creative Process.* New York: Farrar, Straus & Giroux, 1979.

Kundera, M. (1986), *The Art of the Novel.* New York: Grove Press.

Kurzweil, E. (1980), *The Age of Structuralism.* New York Columbia University Press.

—— (1989), *The Freudians: A Comparative Perspective.* New Haven, Conn.: Yale University Press.

Lacan, J. (1977), *Ecrits: A Selection.* New York: Norton.

LaGrange, H. (1995), *Gustave Mahler: Vienna. The Years of Challenge (1897-1904).* New York: Oxford University Press.

Laing, R. (1969), *The Divided Self.* New York: Pantheon.

Landauer, K. (1938), Affect, passions and temperament. *Internat. J. Psychoanal.* 19:388-415.

Langer, S. (1942), *Philosophy in a New Key.* New York: Mentor.

Langs, R. (1982), *Psychotherapy: A Basic Text.* New York: Aronson.

Lasch, C. (1978), *The Culture of Narcissism: American Life in an Age of Diminishing Expectations.* New York: Norton.

Lasch, S. (1985), Postmodernity and desire. *Theory & Society,* 14:1-34.

Lavine, T. (1989), The interpretive turn from Kant to Derrida: A critique. *History and Anti-History in Philosophy,* ed. T. Lavine & V. Tejera. Boston: Kluwer.

Lawrence, J. (1988), Art and philosophy in Schelling. *The Owl of Minerva,* 20:5-19.

Leibniz, G. (1714), *Discourse on Metaphysics, Correspondence with Arnald, Monadology,* trans. G. Montgomery. LaSalle, Ill.: Open Court, 1945.

Levine, M. (1961), Principles of psychiatric treatment. In: *The Impact of Freudian Psychiatry,* ed. F. Alexander & H. Ross. Chicago: University of Chicago Press.

Levy, S. (1985), Empathy and psychoanalytic technique. *J. Amer. Psychiat. Assn.,* 33:353-378.

Lewin, K. (1950), *The Psychoanalysis of Elation.* New York: Norton.

Linder, S. (1970), *The Harried Leisured Class.* New York: Columbia University Press.

Lindley, D. (1993), *The End of Physics.* New York: Basic Books.

Lippman, W. (1953), *The Public Philosophy.* New York: Mentor.

Lipton, S. (1977), The advantages of Freud's technique as shown in his analysis of the Rat Man. *Internat. J. Psycho-Anal.,* 58:255-274.

———— (1979), An addendum to "The Advantages of Freud's Technique as shown in his analysis of the Rat Man." *Internat. J. Psycho-Anal.*, 60:215-216.

———— (1983), A critique of so-called standard psychoanalytic technique. *Contemp. Psychoanal.*, 19:35-46.

Loewald, H. (1978), *Psychoanalysis and the History of the Individual.* New Haven, Conn.: Yale University Press.

———— (1986), Transference-countertransference. *J. Amer. Psychoanal. Assn.*, 34:275-288.

———— (1988), *Sublimation: Inquiries into Theoretical Psychoanalysis.* New Haven, Conn.: Yale University Press.

Lorca, F. G. (1991), *Frederico García Lorca: Collected Poems*, ed. C. Maurer. New York: Farrar, Straus Giroux.

Lorenz, K. (1966), *On Aggression.* New York: Harcourt Press.

———— (1987), *The Waning of Humanness.* Boston: Little, Brown.

Lovibond, S. (1989), Feminism and postmodernism. *New Left Review*, 178:5-28.

Lynn, K. (1987), *Hemingway.* New York: Simon & Schuster..

Lyotard, J. (1984), *The Postmodern Condition: A Report on Knowledge*, trans. G. Bennington & B. Massumi. Minneapolis: University of Minnesota Press.

Macrae, D. (1974), *Max Weber.* New York: Viking.

Magee, B. (1997), *Confessions of a Philosopher: A Journey Through Western Philosophy.* New York: Random House.

Magnus, B., & Higgins, K., Eds. (1996), *The Cambridge Companion to Nietzsche.* New York: Cambridge University Press.

———— Stewart, S., & Mileur, J. (1993), *Nietzsche's Case: Philosophy as/and Literature.* New York: Cambridge University Press.

Maher, A. (1993), Creativity: A work in progress. *Psychoanal. Quart.*, 52:239-262.

Maimonides, M. (1952), *Guide of the Perplexed.* London: Horovitz.

Maker, W. (1994), Reason as revolution. *Philos. Forum*, 26:49-62.

Manchester, W. (1983), *The Lost Lion: Winston Spencer Churchill. Visions of Glory 1874-1932.* Boston: Little, Brown.

Marias, J. (1967), *The History of Philosophy.* New York: Dover.

Maritain, J. (1955), *Creative Intuition in Art and Poetry.* New York: Meridian Books.

Marvell, A. (1681), Definition of love. In: *Andrew Marvell: The Complete Poems*, ed. G. DeF. Lord. New York: Knopf, 1984, pp. 35-36.

Massie, R. (1991), *Dreadnought: Britain, Germany, and the Coming of the Great War.* New York: Random House.

Masson, J. (1980), *The Oceanic Feeling.* Boston: Reidel.

Maugham, S. (1992), *Of Human Bondage.* New York: Penguin.

Mazrui, A. (1986), *The Africans: A Triple Heritage.* Boston: Little, Brown.

McCarthy, T. (1982), *The Critical Theory of Jurgen Habermas.* Cambridge, Mass.: MIT Press.

—— (1991), *On Reconstruction and Deconstruction in Contemporary Critical Theory.* Cambridge, Mass.: MIT Press.

McClelland, D. (1986), Some reflections on the two psychologies of love. *J. Pers.*, 54:334-353.

McCormick, J. (1987), *George Santayana: A Biography.* New York: Knopf.

McDougal, S. (1985), Dreaming a Renaissance: Pound's Dantean inheritance. In: *Among the Poets*, ed. G. Bornstein. Chicago: University of Chicago Press.

McGuinness, B. (1988), *Wittgenstein: A Life.* Berkeley, Calif.: University of California Press.

McLaughlin, J. (1996), Power, authority, and influence in the analytic dyad. *Psychoanal. Quart.*, 65:201-235.

Mead, G. (1962), *Mind, Self and Society.* Chicago: University of Chicago Press.

Meng, H., & Freud, E., Eds. (1963), *Psychoanalysis and Faith: The Letters of Sigmund Freud and Oskar Pfister*, trans. E. Mosbacher. New York: Basic Books.

Michelfelder, D. (1997), Gadamer on Heidegger on art. In: *The Philosophy of Hans-Georg Gadamer.* Chicago: Open Court, pp. 437-456.

Mills, N. (1997), *The Triumph of Meanness: America's War against Its Better Self.* New York: Houghton Mifflin.

Modell, A. (1976), "The holding environment" and the therapeutic action of psychoanalysis. *J. Amer. Psychoanal. Assn.*, 24:285-308.

Money-Kryle, R. (1974), The Kleinian school. In: *American Handbook of Psychiatry* (Vol. 1, 2nd ed.), ed. S. Arieti. New York: Basic Books, pp. 819-827.

Moore, B., & Fine, B., Eds. (1990), *Psychoanalytic Terms and Concepts.* New Haven, Conn.: Yale University Press.

Morgan, G. (1965), *What Nietzsche Means.* New York: Harper.

Mullins, E. (1961), *This Difficult Individual, Ezra Pound.* New York: Fleet.

Nagel, E., & Newman, J. (1974), *Gödel's Proof.* New York: New York University Press.

Natansan, M. (1973), *Edmund Husserl: Philosopher of Infinite Tasks*. Evanston, Ill.: Northwestern University Press.

Newman, J. (1852), *On the Scope and Nature of University Education.* New York: Dutton, 1961.

Newton, P. (1995), *Freud: From Youthful Dream to Midlife Crisis.* New York: Guilford Press.

Niederland, W. (1976), Psychoanalytic approaches to artistic creativity. *Psychoanal. Quart.*, 45:185-212.

Nietzsche, F. (1872), The Birth of Tragedy. In: *Basic Writings of Nietzsche*, trans. W. Kaufmann. New York: Modern Library, 1968, pp. 3-146.

———(1873-1876), *Untimely Meditations*, trans. R. Hollingdale. New York: Cambridge University Press.

——— (1874), *Schopenhauer as Educator*, trans. R. Hollingdale. New York: Cambridge University Press, 1985.

——— (1878), *Human, All Too Human: A Book for Free Spirits*, trans. R. Hollingdale. New York: Cambridge University Press, 1986.

——— (1882), *The Gay Science* (Books 1-4), trans. W. Kaufmann. New York: Vintage Books, 1974.

——— (1883-1888), *The Will to Power*, trans. W. Kaufmann & R. Hollingdale. New York: Vintage Books, 1968.

——— (1884), *Thus Spoke Zarathustra: A Book for All and None.* In: *The Portable Nietzsche*, trans. W. Kaufmann. New York: Viking, 1968, pp. 103-439.

——— (1886), *Beyond Good and Evil,* ed. and trans. W. Kaufmann. In: *Basic Writings of Nietzsche.* New York: Modern Library, 1968, pp. 181-438.

——— (1887), *The Gay Science* (Book 5), trans. W. Kaufmann. New York: Vintage Books, 1974.

Nin, A. (1966), *The Diary of Anaïs Nin: Vol. 1. 1931-1934.* New York: Harcourt Brace.

Noy, P. (1979), Form creation in art: An ego-psychological approach to creativity. *Psychoanal. Quart.*, 48:229-256.

——— (1984-1985), Originality and creativity. *Annual Psychoanal.*, 12/13:421-448.

Ogot, B. (1961), Concept of Jok. *African Studies*, No. 20. Quoted in *The Africans: A Triple Heritage*, by A. Mazrui. Boston: Little Brown, 1986.

Oremland, J. (1997), *The Origins and Psychodynamics of Creativity: A Psychoanalytic Perspective.* Madison, Conn.: International Universities Press.

Ostwald, P. (1997), *Glen Gould: The Ecstasy and Tragedy of Genius.* New York: Norton.

Pao, P. (1979), *Schizophrenic Disorders.* New York: International Universities Press.

Parini, J. (1997), *Benjamin's Crossing: A Novel.* New York: Henry Holt.

Pawel, E. (1984), *The Nightmare of Reason: The Life of Franz Kafka.* New York: Farrar, Straus & Giroux.

Pears, I. (1998), *An Instance of the Fingerpost.* New York: Riverhead Books.

Pelikan, J. (1992), *The Idea of the University: A Reexamination.* New Haven, Conn.: Yale University Press.

Penrose, R. (1992), *Miró.* New York: Thames & Hudson.

Penrose, Roger(1997), *The Large, the Small and the Human Mind.* New York: Cambridge University Press.

Percy, W. (1987), *The Thanatos Syndrome.* New York: Farrar, Straus & Giroux.

Perkins, D. (1976), *A History of Modern Poetry: From the 1890's to the High Modern Mode.* Cambridge, Mass.: Harvard University Press.

——— (1987), *A History of Modern Poetry: Modernism and After.* Cambridge, Mass.: Harvard University Press.

Person, E. (1988), *Dreams of Love and Fateful Encounters: The Power of Romantic Passion.* New York: Norton.

Petzet, H. (1993), *Encounters and Dialogues with Martin Heidegger 1929-1976,* trans. P. Emad & K. Maly. Chicago: University of Chicago Press.

Phillips, J. (1991), Hermeneutics in psychoanalysis: Review and reconsideration. *Psychoanal. Contemp. Thought,* 14:371-424.

Pieper, J. (1952), *Leisure: The Basis of Culture.* New York: Pantheon.

Pine, F. (1985), *Developmental Theory and Clinical Process.* New Haven, Conn.: Yale University Press.

Pipes, R. (1990), *The Russian Revolution.* New York: Knopf.

Pollock, G. (1982), Mourning-liberation process and creativity. *Annual Psychoanal.* 10:333-353.

——— Ed. (1992), *How Psychiatrists Look at Aging.* Madison, Conn.: International Universities Press.

Popper, K. (1994), *Knowledge and the Mind-Body Problem: In Defense of Interaction.* New York: Routledge.

Porteus, H. (1950), Ezra Pound and his Chinese character: A radical examination. In: *An Examination of Ezra Pound,* ed. P. Russell. New York: New Directions, pp. 203-217.

Postman, N. (1985), *Amusing Ourselves to Death: Public Discourse in the Age of Show Business.* New York: Viking.

Pound, E. (1938), *Guide to Kulchur.* New York: New Directions.

——— (1939), *ABC of Reading.* Norfolk, Conn.: New Directions.

——— (1949), *Selected Poems.* New York: New Directions.

——— (1950), *The Cantos of Ezra Pound.* New York: New Directions. (Later editions in 1969, 1972.)

——— (1954), *Literary Essays.* New York: New Directions.

——— (n.d.), *Confucius: The Unwobbling Pivot and the Great Digest.* Washington, D.C.: Square Dollar Press.

Prater, D. (1986), *A Ringing Glass: The Life of Rainer Maria Rilke.* New York: Clarendon Press.

Prosen, H., Martin, R., & Prosen, M. (1972), The remembered mother and the fantasized mother. *Arch. Gen. Psychiatry,* 27:791-794.

Proust, M. (1934), *Remembrance of Things Past,* trans. C. Moncrieff. New York: Random House.

———(1981), *Remembrance of Things Past,* trans. C. Moncrieff & T. Kilmartin. New York: Random House.

Puccini, G. (1956), *Il Tabarro.* Milan: Casa Ricordi-BMG Ricordi. Libretto by G. Adami.

Rank, O. (1932), *Art and Artist.* New York: Knopf.

——— & Sachs, H. (1916), *The Significance of Psychoanalysis for the Mental Sciences.* New York: Nervous & Mental Disease Monograph Publishing.

Reik, T. (1949), *Listening with the Third Ear.* New York: Farrar, Straus.

Reisman, D. (1955), *The Lonely Crowd.* Garden City, N.Y.: Doubleday.

Rescher, N. (1973), *Conceptual Idealism.* Oxford: Basil Blackwell.

——— (1991), Conceptual idealism revisited. *Review of Metaphysics,* 44:495-523.

——— (1992), *A System of Pragmatic Idealism, Vol. 1: Human Knowledge in Idealistic Perspective.* Princeton, N.J.: Princeton University Press.

——— (1993), American philosophy today. *Rev. Metaphysics,* 46:717-745.

Rich, A. (1995), *Dark Fields of the Republic: Poems 1991-1995.* New York: Norton.

Richardson, R. (1995), *Emerson: The Mind on Fire.* Berkeley, Calif.: University of California Press.

Richters, A. (1988), Modernity-postmodernity controversies: Habermas and Foucault. *Theory, Culture Society,* 5:611-643.

Rilke, R. (1962), *Letters to a Young Poet.* New York: Norton.

——— (1984a), *New Poems,* trans. E. Snow. Berkeley, Calif.: North Point Press.

——— (1984b), *The Selected Poetry of Rainer Maria Rilke,* ed. & trans. S. Mitchell. New York: Vintage Books.

Roland, A. (1988), *In Search of the Self in India and Japan: Toward A Cross-Cultural Psychology.* Princeton, N.J.: Princeton University Press.

Rorty, R. (1979), *Philosophy and the Mirror of Nature.* Princeton, N.J.: Princeton University Press.

——— (1982), *Consequences of Pragmatism.* Princeton, N.J.: Princeton University Press.

——— (1989), *Contingency, Irony, and Solidarity.* New York: Cambridge University Press.

——— (1991), *Philosophical Papers: Vol. 2. Essays on Heidegger and Others.* Cambridge: Cambridge University Press.

——— (1997), When work disappears. *Dissent,* 44(3):111-113.

Rose, G. (1996), Necessary Illusion. Madison, Conn.: International Universities Press.

Rosenthal, M. (1966), *A Primer of Ezra Pound.* New York: Grosset & Dunlop.

Ross, N. (1968), Beyond "The Future of an Illusion." *J. Hillside Hospital,* 17:259-276.

Russell, B. (1929), *Marriage and Morals.* New York: Liveright.

——— (1945), *A History of Western Philosophy: And Its Connection with Political and Social Circumstances from the Earliest Times to the Present Day.* New York: Simon & Schuster.

——— (1969), *Unpopular Essays.* New York: Simon & Schuster.

Russell, P. (1950), *An Examination of Ezra Pound.* New York: New Directions.

Ryan, A. (1988), *Bertrand Russell: A Political Life.* New York: Hill & Wang.

Sachs, H. (1942), *The Creative Unconscious.* Cambridge, Mass.: Sci-Art Publishers.

Sadow, L. (1969), Ego axis in psychopathology. *Arch. Gen. Psychiatry,* 21:15-24.

Safranski, R. (1990), *Schopenhauer and the Wild Years of Philosophy,* trans. E. Osers. Cambridge, Mass.: Harvard University Press.

——— (1998), *Martin Heidegger: Between Good and Evil,* trans. E. Osers. Cambridge, Mass.: Harvard University Press.

Sandler, J., Holder, A., Dare, C., & Dreher, A. (1998), *Freud's Models of the Mind: An Introduction.* Madison, Conn.: International Universities Press.

Santayana, G. (1896), *The Sense of Beauty: Being the Outline of Aesthetic Theory.* New York: Dover Books, 1955.

———— (1955), *Skepticism and Animal Faith.* New York: Dover.

Sartre, J.-P. (1938), *Nausea.* New York: New Directions, 1964.

———— (1948), *The Emotions: Outline of a Theory,* trans. B. Frechtman. New York: Philosophical Library, 1973.

———— (1963), *Search for a Method,* trans. H. Barnes. New York: Vintage.

———— (1964), *Nausea.* New York: New Directions.

———— (1973), *Being and Nothingness: A Phenomenological Essay on Ontology,* trans. H. Barnes. New York: Washington Square Press.

———— (1978), *Sartre by Himself,* trans. R. Seaver. New York: Urizen.

———— (1981), *The Family Idiot: Gustave Flaubert 1821-1857* (Vol. 1), trans. C. Cosman. Chicago: University of Chicago Press.

Saul, L. (1958), *Technic and Practice of Psychoanalysis.* Philadelphia: Lippincott.

Saussure, F. (1986), *Course in General Linguistics,* trans. R. Harris. LaSalle, Ill.: Open Court.

Saville, J. (1990), American art. In: *Honolulu Academy of Arts: Selected Works.* Honolulu, Hi.: Honolulu Academy of Arts, pp. 209-248.

Sayen, J. (1985), *Einstein in America.* New York: Crown Books.

Schacht, R. (1983), *Nietzsche.* London: Routledge & Kegan Paul.

———— (1993), *Nietzsche: Selections.* New York: Macmillan.

———— (1996), Nietzsche's kind of philosophy. In: *The Cambridge Companion to Nietzsche,* ed. B. Magnus & K. Higgins. New York: Cambridge University Press, pp. 151-179.

Schafer, R. (1983), *The Analytic Attitude.* New York: Basic Books.

Schiller, F. (1965), *On the Aesthetic Education of Man in a Series of Letters.* New York: Ungar.

Schilpp, P., Ed. (1941), *The Philosophy of Alfred North Whitehead.* Evanston, Ill.: Northwestern University Press.

Schlesinger, A. (1997), Has democracy a future? *Foreign Affairs,* 7:2-12.

Schneider, D. (1954), *Psychoanalyst and Artist.* New York: International Universities Press.

Schopenhauer, A. (1970), *Essays and Aphorisms.* New York: Penguin.

Schulte, J. (1992), *Wittgenstein: An Introduction,* trans. W. Brenner & J. Holley. Albany: State University of New York.

Schur, M. (1972), *Freud, Living and Dying.* New York.: International Universities Press.

Schutte, O. (1984), *Beyond Nihilism: Nietzsche without Masks.* Chicago: University of Chicago Press.

Schwaber, E. (1981a), Empathy: A mode of analytic listening. *Psychoanal. Inquiry,* 1:357-392.

———— (1981b), Narcissism, self psychology, and the listening perspective. *Annual Psychoanal.,* 9:114-131.

———— (1983a), Construction, reconstruction, and the mode of clinical attunement. In: *The Future of Psychoanalysis,* ed. A. Goldberg. New York: International Universities Press, pp. 273-292.

———— (1983b), A particular perspective on analytic listening. *The Psychoanalytic Study of the Child,* 38:519-546.

———— (1983c), Psychoanalytic listening and psychic reality. *Internat. Rev. Psycho-Anal.,* 10:379-392.

———— (1985), *The Transference in Psychotherapy: Clinical Management.* New York: International Universities Press.

———— (1986), Reconstruction and perceptual experience: Further thoughts on psychoanalytic listening. *J. Amer. Psychoanal. Assn.,* 34:911-932.

———— (1987), Models of the mind and data-gathering in clinical work. *Psychoanal. Inquiry,* 7:261-276.

Schwartz, L. (1978), Review of *The Restoration of the Self. Psychoanal. Quart.,* 47:436-443.

Schweitzer, A. (1992), *Letters 1902-1965,* ed. H. Bähr, trans. J. Neugroschel. New York: Macmillan.

Searle, J. (1995), *The Construction of Social Reality.* New York: Free Press.

Searles, H. (1960), *The Nonhuman Environment in Normal Development and in Schizophrenia.* New York: International Universities Press.

Sexton, A. (1981), *The Complete Poems.* Boston: Houghton Mifflin.

Shapiro, G. (1989), Derrida and the question of philosophy's history. In: *History and Anti-history in Philosophy,* eds. T. Lavine & V. Tejera. Boston: Kluwer, pp. 156-187.

Shattuck, R. (1983), *Proust's Binoculars.* Princeton, N.J.: Princeton University Press.

Silver, I. (1994), *Socialism: What Went Wrong? An Inquiry into the Theoretical and Historical Sources of the Socialist Crisis.* Boulder, Col.: Pluto Press.

Silverman, M., & Will, N. (1986), Sylvia Plath and the failure of emotional self-repair through poetry. *Psychoanal. Quart.,* 55:99-129.

Skinner, B. (1948), *Walden Two.* New York: Macmillan.

Smith, G. (1996), *Nietzsche, Heidegger, and the Transition to Postmodernity*. Chicago: University of Chicago Press.

Solomon, R. (1988), Introduction: Reading Nietzsche. In: *Reading Nietzsche*, ed. R. Solomon & K. Higgins. New York: Oxford University Press, pp. 3-12.

———— (1996), Nietzsche *ad hominem:* Perspectivism, personality and *ressentiment.* In: *The Cambridge Companion to Nietzsche*, ed. B. Magnus & K. Higgins. New York: Cambridge University Press, pp. 180-222.

Spence, D. (1982), *Narrative Truth and Historical Truth*. New York: Norton.

Spender, S. (1976), *T. S. Eliot*. New York: Viking.

Spengler, O. (1926), *The Decline of the West: Vol. 1. Form and Actuality*, trans. C. Atkinson. New York: Knopf.

———— (1928), *The Decline of the West: Vol. 2. Perspectives of World-History*, trans. C. Atkinson. New York: Knopf.

———— (1962), *The Decline of the West* (abridged ed.), trans. C. Atkinson. New York: Knopf.

Spinoza, B. (1955), *Ethics*. New York: Dover.

Spitz, R. (1965), *The First Year of Life*. New York: International Universities Press.

Stambaugh, J. (1994), *The Other Nietzsche*. Albany: State University of New York Press.

Starr, P. (1982), *The Social Transformation of American Medicine*. New York: Basic Books.

Stein, G. (1940), *Paris France*. New York: Scribner.

Stein, R. (1995), Reply to Chodorow. *Psychoanal. Dial.*, 5:301-310.

Steiner, G. (1989), *Real Presences*. Chicago: University of Chicago Press.

———— (1997), *Errata: An Examined Life*. New Haven, Conn.: Yale University Press.

Steiner, W. (1995), *The Scandal of Pleasure: Art in an Age of Fundamentalism*. Chicago: University of Chicago Press.

Stekel, W. (1950), *Autobiography*. New York: Liveright.

Stern, D. (1983), Unformulated experience. *Contemp. Psychoanal.*, 19:71-99.

———— (1988), Not misusing empathy. *Contemp. Psychoanal.*, 24:598-611.

———— (1991), A philosophy for the embedded analyst. *Contemp. Psychoanal.*, 27:51-80.

———— (1992), Commentary on constructivism in clinical psychoanalysis. *Psychoanal. Dial.*, 2:331-363.

———— (1994), Empathy is interpretation (and who ever said it wasn't?). *Psychoanal. Dial.*, 4:441-471.

―――― (1996), Dissociation and constructivism: Commentary on papers by Davies and Harris. *Psychoanal. Dial.*, 6:251-266.

Stern, J. (1979), *A Study of Nietzsche.* New York: Cambridge University Press.

Stevenson, R. (1988), *The Lantern-bearers and Other Essays,* ed. J. Treglown. London: Chatto & Windus.

Stock, N. (1966), *Reading the Cantos: The Study of Meaning in Ezra Pound.* New York: Minerva Press.

―――― (1970), *The Life of Ezra Pound.* New York: Pantheon.

―――― (1976), *Ezra Pound's Pennsylvania.* Toledo, Ohio: University of Toledo Libraries.

Stolorow, R., & Atwood, G. (1992), *Contexts of Being.* Hillsdale, N.J.: Analytic Press.

Stone, L. (1981), Notes on the noninterpretative elements in the psychoanalytic situation and process. *J. Amer. Psychoanal. Assn.*, 29:89-118.

Straus, E. (1958), Aesthesiology and hallucinations. In: *Existence: A New Dimension in Psychiatry and Psychology,* ed. R. May, E. Angel, & H. Ellenberger. New York: Basic Books, pp. 139-169.

Sullivan, H. (1947), *Conceptions of Modern Psychiatry.* Washington, D.C.: White Foundation.

―――― (1953), *The Interpersonal Theory of Psychiatry.* New York: Norton.

Sutton, N. (1996), *Bettelheim: A Life and a Legacy,* trans. D. Sharp. New York: Basic Books.

Tallchief, M. (1997), *Maria Tallchief: America's Prima Ballerina.* New York: Henry Holt.

Tanner, M. (1996), *Nietzsche.* New York: Oxford University Press.

Tausk, V. (1933), On the origin of the influencing machine in schizophrenia. *Psychoanal. Quart.*, 2:19-56.

Taylor, C. (1975), *Hegel.* New York: Cambridge University Press.

―――― (1985), *Philosophy in the Human Sciences.* Cambridge, Mass.: Cambridge University Press.

―――― (1989), *Sources of the Self: The Making of the Modern Identity.* Cambridge, Mass.: Harvard University Press.

Tennov, D. (1979), *Love and Limerence: The Experience of Being in Love.* New York: Stein & Day.

Tennyson, A. (1886), *The Poems of Tennyson in Three Volumes* (Vol. 3), ed. C. Ricks. Berkeley, Calif.: University of California Press, 1987.

Todorov, T. (1984), *Mikhail Bakhtin: The Dialogical Principle,* trans. W.

Godzich. Minneapolis: University of Minnesota Press.

Tolstoy, L. (1868), *War and Peace*, trans. L. & M. Maude. New York: Simon & Schuster.

———— (1947), *Resurrection*. London: Hamish Hamilton.

Tomkins, C. (1996), *Duchamp*. New York: Henry Holt & Co.

Tomlin, E. (1952), *The Great Philosophers of the Western World*. New York: A. A. Wyn, Inc.

Torrey, N. (1938), *The Spirit of Voltaire*. New York: Russell & Russell, 1968.

Toulmin, S. (1990), *Cosmopolis: The Hidden Agenda of Modernity.* New York: Free Press.

Tracy, S. (1990), *The Story of the Odyssey.* Princeton, N.J.: Princeton University Press.

Trilling, L. (1939), *Matthew Arnold*. New York: Harcourt Brace Jovanovich.

———— Ed. (1949), *The Portable Matthew Arnold*. New York: Viking.

———— (1955), *Freud and the Crisis of Our Culture*. Boston: Beacon Press.

Trosman, H. (1974), T. S. Eliot and *The Wasteland. Arch. Gen. Psychiatry,* 30:709-717.

———— (1990), Transformations in unconscious fantasy in art. *J. Amer. Psychoanal. Assn.,* 38:47-60.

Turgenev, I. (1948), *Fathers and Sons*. New York: Rinehart.

Twemlow, S., & Gabbard, G. (1989), The lovesick therapist. In: *Sexual Exploitation in Professional Relationships,* ed. G. Gabbard. Washington, D.C.: American Psychiatric Press.

Tytell, J. (1987), *Ezra Pound: The Solitary Volcano*. New York: Doubleday.

Updike, J. (1963, August 24), More love in the western world. *The New Yorker,* 39:90-104.

Varnedoe, K. (1998), *Jackson Pollock*. New York: Museum of Modern Art.

Verhulst, J. (1984), Limerence: Notes on the nature and function of passionate love. *Psychoanal. Contemp. Thought,* 7:115-138.

Vico, G. (1744), *The New Science of Giambattista Vico,* trans. T. Bergin & H. Fisch. Ithica, N.Y.: Cornell University Press, 1984.

Viederman, M. (1988), The nature of passionate love. In: *Passionate Attachments: Thinking about Love,* ed. W. Gaylin & E. Person. New York: Free Press, pp. 1-14.

Wallerstein, R. (1995), *The Talking Cures: The Psychoanalyses and the Psychotherapies*. New Haven, Conn.: Yale University Press.

Weber, M. (1930), *The Protestant Ethic and the Spirit of Capitalism,* trans. T.

Parsons. New York: Routledge, 1992.

Weissman, P. (1967), Theoretical considerations of ego regressions and ego functions in creativity. *Psychoanal. Quart.*, 36:37-50.

Werman, D. (1986), On the nature of the oceanic experience. *J. Amer. Psychoanal. Assn.*, 34:123-140.

———— Jacobs, T. (1983), Thomas Hardy's *The Well-Beloved* and the nature of infatuation. *Internat. Rev. Psychoanal.*, 10:447-457.

White, S. (1991), *Political Theory and Postmodernism.* Cambridge: Cambridge University Press.

Whitehead, A. (1929a), *The Function of Reason.* Boston: Beacon Press.

———— (1929b), *Process and Reality.* New York: Social Sciences Publishers, 1941.

———— (1933), *Adventures of Ideas.* New York: Free Press.

Wilde, O. (1982), *The Artist as Critic: Critical Writings of Oscar Wilde*, ed. R. Ellman. Chicago: University of Chicago Press.

———— (1988), Lady Windermere's fan. In: *The Plays of Oscar Wilde.* New York: Vintage, pp. 1-82.

Wilhelm, J. (1977), *The Later Cantos of Ezra Pound.* New York: Walker.

Wilson, E. (1931), *Axel's Castle.* New York: Scribner.

Wilson, W. (1996), *When Work Disappears: The World of the New Urban Poor.* New York: Knopf.

Winnicott, D. (1965a), *The Family and Individual Development.* London: Tavistock.

———— (1965b), *The Maturational Processes and the Facilitating Environment: Studies in the Theory of Emotional Development.* New York: International Universities Press.

Wittgenstein, L. (1961), *Tractatus Logico-Philosophicus,* trans. D. Pears & B. McGuinness. New York: Humanities Press.

———— (1972), *On Certainty,* trans. D. Paul & G. Anscombe. New York: Harper.

Wolf, E. (1985), The search for confirmation: Technical aspects of mirroring. *Psychoanal. Inquiry,* 5:271-282.

Wolheim, R. (1993), Danto's gallery of indiscernibles. In: *Danto and His Critics,* ed. M. Rollins. Cambridge, Mass.: Blackwell, pp. 28-38.

Wood, R. (1995), Six Heideggerian figures. *American Catholic Philos. Quart.,* 69:312-331.

Young-Bruehl, E. (1991), *Creative Characters.* New York: Routledge.

Zimmerman, M. (1981), *Eclipse of the Self: The Development of Heidegger's Concept of Authenticity.* Athens: Ohio University Press.

NAME INDEX

SUBJECT INDEX

459

ABOUT THE AUTHOR

Richard D. Chessick, M.D., Ph.D., is Professor of Psychiatry and Behavioral Sciences at Northwestern University, training and supervising analyst at the Chicago Center for Psychoanalytic Study, and Senior Attending Psychiatrist at Evanston Hospital. Dr. Chessick is the 1989 recipient of the American Society of Psychoanalytic Physician's Sigmund Freud Award for outstanding contributions to psychiatry and psychoanalysis, and he was elected president of that organization in 1996–1997. He is a Fellow of the American Academy of Psychoanalysis (where he serves as vice-chair of their committee on human rights and social issues and as a member of the committee on psychoanalysis and women, among other assignments), a Life Fellow of the American Psychiatric Association and the American Orthopsychiatric Association, a Fellow of the Academy of Psychosomatic Medicine and the American Society for Adolescent Psychiatry, a Councillor of the American Association for Social Psychiatry, a corresponding member of the German Psychoanalytic Society, and a member of eighteen other professional societies. His Ph.D. is in philosophy, and he taught as Adjunct Professor of Philosophy at Loyola University of Chicago for several years. Northwestern University residents in psychiatry have repeatedly awarded him their "teacher of the year" certificate over his thirty-eight years of donated teaching at the university.

Dr. Chessick is on the editorial board of four major journals: *Journal of the American Academy of Psychoanalysis, American Journal of Psychoanalysis, Psychoanalysis and Psychotherapy,* and *American Journal of Psychotherapy;* he also serves the latter as Associate Editor in charge of the International Editorial Board. He has pub-

473

lished more than two hundred papers since 1953 in the fields of neurology, psychiatry, philosophy, and psychoanalysis. An international lecturer, he is the author of fourteen books. Dr. Chessick is in the private practice of psychiatry and psychoanalysis in Evanston, Illinois.